101 Q&A
ACUPRESSURE
&
REFLEXOLOGY

101 Q & A
ACUPRESSURE
&
REFLEXOLOGY

Dr. A.K. Saxena

Dr. Preeti Pai

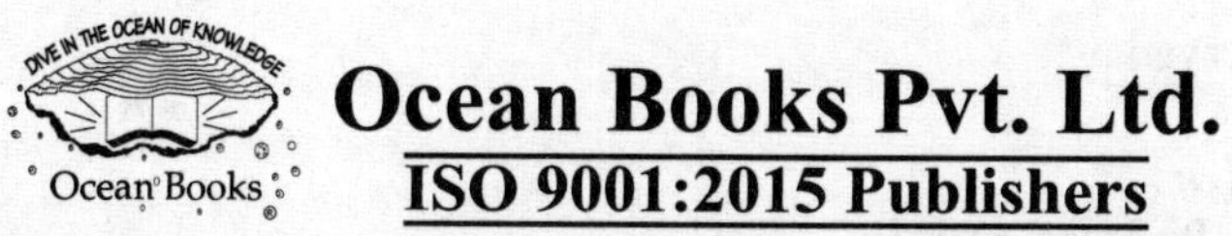

Ocean Books Pvt. Ltd.

ISO 9001:2015 Publishers

Published by
Ocean Books (P) Ltd.
4/19 Asaf Ali Road,
New Delhi-110 002 (INDIA)
e-mail: info@oceanbooks.in

ISBN 978-81-8430-151-9
100 Q & A ACUPRESSURE & REFLEXOLOGY
by Dr. A.K. Saxena/Dr. Preeti Pai

Edition
2024

Paperback Price
₹ 350.00 (Rupees Three Hundred Fifty only)

Printed at
Narula Printers, Delhi

Dedication

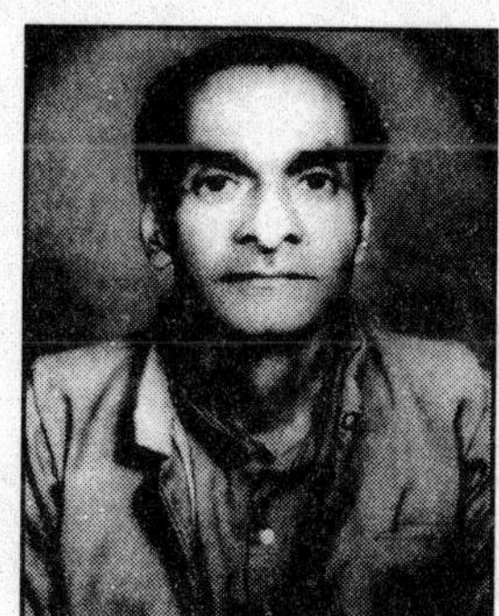

(Late) Shri Vidya Dhar Saxena

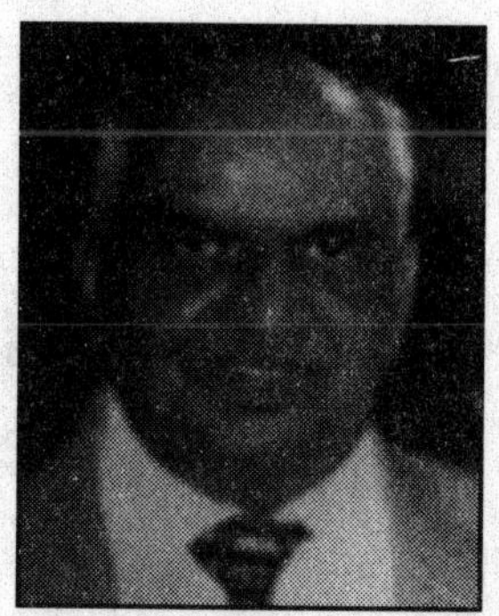

Padamshree (Late) Dr. L.C.Gupta

This book is dedicated to my respected father (Late) Shri Vidya Dhar Saxena who led a saintly life. He always inspired me to learn to live for others and work selflessly. He left for his heavenly abode on 13th January, 1968 when I was about 19 years old. His noble soul has always been with me, inspiring me to do something which could be of some use to the people for times to come.

I also dedicate this book to my 'Friend, Philosopher and Guide' Padamshree (Late) Dr. L.C. Gupta, former Inspector General of Police and Director(Medical), B.S.F, and my co-author in my earlier books 'Miraculous Effects of Acupressure' and 'Acupressure aur Swasth Jeevan'. Dr. Gupta held the world record of writing 112 books on medical science. He was 'an institution in himself.' He had an open mind, vast knowledge and a great sense of humor. His mere presence used to be a great source of inspiration for me, whether it was writing a book or holding a workshop. The idea to bring out this book was also conceived by him and he helped me greatly in jotting down probable questions that pester the minds of people about this 'Art and Science'. I am grateful to the Almighty and my publishers Dr. Piyush Agarwal in providing me the opportunity of bringing out this book, thus accomplishing the work left half way by Padamshree (Late) Dr. L.C. Gupta.

A.K. Saxena

Acupressure Training and Healing Centre

Acupressure is not only curative; it is preventive and diagnostic to a large extent. It removes the root cause of the disease. It is non-conventional, non-interventional and non-invasive. Moreover it is simple to learn and easy to practice and is free from any side effects.

Anyone can learn how to heal by using this technique. Qualification is no constraint and even if one can understand spoken English or Hindi language, has willingness to do hard work with dedication he/she can be trained to help himself/herself. Even house-wives can learn to heal using this technique. In case you want to avail this opportunity, please contact:

Director, Acupressure Training and Healing Centre,
B-702, Shramdeep Apartments, Plot B-9/1-B,
Sector-62, NOIDA-201301 (Uttar Pradesh), INDIA
Phone: 09810484242 / 09810430343
Web: acupressureguide.org
e-mail: saxenaashokk@yahoo.com

Highlights:

- Training is given by Dr. A.K. Saxena himself
- Three months/Crash* Courses (One month) available
- Reasonable Fees (Rs. 5000/=) only*
- Practical Training Compulsory

---

* For Indians.

Message-1

06.11.08

I came to know Dr. A.K. Saxena personally when we took his help in comanaging a critically ill patient in 2006. This was a 45 years old gentleman with critical coronary artery disease who developed a cardiac arrest post angiography and was taken up for emergency bypass surgery while continuing CPR. Post surgery, patient developed signs of severe Hypoxic encephalopathy and critical illness myoneuropathy. He was comatose and could not move any of his limbs. MRI Scan suggested poor prognosis. In addition to conventional therapy, Dr. A.K. Saxena performed acupressure therapy on the patient regularly. To our surprise, there was a dramatic sustained improvement in his neurological status after Dr. Saxena's therapy and patient gradually recovered completely; was discharged, has resumed regular work and is doing fine on follow up. We had another similar patient with post cardiac arrest Hypoxic encephalopathy and critical illness myoneuropathy this year who also did reasonably well with comanagement using Dr. A.K. Saxena's acupressure therapy. I look forward to Dr. A.K. Saxena's continued association in comanaging critically ill patients.

I wish him success in all his endeavors.

Dr. Pradeep Jain
M.D. Medicine (PGI)
D.M. Cardiology (AIIMS)
Fellow, Indian College of Cardiology
Fellow, Cardiological Society of India
Sr. Cons. Interventional Cardiology
Indraprastha Apollo Hospitals
Delhi

Message-2

29-11-2011

I had developed disc prolapsed at L_5 S_1 level in January, 2008 for which all types of treatment, including Allopathy, Homeopathy and Physiotherapy failed to relieve the pain permanently. It was in July, 2008 that I took my first course of Acupressure Therapy from Dr. Saxena, followed by intermittent therapy for 3 months. There was complete pain relief without any medication. He was very confident about his therapy and it really showed results for me. I was very thankful to him. I remained pain free till June, 2011; however, the pain recurred with gradually increasing intensity especially in the left leg. By October it had become unbearable, even disturbing sleep at night. I again talked to Dr. Saxena and he and his team were kind enough to give me appointment immediately inspite of his busy schedule.

I have completed my 10 sitting course. As expected I am already better with about 70% improvement in pain without any pain killers. I am not disturbed by pain at night and the sense of well being is returning back. He is now planning an intermittent follow up every week for me, and I am confident that very soon I will be completely free of pain. I feel that not only this therapy is excellent, the dedication and knowledge of Dr. Saxena is remarkable. I sincerely thank him for his effort and concern about my health.

Rohatgi

Dr. (Mrs.) Jolly Rohatgi
M.S. (Ophthalmology)
Professor of Ophthalmology
Deptt. of Ophthalmology
UCMS & GTB Hospital
Delhi-95.

Message-3

26.05.2011

I extend my sincere gratitude to Dr. Saxena, who has diligent devotion and dynamic co-operation to all his patients attending him for cure through acupressure techniques. I wholeheartedly give my appreciation to Dr. Saxena for his regular dynamic assistance in curing me for my 'sciatica' and backache. Not only he is a successful therapeutist but he practices the medical science with humanity. I have great respect for him and pray to God for his long life and happiness.

His contributions for all these practitioners and his thoughts on this ancient practice have been put in the form of the book "Miraculous Effects of Acupressure"and can help to cure the patients by understanding the techniques. It would be a real pleasure to see this effort being translated in other languages to promote the practice and nuances of holistic medicine.

Dr.saxena is an asset for the suffering millions.

(DR.R.L.TRIPATHI)
PhD (FMS)
Associate Professor & Coordinator,
Hospital Lab Services
Department of Biochemistry
University College of Medical Sciences
(university of Delhi)
& Guru Teg Bahadur Hospital
Delhi-110095

Preface

Since putting out my first book on acupressure viz. 'Miraculous Effects of Acupressure' which I authored along with Padma Shree Dr. L.C. Gupta on the insistence of my Revered Guru Dr. Attar Singh in English language, I have been receiving numerous letters and calls complementing in bringing out the book in a very simple language without using too many technical words. As a matter of fact what prompted me to make such an attempt was our desire to reach out to the people at the grass root level, suffering from various ailments. I had seen people spending a good deal of money and time in undergoing plathora of blood tests, getting x-rays, Ultra Sonic examinations & other tests done & there after leaving the treatment in between for the reason, (i) exhorbitent cost of the medicine or (ii) because of the heavy cost of the recommended surgery. I observed that a good number of these cases could have been taken care of without medicine or surgery, in case recourse would have been taken of getting cured using various therapies available in Nature Cure treatment e.g. taking acupressure treatment. The hassle of entering into never ending chain of blood tests, x-rays, ultrasonic examination or even MRIs, etc., which are being recommended these days as a routine. No doubt these tests become necessary in case the disease is prolonged. However, to send a patient to get MRI done who is suffering from cervical spondylitis, knee pain, migraine, sinusitis or sciatica, etc., which are in no way life threatening conditions, makes no sense to me, since such conditions can be taken care of very easily using acupressure technique.

My readers as well as my students have also been making a persistent demand that they would like to be exposed to the trigger points used by the practitioners of acupuncture. There was demand from another quarter for having a book in question and answer forın, answering the questions that generally trouble the mind of learners/readers about the efficacy and usefulness of this therapy.

This third book of mine i.e. '101- Questions on Acupressure and Reflexology', the idea of which was conceived by my senior colleague Padma Shree (Late) Dr. L.C .Gupta is being brought out to fulfill the long standing demand. As the title of the book itself suggests, an attempt has been made to answer probable questions that may come to the mind of the reader. All possible efforts have also been made to explain the precise location of the trigger points shown in the figures with as much clarity as possible. Dr. Preeti Pai who has been practicing acupuncture and acupressure for over 10 years has helped me immensely in this endeavour.

Before offering an apology for anything that may be lacking, I invite positive suggestions, criticism for further improvement and wish that our work is put to use for the benefit of mankind for the times to come. I conclude with the famous quote, 'A good start in the right direction is an immense advantage to the end of the race'.

—A.K. Saxena

Introduction

Acupressure is perhaps one of the oldest healing arts based on the technique of stimulating various key points on the surface of the body, by applying pressure on these acu-points/trigger points (also called reflex points) with the primary objective of relieving pain or discomfort. It is believed that the human body has immense self-curing capability. As and when pressure is given on the reflex points relating to the vital organs(s) of the body, they get stimulated and the pain and discomfort, which is considered to be a sign of energy imbalance, is corrected and the patient feels relieved. How is all this achieved? In simple terms, it can be said that when the pressure is given on the selected reflex points, it releases muscular tension and promotes circulation of blood, thereby stimulating body's life force/vital force to aid the healing.

Over a period of time, acupressure has gained a lot of prominence for the precise reason that it is free from any side effects since no medication/surgery is required. It is totally non-conventional, non- invasive and non- interventional. Moreover, my experience of over 22 years with various patients shows that this therapy is very effective in helping patients suffering from cervical/ lumber spondylitis; sinusitis; backaches; knee pain; heel pains; sciatica; prolapsed disc; constipation; indigestion; IBS; PMS; insomnia; depression; tennis elbow; asthma; hypertension, migraine; neuro problems, etc., to name a few.

Looking into the efficacy of this easy to learn and simple to perform therapy, even orthodox practitioners of conventional medicine have started opening out. In my association of more than five years with various hospitals of repute, where I have been attending critically ill patients on call in the ICUs, it has been established beyond doubt that in case treatment through acupressure is given along with any other conventional branch of medicine (i.e. co-managing patients), the results are quicker, effective and at times, unbelievable. Another advantage is that one can be trained in healing using this simple and inexpensive therapy as a home remedy, without fear of any side effects. In their present form, acupressure and acupuncture are attributed to Chinese origins where intensive research and significant work has been done to make these systems more effective and popular. During their historic visit to China in 1972, the U.S. President, Richard M. Nixon and his wife Pat, showed deep interest in acupuncture which became instrumental in bringing greater attention to this system in USA and in some other countries. Today, it is being practiced widely in Sri Lanka, Korea, Japan, Indonesia, Malaysia, India, etc.

Acupressure or reflexology or zone therapy, in fact, received a scientific approach during the early years of the twentieth century when an American doctor William H. Fitzgerald, M.D. (1872-1942), a reputed medical physician and surgeon, who was the Head of Nose and Throat Department of St. Francis Hospital in Hartford, Connecticut, developed the modern zone therapy.

Dr. Edwin F. Bowers, M.D. and George Starr White are two other great physicians of this period who also did remarkable work in elaborating this unique theory of healing. Dr. Joe Shelby Riley and his wife Elizabeth Ann Riley were two other stalwarts who tried out this system on a large number of their patients and made an unmatched contribution towards its development. Dr. Riley wrote twelve books on zone therapy, the first being copyrighted in 1917 and the last in 1942. Of late within a span of a decade or so a good number of alternative therapies e.g. acupuncture without needles (a new name given to acupressure – pressure point therapy), zone therapy, reflexology, shiatsu, massage, magneto therapy, hydro therapy and so on have emerged. However, it would be better to call them complementary therapy since the term alternative therapy may miss-communicate and give rise to the feeling that conventional medicine and alternative remedies are at odds with each other. The idea is to complement each other for the benefit of the patients, rather than to provide an alternative. The word complementary also has the right connotations which also suggest that there is a sense of acceptance which suggests that conventional medicine and complementary therapy treatments have a common goal to achieve and both of them must be allowed to play their respective roles amicably and supportively. There should be only one goal for the patient and the doctor — that is to get rid of the disease, as quickly as possible.

Perhaps this is the right time for the practitioners of medicine and complementary therapies to work together for the benefit of their patients. This point of view is gaining momentum with an increasing number of doctors, qualifying in complementary therapies. Few doctors of conventional medicine would disagree with an emphasis on body, mind and soul; eating for health and vitality; growing awareness amongst masses about exercise, self-help measures to enhance and improve the physical, emotional, mental and spiritual health and wellbeing. Two undisputed advantages of complementary therapies are that the practitioner has more time to devote to you and your problems than most doctors of medicine have. Moreover, complementary therapies are much in demand these days, perhaps the reason behind it is the growing consciousness amongst the masses about the side effects of medicine and the cost factors for some of the medicines prescribed are beyond the reach of the common man. Yet another cause of complementary therapies being in demand is that emphasis is placed on health rather than on illness, on prevention as well as on cure. Yet another cause of attraction is the emphasis on self-healing life forces, which can be balanced and remarshaled with minimal effort? Moreover it is simple to learn and easy to practice without the fear of any side effect, since no medication is required. It is totally non-invasive. No major gadgets are required thereby reducing the cost to almost zero. Another major advantage is that this therapy concentrates on prevention rather than the cure. The simple theory 'Prevention is better than cure'is the essence. Yet another advantage is that this therapy is partially diagnostic too. A good and experienced acupressure therapist will seldom refer you for an x-ray.

In case a person practices the daily work out programme, just by pressing 12 points over his body, he can stay fit and keep himself away from disease and medicine. Since by pressing these points, you stimulate your immune system and other important systems in your body that helps keep you fit in a natural way.

The ancient healers recognized the vital energy, a life force that animates every living being. They perceived that life energy permeates all the elements of the material world. The ancient physicians observed that this life energy circulates in the body along specific channels called meridians. Along each of these channels are numerous points. These are the points (also known as acu-points or trigger points) at which the flow of life force can be most effectively influenced.

At any given point of time, the flow of energy through the meridians of the body determines our health. When the flow is smooth, balanced and unobstructed, we are in good health. Pain and disease can occur when there is disturbance in the flow of vital force. By learning to apply gentle pressure with your thumb or finger tips on the key pressure points, these imbalances can be corrected to restore health and to overcome pain.

Acupressure therapy is based on the principle of keeping the Ch'i or Prana flowing in a balanced and harmonious way. Lack of exercise or faulty diet can also disrupt our system. Stomach disorders, colds, allergies, fatigue, etc., are a few ailments which caution us that there is something wrong with the flow of vital energy i.e. it is disturbed or blocked. If these minor imbalances are not corrected timely more serious health problems may occur.

There is substantial evidence now to show that acupressure is capable of regulating the nervous and circulatory system. Increasing circulation helps in flushing out the toxins from the body and brings nutrients and oxygen to all our cells. It also triggers the brain to release endorphins, a chemical known to reduce pain and bring a feeling of wellbeing.

The ancient healers felt that as long as there is coordination and cooperation among various organs in the body, we remain in good health. When this natural equilibrium is disturbed in the body for one reason or the other, one or more ailments take place depending upon the proportion and nature of imbalance or disturbance. Acupressure has been found to be the best method to restore normal functioning of the body in a natural way. Acupressure cleanses the body of toxins and impurities which accumulate at the nerve endings leading to many ailments. These toxins obstruct the normal flow of energy to various organs which in turn disturbs the balance of the whole body. When acupressure is given at the reflex centers of various organs, toxins, calcium, urea deposits accumulated in crystalline form, at the nerve endings in the palms and soles get crushed and are thrown out of the body through various outlets.

To summarize, it is an established fact that human body possesses immense natural strength to heal itself of any disease. All that is required is to tap this natural force to rejuvenate its energy. Acupressure has emerged as one of those few natural systems which are capable of reviving and revitalizing the hidden strength within the body to cure all kinds of ailments.

Foreword

Acupressure is an ancient 'healing-art' developed in Asia over 5000 ago , using fingers to press 'key-points' (energy centres, also called 'acu-points') on the surface of the skin to stimulate the body's natural self-curative abilities. These energy centres or acu-points are found on energy 'pathways' called meridians (carrying the energy 'chi'). Acupressure treats the body as an energy system and works to remove person's individual symptoms by identifying and releasing 'blocked' or 'congested' energy centres in the body.

Acupressure points on the body are generally massaged using finger or thumb and sometimes with a blunt object bringing relief to the person undergoing acupressure. Now this therapy is coming up in a big way globally, as one of the ancient Asian alternative therapies e.g. acupuncture without needles (a new name given to acupressure – pressure point therapy), reflexology, zone therapy, shiatsu, massage, magneto therapy, hydro therapy, etc.

These alternative/complementary therapies are much in demand these days, possibly on account of the growing consciousness amongst the masses about the side effects of the allopathic medicine, its cost factor, for some of the medicines are beyond the reach of the common man. Yet another cause of complementary therapies being in demand is that emphasis is being placed on 'Health' rather than on 'illness', on 'prevention' rather than on 'cure', as a part of the holistic healing. This point of view is gaining momentum with an increasing number of doctors, qualifying in alternative/complementary therapies.

Few doctors of conventional medicine would disagree with an emphasis on body, mind and soul; eating for health and vitality; growing awareness amongst masses about exercise/yoga, self-help measures to enhance and improve the physical, emotional, mental and spiritual health and wellbeing.

The authors have been working on patients for many years in various hospitals of repute, where they have been attending even critically ill patients. It is, by now, well established, that in case treatment through acupressure is given along with any other conventional branch of medicine (i.e. co-managing patients); the results are quicker and effective.

A.K. Saxena has already authored two books on acupressure, a pioneering work indeed, one by the name 'Miraculous Effects of Acupressure' in English (Gujarati and Marathi versions are in print) and the other 'Acupressure aur Swasth Jeevan' in Hindi, which has a large readership.

The present work '101-Questions on Acupressure and Reflexology' in question and answer form, would be of immense value to the aspiring students of the science and art of acupressure and reflexology, as it aims to address many queries in the mind of a person about the usefulness of alternate/ complimentary therapies.

Dr A.K. Saxena and Dr. Preeti Pai have taken care to answer all possible questions that bother the minds of learners and their effort is appreciable.

I hope that this work shall go on to achieve the objective, which drove the experienced, knowledgeable and committed authors to undertake this enterprise.

I wish them all the success.

(Brij K Taimni)
IAS (Retd)

Contents

101 Q&A Acupressure & Reflexology

Q. 1: What do you understand by the term acupressure? Throw some light on its advantages.

A. 1: Acupressure is perhaps one of the oldest healing arts based on the technique of stimulating various key points on the surface of the body, and by exerting pressure on these acupoints/trigger points with the primary objective of relieving pain or discomfort. It is believed that the human body has immense self curing capability. As and when pressure is applied on the reflex points relating to the vital organ(s) of the body, they get stimulated and the pain and discomfort considered to be a sign of energy imbalance gets corrected and the patient feels relieved. How is all this achieved? In simple terms, it can be said that when pressure is given on the selected reflex points, it releases muscular tension and promotes circulation of blood thereby stimulating body's life force/vital force to aid healing.

Acupressure is a Latin word wherein Acu stands for the word thumb while the word pressure is self explanatory. As the name itself suggests, while giving treatment through this technique, pressure has to be given on various selected reflex points using the thumb or fingers. However, in case a lot of patients have to be attended at a time, with a view to conserve energy of the therapist, pressure can also be applied with the help of certain instruments devised for the purpose. Reflex points pertaining to various organs of the body have been identified primarily in the palms and soles based on research/observations of over 5000 years. These acupoints generally occur in pairs except in the case of the heart and liver. The reflex points in respect of the heart are found in the left sole and left palm and in respect of liver they are found in the right palm and right sole.

Over a period of time, acupressure has gained prominence

for the simple reason that it is free from any side effect since no medication or surgery is required. It is totally non-conventional, non-invasive and non-interventional. Moreover, my experience of over 20 years with various patients shows that this therapy is very effective in helping patients suffering from cervical/ lumbar spondylosis; sinusitis; backaches; knee pain; heel pains; sciatica; prolapsed disc; constipation; indigestion; irritable bowel syndrome; insomnia; depression; tennis elbow; asthma; migraine; neuro problems, etc. to name a few. Looking into the efficacy of this easy-to-learn and simple-to-perform therapy, even orthodox practitioners of medicine have started opening out. In my association of about three years with various hospitals of repute, it has been established beyond doubt that in case treatment through acupressure is given along with any other conventional branch of medicine, the results are much faster, and at times unbelievable. Another advantage is that a person with average intelligence can be trained in using this inexpensive therapy as a home remedy, without fear of any side-effect.

Q. 2: What is the historical background of acupressure?

A. 2: There are claims and counter claims about the origination of this ancient healing art, which is also known by the names Acupuncture without needles, Zone therapy, Reflexology, Shiatsu, Pressure Point Therapy, etc. However, there is no denial to the fact that perhaps this is one of the oldest systems of nature cure in the world, based on the technique of massage or pressure. Earlier, it was assumed by people that perhaps this system originated in China, However, another school of thought held the view that this concept was conceived by Indian thinkers in ancient times. It was from here that this art and science was carried to other parts of the world by scholars, pilgrims, etc. Russians have also endorsed this view through their research that this art and science originated in India. To this effect an article was published in *'Indian Medicines in Ancient Russian Treatment of Diseases'* by N.A. Bogoyavlensky in 1956 by the State Publishing House of Medical Literature, Leningrad Department.

If we carefully look at the Indian tradition of wearing jewellery, it becomes apparent that perhaps our ancestors were aware of the importance of pressure technique; and that is why the Indian tradition of wearing heavy jewellery in the fingers in the shape of rings, bangles (thin as well as thick made of heavy silver/gold) around wrists and at the ankles, as these are the areas where the reflex points of the lymphatic system as well as the genitals are located and are stimuled by the weight of the jewellery. Similarly, the tradition of piercing ears and nose has something more to it than mere beautification.

Another prominent 8th Century scholar from China, Hieun Tsang spent many years at Nalanda University in India. On his return to his country, he wrote a book in which he described in detail what was taught in Medical Science at Nalanda University. Another prominent scholar from China, Ia Tzin, who visited India in 673 AD and also studied in Nalanda University for many years, has in his writings described how Indians imparted knowledge about the science and art of medical treatment by pricking needles, now known as acupuncture. He has also mentioned about various branches of medical sciences flourishing in India. Chinese translations of many Indian manuscripts on philosophy, astronomy, mathe-matics and medical science have been preserved in various libraries in China till date. From China, Indian knowledge of medicine also circulated to Tibet and many other countries.

Bogoyavlensky's book also contains an interes-ting and revealing illustration which shows various points and areas in the human body for the purpose of curative cauterisation and acupuncture. This illustration dates back to the first century A.D. and was procured from Eastern India. These writings undoubtedly establish India's pioneering role in the field of acupressure and acupuncture. reflexology historian Christine Issel has mentioned that certain traditional paintings of the feet of Hindu god Vishnu are covered in symbols coinciding with the reflex points, which further corroborates that acupressure, was widely practiced in earlier times in India. Stanley Burroughs in his book *'Healing for the Age of Enlightenment'* has tried to authenticate that this sort of medical treatment was known and practiced in many parts of ancient India. On the basis of certain tomb drawings which depict feet being massaged in a particular position, Egyptians are also believed to have been practicing an acupressure-like system in ancient times. With the advent of certain new pathies, acupressure and acupuncture suffered some setback but these systems could not be ignored altogether for a long time. Their enduring qualities again attracted the attention of men in the medical profession as well as others. During the year 1582, two distinguished European physicians, Dr. Adamus and Dr. A'tatis, brought out a book on Zone Therapy which gave eminence to this primitive system of treatment.

acupressure or reflexology or zone therapy, in fact, got scientific approach during the early years of the twentieth century when an American doctor William H. Fitzgerald, M.D. (1872-1942), a reputed medical physician and surgeon, who was the Head of Nose and Throat Department of the St. Francis Hospital in Hartford, Connecticut, developed the modern Zone Therapy. Dr. Edwin F. Bowers, M.D. and Dr. George Starr White are two other great physicians of this period who also did remarkable work in elabourating this unique theory of healing. Dr. Joe Shelby Riley and his wife Elizabeth Ann Riley were two other stalwarts who tried out this system on their vast number of patients and made an unmatched contribution towards its development. Dr. Riley wrote twelve books on zone therapy, the first being copyrighted in 1917 and the last in 1942.

Eunice D. Ingham, a member of New York State Society of Medical Masseurs, also did creditable work in popularising this therapy by benefitting her numerous patients and by bringing out certain good books on Reflexology including 'Stories The Feet Can Tell' and *'The Stories The Feet Have Told'*. From the early 1930s until her death in 1974, Eunice worked zealously to make it a perfect branch of medical science.

In their present form, acupressure and acupuncture are attributed to China where intensive research and significant work has been done to make these systems more effective and popular. During the historic visit of U.S. President, Richard M. Nixon and his wife Pat, to China in 1972, they showed deep interest in acupuncture which became instrumental in drawing greater attention to this pathy in the U.S. and in some other countries. In Denmark too, reflexology is the most popular of all complementary therapies.

Japan has taken a lead in developing and popularising a distinct type of pressure therapy called 'Shiatsu', which is also based on the principles of acupressure. In Japanese language, 'Shi' means finger and 'atsu' means pressure. Prof. Sir Park Jae Woo, a South Korean by birth, who has set up his academy in Moscow, gave Su Jok system of the treatment to the world in the year 1986, which has its roots in acupressure.

In recent times, immense interest has been shown in reflexology by certain highly qualified health professionals in Europe, U.S.A., Canada, Germany and many other countries including India, the place of its origin. Stephanie Rick in his book *'The Reflexology Workout'* has mentioned that in Europe nearly six thousand medical personnel combine reflexology as a part of their healing process these days. The number of such practitioners is on the rise. More and more people are now taking a deep interest in this system in view of its efficacy. It would thus be correct to conclude that acupressure has now become one of the most popular systems of natural treatment in many countries across the globe.

Q. 3: What do you understand by alternative/ complementary therapy? Why is this therapy becoming so popular?

A. 3: Of late, within a span of a decade or so, a good number of alternative therapies, e.g. acupuncture without needles (a new name given to acupressure – pressure point therapy), Zone therapy, Reflexology, Shiatsu, Massage, Magnet therapy, Hydro therapy, etc. have emerged. However, we shall try to use the term complementary therapy since the term alternative therapy may miscommunicate and give rise to the feeling that practitioners of medicine and alternative remedies are at odds with each other, whereas the idea is to complement each other for the benefit of the patients than to provide an alternative. The word complementary also has the right connotations which suggests that there is a sense of acceptance; which also suggests that conventional medicine and complementary therapy treatments have a common goal to achieve and both must be allowed to play their roles amicably and supportively for there is only one goal for the patient and that is to get well as quickly as possible. How and using which medium is none of his concern.

Perhaps this is the right time for practitioners of medicine and complementary therapies to work together for the benefit of their patients. This point of view is gaining momentum by an increasing number of doctors qualifying in complementary therapies. Few doctors of conventional medicine would disagree with an emphasis on the positive aspect of holistic healing systems that place equal emphasis on body, mind and soul; eating for health and vitality; growing awareness amongst masses about exercise, and self-help measures to enhance and improve physical, emotional, mental and spiritual health and well-being.

Two undisputed advantages of complementary therapies are that the practitioner has more time to devote to you and your problems than most doctors of medicine have. Moreover, complementary therapies are much in demand these days, owing to the growing consciousness about the side-effects of medicine and the cost factor, for some of the medicines are beyond reach of the common man. Yet another cause of complementary therapies being in demand is that emphasis is placed on health rather than on illness. Yet another cause of attraction being the emphasis on self-healing life forces, which can be balanced and remarshalled with minimal effort. Moreover, it is simple to learn and easy to practice without the fear of any side effect, since no medication is required. It is totally non-invasive. No major gadgets are required thereby reducing the cost to almost zero. Another major advantage is that this therapy concentrates on the preventive part than the cure. The simple theory 'Prevention is better than cure' is the motive. Yet another advantage is that this therapy is partially diagnostic too. A good and experienced acupressure therapist will seldom refer you for an x-ray. The reason, by touching the reflex point pertaining to a particular part/organ of the body, he can reveal to you the internal status of the organs. In case a person is suffering from cervical pain, the therapist would just press certain pressure points on the big toe and let you know almost the exact location of the problem area, i.e. the exact number of vertebra viz. C-1 to C-7 that an X-ray would have otherwise revealed, which is expensive as well as hazardous to our health. Similarly, by touching the points on the wrist, an experienced therapist can tell about the status of the internal organs, e.g. ovaries, uterus etc.; by touching the pressure points over the Heart meridian, one can tell if a person is suffering from blood pressure and so on.

In case a person practices the daily workout programme discussed in this book, just by pressing 12 points over your body, you can stay fit and keep yourself away from disease and medicine. Since by pressing these points, you stimulate your immune system and other important systems in your body that helps you to keep fit in a great natural way.

Q. 4: How does Acupressure work?

A. 4: The Chinese recognised a vital energy, a life force that animates every living being. The ancient healers perceived that life energy permeates all the elements of the material world. In China this life energy is called Ch'i, Ki in Japan and Prana in Indian Yoga. All these words are the names for the same thing and are known as life energy or life force in the West. The ancient physicians perceived that this life energy circulates in the body along specific channels called meridians. Along each of these channels are numerous points. These are the points (also known as acupoints or trigger points) at which the flow of life force can be most effectively influenced.

At any given point of time, the flow of energy through the meridians of the body determines our health. When the flow is smooth, balanced and unobstructed, we are in good health. Pain and disease can occur when there is disturbance in the flow of vital force. By learning to apply gentle pressure with your thumb or finger tips on the key pressure points, these imbalances can be corrected to restore health and to overcome pain. Acupressure therapy is based on the principle of keeping the Ch'i or Prana flowing in a balanced and harmonious way. Lack of exercise or faulty diet can also disrupt our system. Stomach disorders, colds, allergies fatigue, etc., are a few ailments which caution us that there is something wrong with the flow of vital energy, i.e. it is disturbed or blocked. If these minor imbalances are not corrected in time, more serious health problems may occour.

There is substantial evidence now to show that acupressure is capable of regulating the nervous and the circulatory systems. Increased circulation helps in flushing out toxins from the body and takes nutrients and oxygen to all our cells. It also triggers the brain to release endorphins, a chemical known to reduce pain and bring feeling of well-being.

Ancient healers felt that till there is coordination and cooperation among the various organs in the body, we remain in good health. When this natural equilibrium is disturbed for one reason or the other, ailments develop depending upon the proportion and nature of imbalance or disturbance. Acupressure has been found to be the best method to restore normal functioning of the body in a natural way. Acupressure cleanses the body of toxins and impurities which accumulate at the nerve endings leading to many ailments. These toxins obstruct the normal flow of energy to various organs which in turn disturbs the balance of the whole body. It is through acupressure that various crystal like calcium and urea deposits accumulated at the nerve endings in the palms and soles get crushed slowly when pressure is given at the reflex centres of various organs, and are thrown out of the body through various outlets.

To conclude, it is an established fact that the human body possesses immense natural strength to cure itself of any disease. All that is required is to tap this natural force to rejuvenate its energy. Acupressure has emerged as one of those few natural systems which are capable of reviving and revitalising the hidden strength within the body to cure all sorts of ailments. Many theories exist about its working as to how such remarkable results are achieved in overcoming even certain terminal diseases in conjunction with conventional medicine. However, we have to accept that it is still a mystery as to how this system works inside the body in curing various diseases.

Q. 5: Define the terms acupressure, reflexology and acupuncture. Highlight the difference, if any, between them.

A. 5: Acupressure is a natural way to provide health and well-being using the thumb or the fingers of our hands to stimulate specific key points also called trigger points on the body in general and on the palms and the soles in particular with a view to overcome pain and discomfort. As a matter of fact, pain or discomfort in any part of the body is the natural way of the body to sound an alarm bell indicating that some energy imbalance has taken place and pain is a sort of caution to us about any ensuing ailment. In acupressure various acupoints also called trigger points, are stimulated with an objective to restore the energy imbalance. These acupoints are located on the pathway of the meridians or the channels that run throughout our body and connect all parts of the body together as a whole. These pressure points pain a lot on being pressed, and give a feeling as if something is being pierced into. They act as remote control since by giving pressure on a point on the big toe or the thumb, the pain in the neck or headache can be cured. These points also help us restore any imbalance in the energy flow in our body.

Reflexology is similar to acupressure in basic principle. In this system too, healing is based on balancing energy by stimulating certain defined areas in the soles and palms. These areas relate to various organs and parts of our body. Both the systems, viz. acupressure and reflexology work towards restoring imbalances in the energy force by exerting pressure or giving massage like pressure on certain specific areas which relate to the affected organ(s). Applying pressure on specific reflex areas results in adjustment in the flow of energy in the body thereby creating positive response, i.e., proper functioning of an organ or reduction of pain, and we say that the patient has been treated.

Acupuncture, which is said to be in use in China for about 5000 years, is also based on the principle that good health depends upon the balance in energy flow in our body which the Chinese call Qi or Ch'i and pronounce it as 'chee'. It is believed that Ch'i flows throughout the body and is concentrated in the channels also known as meridians. 14 meridians run from the hands and feet to the body and head. The aim of acupuncture is to maintain health and to restore the balance among the physical, emotional, mental and spiritual aspects of an individual by maintaining a harmonious balance between the equal and opposite qualities of Ch'i, viz. the Yin (passive) and the Yang (active). As per theory of Chinese medicine, many factors, e.g. anxiety, fear, grief, stress, undereating/overeating, environmental or occu-pational conditions, hereditary factors, infections and shock or trauma may upset the balance of Yin and Yang which results in disharmony or ill health. Acupuncture helps in restoring the Yin-Yang balance, thereby helping in attainment of natural state of health and harmony. Acupuncture needles are so thin and fine that in the hands of the skilled practitioners the amount of discomfort is very little. Moxibustion compliments acupuncture. In the process, the patient receives warmth, either directly through the heating of acupuncture needles or indirectly through the warming of certain points or areas on the skin. The combination of acupuncture and moxibustion is known as Zhen Jiu which means 'poking and burning'.

From above it would be seen that primarily all the three forms, i.e., acupressure, reflexology and acupuncture are more or less similar. The underlying principle of all the three forms is to restore the imbalance, if any, in the flow of energy with a view to overcome pain and discomfort. However, there is some difference between them. Acupressure is simple to perform and can be considered to be a home remedy since any person with basic intelligence can learn to do it as it does not require much precision to get benefit out of it. Moreover, it is inexpensive and with a little effort one can treat himself/herself to get the benefit sitting at home.

As for Reflexology, whereas it is similar to acupressure in principle, but the two have some differences as well. While acupressure involves meridians and acupoints, reflexology relies on pathways called reflex zones, Moreover, the reflexologist restricts his healing work primarily to the feet and he lays only a secondary emphasis on the hands. According to them, giving a thorough workout to your feet can invigorate or relax your entire body. The focus of a reflexology treatment is basically on the reflex zones which are more generalised areas than the specific points used in acupressure. Yet since many of the meridians run through the foot, perhaps that is why reflexology is so effective. Moreover, foot massage is a universal and time tested practice. Reflexology has roots in the ancient Asian pressure point systems, though it was rediscovered and redeveloped in late 19th and early 20th centuries. William Fitzgerald, a physician, discovered that he could do minor surgeries after applying pressure on certain points on the hand to prevent pain. He identified them as reflex zones of the body and called his work 'Zone Therapy'.

Coming to Acupuncture, whereas this therapy also follows reflexology and also strives to re-establish the balance of flow of energy through various meridians, its methodology is quite different. First of all, not all can use this therapy as a home remedy for it requires lot of precision in inserting needles. It would not be wrong to say that the extent of precision required is more than that of a surgeon. Secondly, not many practitioners are easily available. Further, it is an expensive treatment and can in no way be compared with acupressure. A separate set of needles (disposable/otherwise) is required which becomes quite expensive. The fees of the acupuncture therapist is obviously high because of their scarcity. Thirdly, there may be least pain while pricking needles in expert hands, yet the fear of needles being pricked is another deterrent.

Q. 6: Is it necessary to have thorough knowledge of meridians before beginning using pressure points for healing?

A. 6: Meridians are channels or pathways through which Ch'i circulates and is similar to our circulatory or nervous systems. These channels can be compared as the wiring in the body's electrical system, carrying the vital force.

It is not essential to have a detailed under-standing of the meridians (heart/lungs etc.) to begin using pressure points for healing. However, basic knowledge of the principles involved, will make us more confident of what we are doing and why.

In short, there are twelve main meridians which carry the vital life energy throughout the body. Each meridian traverses a specific path through the body and links specific organs. For example, the Heart meridian runs from the side of the chest from under the armpit down to the inside of the arm to the little finger.

This is the path pain follows during a heart attack.

The twelve meridians are divided into pairs, i.e. the meridians on the right and left sides of the body are mirror images of each other. Six pairs run over the arms to torso and another six pairs run up and down the legs to the trunk.

These twelve pairs of meridians influence and reflect the functioning of major organs in the body.

The Six Arm Meridians:

Li.......Large Intestine

Si.......Small Intestine

H........Heart

Pc.......Pericardium

TW......Triple Warmer (the abdominal cavity which maintains internal heat.)

L.........Lung

The Six Leg Meridians:

Gb.......Gall Bladder

B.........Urinary Bladder

K.........Kidney

Lv........Liver

St.........Stomach

Sp........Spleen and Pancreas.

In addition, there are two unpaired meridians not associated with any particular organ but are reservoirs of Yang and Yin energy. The Governing Vessel (GV) links the spinal column, brain and the nervous system. It runs from the tail bone straight up the back and over the top of the head to the centre of the upper lip. Its main function is to govern all the Yang meridians in the body. Points along this meridian can help alleviate stiffness of the spine, fever, irritability and muscle spasms of the back. The second unpaired meridian, the Conception Vessel (CV), is the Yin partner to the Governor Vessel. This meridian is responsible for all the Yin pathways. It is linked to the digestive and reproductive systems and flows up the front of the body from the perineum (a point between the anus and genitals) to the lower lip. Ailments such a cough, asthma, urinary or genital problems can be treated from key points along this meridian.

Let us look at just one of the important meridians, i.e., the Kidney meridian:

The kidneys are considered to be the store house of Ch'i. They govern the sexual energy, the urinary system and the bones being linked with the brain. When the kidneys have energy in abundance, the functioning of the vital organs is strong, vitality and creativity are high. On the other hand in case you feel exhausted, it implies that your store of Ch'i in the kidneys may be low or the kidney meridian may be blocked.

The kidney meridian goes from the little toe to its first pressure point on the sole of the foot. It passes the heel, reaches the ankle bone on the inner side and flows up the inside of the leg past the knee and up the thigh to the coccyx. From there it goes up to the kidneys, then through the liver, diaphragm and lungs as far as the throat and the root of the tongue. Along this meridian there are 27 main pressure points.

Some symptoms one might experience owing to the imbalance along this meridian are asthma, breathlessness, dryness of the tongue, throat pain, oedema, diarrhoea, weakness of the legs, lower back pain, and diminished sex drive. If points on the kidney meridian are painful to touch it does not necessarily mean that the kidney itself is weak, but that the energy in that meridian is blocked, excessive or unbalanced. Working various points along the meridian can unblock the energy flow and help to heal various conditions. For example, pressing on K1 can help relieve impotence and hot flushes, and is rejuvenating. Working on K 2 can relieve irregular menstruation and foot cramps. Pressure on K 6 may help relieve insomnia and so on.

Q. 7: It is said that acupressure can also be used as a home remedy. Apart from the professionals who have knowledge of reflex points and meridians, how can a layman locate the points to be pressed for achieving the desired result?

A. 7: Yes, it is correct to say that acupressure can be used as a home remedy. Though it would be appropriate that at the beginning of the session(s), the patient consults a professional therapist to know the reflex points to be pressed in a particular median and their position on the sole or palms or on other parts of the body in respect of a condition peculiar to him. This is generally done by the professional therapists by marking a chart and handing it over to the patient(s) who can ill afford to visit a professional time and again. As already stated earlier, an average intelligence and understanding of a language commonly used, i.e. English or Hindi is essential.

Once the points to be pressed are known, one can easily reach out to these points by following the directions given below:

Give a thorough rolling, say for a period of 30 seconds to a minute, to the area where the points to be pressed are located. These may generally be in the soles and palms. By rolling, that specific area gets stimulated to get pressure. Start giving pressure either with the help of your thumb or by placing the index finger or middle finger on the point and pressing it with the thumb of the other hand. This way the extent of pressure gets doubled. Gradually, one can learn to adjust the extent of pressure to be exerted. While doing so one has to watch out for the reaction of the pressure point which is being pressed. In case you are putting pressure on the right spot, it will hurt in a peculiar manner as if some needle or a piece of glass is being pierced. The reason behind this sort of feeling, which is absolutely different from the one in case you are not pressing at the right spot, is that if a particular organ say kidney or liver is not functioning properly because the flow of energy to that organ is being obstructed for one reason or the other, it hurts making it feel like the prick of a needle because of some crystal like formation at the trigger/ pressure point relating to that organ which gets crushed slowly when pressed and the blockage from the path of meridian is cleared. Once the blockage is cleared and the flow of the vital force/energy/life force whatever name you give it, is restored, the particular organ gets fully stimulated and starts functioning with full vigour and we say that the disease has been eliminated. In case, however, despite pressing on a point with sufficient pressure no feeling of that prick-like pain is felt, it means that you are not pressing at the right spot and must look for the place that hurts. Be sure that you will find it very close, say a few millimetres from the point where you are pressing. Slowly you will be able to locate the point to be pressed without any problem. Pressure can also be given with the help of some instrument(s) specially designed for the purpose so that one can conserve his/her energies to attend to more than one patient in a row.

Another important factor is to keep your expectations realistic. In case you do not get immediate results, do not be disappointed and feel like giving it up before you make really good progress. After all, chronic ailments do not show up overnight so it would be unrealistic to assume that they can be cured overnight. Rest assured that you will be benefitted even if there is a gradual progress in the beginning, i.e. you get even partial relief at the end of a session say even for an hour or two, and do not get demoralised in case the pain recurs after an hour or so after the sitting. Gradually the pain will be cured completely.

Have faith in the therapy and be sure that you will attain the goal since ultimately it is your own body which is going to get you the results. Never forget that our body has immense natural power to fight disease and all that is required is to direct the body force in the right direction to get rid of an ailment. Through acupressure, we strive to revitalise the life force in our body by giving pressure on the trigger points of vital organs in our body. Remember, nature can never fail and as such despite giving a fair trial, in case you are not able to get relief, consult a professional. In other words, our approach should be, 'Blame the therapist not the therapy'. However, as a word of caution, one must not use this technique as a substitute for medical care and treatment, particularly when the disease involves vital organs. It would be safer to use it in conjunction with medical treatment (i.e co-management) and not in place to get better results.

Q. 8: What type of knowledge is required to learn acupressure technique for healing? Is formal training essential to enable one to use it as a home remedy?

A. 8: This simple question is really a tough one to answer. We all know that there is no substitute to knowledge. The more knowledge we have the better it is. Especially, when we talk of healing others, it goes without saying that a person without adequate basic knowledge of anatomy, disease, physiology, etc., cannot and should not think of becoming a professional healer of acupressure.

Although it is said that acupressure is simple to learn and easy to perform, yet, one should be conversant with the functioning of various systems in our body, e.g., digestive, circulatory, excretory, respiratory, skeletal (bone), reproductive systems, etc., the role and functioning of various endocrine glands, for the reason that our body is an inter-related cohesive system in which every vital organ has an important role to play. Lack of knowledge could be disastrous. However, one can manage to learn this technique as a home remedy in case he has some basic knowledge of the working of the body, the position of various organs in the body and their functions, some understanding of the zone therapy and location of reflex points in the palms, soles and other parts of the body and their relation to various organs of the body. He/she should keep in mind that it would be safer for the patient if before getting on to the technique of acupressure healing, to consult a professional practitioner of medicine for a proper diagnosis of the ailment and only then resort to acupressure healing. In such a situation also it would be advisable to first contact an acupressure therapist to get a fair knowledge of the points to be pressed in a particular situation. In case this is not done, there is a fear that a major symptom, i.e., pain which is given by the body at the beginning of some ailment to draw our attention towards it, may get suppressed and deprive us of the attention the disease should have otherwise gained. It is always safer to first get a diagnosis done at the hands of a professional medical practitioner and to then start the healing through acupressure.

Other factors to be kept in mind to get best results are:

(i) Where to press,
(ii) How long to press,
(iii) How much to press,
(iv) How frequently, etc.

As for the first part as to where to press, this has been discussed in the earlier question at length. The only thing that needs to be elaborated here is that the patient should be made to sit or lie in a very cosy and comfortable position, free from any distraction, and he/she should be properly explained what is going to be done and what benefits the patient can expect. Over the years of experience with the patients, it is felt that it is extremely important to remove the fear factor from the mind of the patient. Since some therapists believe in giving very strong pressure which makes the patient cry out in pain, that fear does not allow the patient to keep a cool mind. In case the patient is explained that at no point of time the therapist is going to cross the limit of the pain threshold of the patient and that at the slightest indication of pain the extent of pressure would be reduced to match the pain-bearing capacity of the patient, the fear factor shall be overcome. If possible, some light music can be played, this too will have a soothing effect on the mind and body of the patient. As for the duration of the pressure, it can be 10 seconds at a time on one point and this can be repeated thrice on a point that is 30 seconds in total at one point. As for the extent of pressure, as already discussed above, we should begin with rolling pressure to mild pressure and then go towards moderate pressure. Under no circumstances should the pressure be severe . The frequency of giving pressure should be decided on a case to case basis. Generally, it would be preferable to give first three sittings consecutively. Thereafter, it could be twice or thrice a week depending upon the body's response and requirement of the patient as also the ailment as well as the time available at the disposal of the patients, since some patients who come from far off cities or a different country have only a few days/weeks at their disposal and can ill afford gaps between two sittings. Similarly, patients suffering from sciatica or prolapsed disc may need two sittings at times in a day, depending upon the severity of the pain.

In general, 10 to 15 sittings are enough for healing conditions like cervical/ lumbar spondylosis; heel/knee/back pain; sinusitis; piles; migraine; insomnia; tennis elbow; hiccups; acidity; constipation; female/male problems; bed wetting; prostate, etc.

It may take even longer in case of conditions like paralysis; arthritis; frozen shoulder and at times depression in cases where the patient has been under the influence of drugs for a prolonged time.

In short, a person desirous of learning this art and science of healing through the technique of acupressure can be trained within a short spell to use it as a home remedy and not for professional purposes, even if he considers himself to be having an average level of intelligence, knowledge of language (English/Hindi).

Q. 9: What are the basic tools required to practice acupressure?

A. 9: The word Acupressure itself comprises of two words, i.e., Acu which means 'thumb' and the word Pressure is self explanatory. Generally acupressure can be done without the help of any tools. However, while giving pressure in certain parts of the soles say heels, the necessity of some tool is felt in view of its thickness and strength. One has to apply a lot of strength to give pressure on or behind some important pressure points on the heel. Similarly, when you have to give pressure to a good number of patients at a stretch, you start feeling exhausted after attending to two or three patients. At such a time you feel the necessity of some tools that may come handy in conserving your energy. With this in view, some instruments have been devised and are easily available in the market. They are being described here, but the authors would like to clarify here that there is no point in procuring these tools, which are as yet not too expensive, till you seriously intend to use them. The reason being that they will be of use to you only if you use them. Simply buying them as a showpiece serves no purpose. We come across a good number of patients every day who make a mention of a good number of tools they have purchased from the market, but when asked to show them or how they use them, they inform that they must be lying somewhere in the house. So you can well imagine how useful they could be to you lying in some remote corner of your house.

Here are the names of some tools that are frequently seen in the markets:

(i) Jimmy;
(ii) Magic Massager,

(iii) Foot Roller
(iv) Pyramid Plate
(v) Twister,
(vi) Spine Roller, etc.

Of these the first three, i.e., Jimmy, Magic Massager and Foot Roller are enough for home use as described below:

Jimmy is used for giving pressure on self and on others. This is generally made of hard rubber. However, those made of wood are also available in the market. Jimmy can also be used for giving rolling pressure to stimulate the area where pressure on various trigger points needs to be given.

Magic Massager is yet another tool which is very-very useful if properly used. This is also made of hard rubber and has fourteen protrusions as against only one in the jimmy. This has been a boon to the patients who cannot visit a therapist on a regular basis on their own, particularly elderly persons or those who are bed ridden. As the name itself suggests, out of its 14 protrusions at least 8 to 10 touch reflex points of various organs in our palms at one time and once we press this magic massager between both our palms, at least 16 to 20 points are getting pressure at a time. This stimulates trigger points of various organs/parts of our body. By regularly using this massager, we take care of our organs and use this as a preventive therapy to keep ourselves fit. This massager can be used two to three times in a day for about three minutes on each occasion. The only care to be taken is that it should not be used till two hours or so have elapsed after lunch or dinner.

Foot roller made from fine quality wood, having uniform spikes has been found to be very useful, for the purpose of using acupressure as a home remedy. It has multi purpose utility. In case you want to use it for taking away that tired feeling, after the day's work, just sit on a chair in a relaxed posture, keep both your soles on it in the middle of the arch of your foot. Roll your soles slowly over it from the tip of the toes to the heel of your foot. Within two-three minutes of rolling you will feel that the circulation of blood in your body has improved tremendously, the feel of exhaustion has gone and you start feeling fresh. In case you want to take care of some problem in the lower part of your body say below the waist, roll the portion of the heel over this roller putting some pressure over the heels for two-three minutes. For problems in your abdominal area, roll the portion of the arch of your foot over the roller for the same period of three minutes or so and for overcoming any problem above your neck, roll the area of upper soles on this roller.

In case, however, it has to be used for reducing weight, the main function of this roller for which it is used, one should sit comfortably on a dining chair at its edge, in such a manner that one does not fall. Place both the feet over the roller in such a position that the middle of the arch of the foot rests on it. Put your body weight over it to the extent you can tolerate. Start rolling your feet over the roller briskly. Initially you may cover just the middle portion of the feet and then slowly try to cover the heel portion too. By brisk rolling for a period of three minutes in the morning and three minutes in the evening, we can think of reducing 2-3 kg of our weight in a month without resorting to dieting. However, to achieve this target normal dietary restrictions, e.g., minimal use of chocolates/ice creams/dry fruits/ sweets/ oils and fats have to be observed. Another important thing to be kept in mind is not to try to do it for three minutes on the First day itself. Begin with one minute or so depending on your stamina and age and gradually increase the usage time by half a minute to one minute so that you reach the target duration of three minutes at a time in a period of one week or even two, lest the muscles of the thighs and calves get overstretched and hinder simple movements. Gradually you may increase this duration to five minutes at best. Once you have achieved the target weight, you may do it only once or twice a week to maintain it.

The Pyramid plate can be used for about three minutes on each occasion and has more or less similar use as that of a roller. You can tilt the weight of your body on the heel portion of your body in case you have a problem in the lower part of your body, towards the tip of the toes in case the problem is above the shoulder area and in the middle, i.e., arch of the foot in case you want to address any problem in the abdominal area of the body.

Twister has more of cosmetic value. It can be used by obese people to shape their body. But one has to be careful while using it and in case one finds it difficult to maintain the balance of body, no harm in holding something, i.e. the handle of a door, etc. It helps in strengthening/tightening the loose muscles/fat that gets accumulated around the waist /hips or thighs in the shape of tyres because when one swings the body in a to and fro motion, the muscles in this zone get stretched and persistent use helps in burning fat also. This ultimately results in body shaping too.

Q. 10: What will happen if you press at wrong points?

A. 10: If we have a re-look at the answer to question 7, it has been clearly stated that as and when we press a reflex point which pertains to some organ or part of our body, it hurts as if a needle or piece of glass is being pierced. When we press on a pressure point, if it does not give a feeling of a peculiar sort of prick, we have to look for the right spot where it hurts. So there is very little scope of pressing a wrong point if either of the persons, i.e., who is giving pressure or the one who is receiving pressure is a little observant.

Even assuming that none of them come to know that they are not pressing at the right spot, which again is a remote possibility since it would be purely hypothetical to think of a situation that out of a set of five or six pressure points being pressed, none is being pressed properly or at the right place. But as said earlier, even out of the set of 5-6 pressure points to be pressed, even if 3-4 are being pressed correctly at the right place, at least it will help us stimulate some organs fully and a partial relief in respect of the points being pressed wrongly for the reason that before applying pressure, the area to be treated has to be stimulated by rolling the jimmy over that area. As such, while rolling, the reflex points falling in that area get some stimulation, though not to the extent they would have got in case proper pressure would have been applied on those points. In other words, the patient will take time in recovering should he be getting even partial/indirect pressure in the required zone/area.

In case, however, assuming that a person has to be treated for jaundice and in that situation the most important organ that needs stimulation is the liver. But, the person who administers the therapy at home is not aware of the disease nor conversant with the reflex point of Liver, and he has just been told to press at certain areas. As a layman, he gives pressure on the left palm instead of the right palm. Now the same pressure point on the right hand belongs to the liver and the same on the left hand belongs to the heart. That means the patient is getting his heart stimulated in place of the liver. Obviously, the patient is the gainer so far as his heart is concerned but is losing to the extent that he is not getting pressure on the liver point which requires a boost. As such his main ailment is bound to suffer a setback. But perhaps you will be astonished to know that the loss would be only partial for the reason that in the set of points to be pressed there will be other pressure points also which will have curing/ stimulating effect on the liver. Some results, though slow, would be forthcoming when those pressure points are pressed during the process. Further, in all probability we assume that the person adminis-tering the therapy the next time will not repeat the same mistake and the loss is cut short.

Yet another example to clarify this important aspect is that in case a diabetic patient is not given pressure on the pressure points pertaining to the pancreas (though it is again a rare possibility for the reason that pressure has to be given in both the palms and both the soles; and that the person giving the pressure forgets to give pressure on either of the four areas does not sound convincing). Anyway the loss in terms of the treatment shall be partly overcome in case the person giving pressure at least gives rolling pressure over the area, i.e., middle of the palm and arch of the foot and on at least two places out of four in the palms and the soles and proper pressure on the pressure point that belongs to the pituitary gland, the master gland of the endocrine system.

Q. 11: What side effects can this therapy cause? Are there any known side effects?

A. 11: In the context of modern medicine, the term side effect has assumed an alarming dimension. Almost everyone, even with an average knowledge about health and well-being is apprehensive that whatever medicine he is taking is going to have a side effect. They become suspicious even about certain medicines that have no side effects, or have not yet come to light or are not known to one and all. Any way, perhaps every citizen has a right to know about the side effect, if any, of any medicine or therapy he is about to undergo in the best interest of his health.

So far as pressure point therapy, i.e, acupressure and reflexology are concerned, based on our experience of about twenty years in practice, we can safely say that there are no known adverse side effects of this therapy. However, we would like to share with you certain situations which we came across while handling patients from different age groups for different ailments.

As mentioned in earlier pages, before beginning to give pressure to a patient, the foremost requirement is an understanding between the therapist and the receiver about the extent of pressure to be given/taken. In case a clear understanding is there in the mind of the therapist about the pain threshold of the patient and the patient is clear that no good purpose would be served by taking more pressure beyond the pain threshold (there is a possibility that the patient tends to accept more pressure in a bid to get well soon). This becomes counter-productive in the sense that the area where a particular point falls will become oversensitive/tender and at the slightest touch, even of a the cloth at times, will hurt. This is why we have used the term counter-productive since on the next sitting the patient will not be able to receive pressure on that point or area and that will result in terms of loss of time in recovering. Though not a side effect, we consider it non-productive since it will take about 2-3 days for the tenderness to vanish.

Similarly, at times in case excessive pressure is given which exceeds the pain-bearing capacity of the patient, some weak/fragile patients may faint. Though, on the face of it, this may sound like a serious situation, yet it is equally simple to bring the patient out of it. To achieve this, massage-like pressure is given on the little finger and the ring fingers of both the hands (to and fro movement). Within a spell of thirty seconds to one minute the patient will revive.

Yet another situation could be that one out of about 500-1000 patients complains of a feeling of weakness at the end of a session. What we found was that at times a patient is too scared to undergo this therapy for some reason. Most of the times it is found that the patient was too terrified owing to some earlier experience on himself/herself or of some relation/friend, at the hands of a therapist who might be giving too harsh a pressure to his patients. But in such cases, the best way is to reassure the patient that under no circumstances the pressure to be given will exceed his/her pain-bearing capacity. If necessary, the treatment can be discontinued and the patient told to come back as and when he feels confident. This, at times, inspires confidence in the mind of the patient and he soon returns and gets beneficial results.

Q. 12: Do pressure points for different diseases overlap?

A. 12: Yes, pressure points for different diseases will at times overlap. The reason being that most of the time when a patient approaches you he/she comes with a long list of ailments that he is suffering from. Although acupressure therapy has become very popular now, yet the fact remains that by and large people come for this therapy after having tried most of the other options available to them without much success. And at the end of the day when the patient approaches a non-conventional therapist, the expectations are too high and his/her patience is almost exhausted. The nett result is that the therapist has to put in his best effort to ensure that the confidence of the patient is not shattered and another important factor, i.e. the results do not send a wrong signal in the mind of the patient and through him to people about the capability of the therapy as such.

The first thing to be told to the patient in such cases is that at a time, if possible we have not to address more than two or at best three ailments, otherwise the results get cluttered. Now, to understand the overlapping part, let us assume that a patient is suffering from arthritis, prostate, and diabetes. Since in the disease of arthritis the level of urea is increased, we have to stimulate the reflex point(s) relating to the kidney, the vital most organ in the excretory system besides other reflex points; now in case we look at the prostate problem, again in this urological problem kidneys need to be stimulated and as such pressure needs to be given on the reflex points relating to the kidneys;

now going to the next disease, i.e. diabetes for which the patient has to be treated, though kidneys have nothing to do with the treatment of diabetes, yet as the sugar goes into the urine once the sugar level in the blood goes beyond 170, as such kidneys have to do a lot of work in diabetics and to protect kidneys from any kind of damage, they need to be stimulated. Thus we see a clear overlapping of the same organ or same pressure points for three different diseases.

Similarly, in case a patient suffering from jaundice also has constipation and other problems with the digestive system have to be attended, reflex points relating to liver have to be stimulated in respect of all the ailments. Again it is a case of overlapping of the reflex points. However, this in no way causes any problem in handling a patient, rather it saves the time of the therapist as by stimulating a reflex point he is able to address more than one problem in one go.

In this context, it would perhaps be relevant to clarify that as per the principle of zone therapy, all those organs that fall in a particular zone of the body, the reflex points pertaining to them also become tender to touch in case any organ in that zone develops any sort of problem. This happens for the reason that all the organs falling in that zone are linked to the same life force. For example, in case some problem develops in the eye, the reflex points of all the organs falling in the same zone, i.e. the reflex points of eyes, kidneys, liver and small intestines will also become tender to touch. As such for the treatment of the eyes, we shall have to give pressure on the reflex points of kidneys, liver and small intestines also besides pressing the points related to the eyes with a view to restore the energy flow in the entire zone and the organs falling in that zone. The same procedure will have to adopted in respect of all the diseases and this is why also the pressure points overlap.

Q. 13: Can this therapy be applied along with the allopathic line of treatment or should allopathic drugs be discontinued?

A. 13: In case a patient is undergoing allopathic treatment for the same disease or some other disease, he need not discontinue the use of allopathic drugs since it does not in any way infringe the functioning of the other. However, if the patient is undergoing treatment for some painful condition, say sciatica or simple back pain and is getting only painkillers, it is always in the interest of the patient to cut down on medicine as recovery starts, and gradually increase the duration time of the medicine from 6 hrly to 8 hrly and then to 12 hrly dose. Once the patient has taken about 4-6 sittings, generally the use of the medicine can be restricted to SOS dose. However, suppose a patient undergoing treatment for a painful condition is suffering from hypertension as well as diabetes, it would be foolish to suggest withdrawal of the medicine. He can, without the least doubt, continue the use of medication on a regular basis while undergoing acupressure treatment.

As a matter of fact, it has been found that patients undergoing treatment for chronic ailments respond better and faster in case they are given acupressure treatment along with the conventional medical treatment.

Q. 14: How many minimum sittings are generally required for treatment of a disease? On an average, how much time will the practitioner take in one sitting?

A. 14: It is difficult to say with certainty as to how many sittings would be required for the treatment of a disease. It all depends upon the age, disease from which the patient is suffering, for how long the disease has been persisting, etc. Even more important is the body's response and the pain-bearing capacity also referred to as pain threshold of the patient. At times you come across a patient who would cry at the slightest touch and would not tolerate even rolling pressure. In such cases, the number of sittings could be much more as compared to a patient who is able to accept mild to even moderate pressure. In general, based on our experience with various types of patients coming from all age groups and stature, on an average the number of sittings required may vary from 10 to 15 in respect of most of the diseases with an exception to diseases like paralysis, frozen shoulder, arthritis, depression, etc., in which case much depends upon the duration of the disease, willpower of the patient and the pain threshold. However, in these diseases the number of sittings can swell up to 30 to 50 sittings or even more. In case of diseases like diabetes, hypertension, etc., the patient should be given only 3-4 sittings, and during these sittings effort should be to make him conversant with what to do. However, they have to continue to take pressure at home on a regular basis, say for a month or two, in the beginning on a daily basis or even twice a day, and there-after at least 2-3 times in a week.

Similarly, the time taken by the practitioner shall depend up on the disease being treated. In case of paralytic or arthritic patients, the number of pressure points to be pressed are much more. Moreover, such patients have little or no control over their limbs, so one sitting may even take something between 40 to 50 minutes. Otherwise, in general cases, the duration of a sitting may vary from 10 to 30 minutes depending upon the nature of the ailment(s) being addressed.

Q. 15: Should the patient be empty stomach before starting the treatment?

A. 15: No, it is not necessary to be empty stomach before taking the treatment. One can take light breakfast before the sitting. Taking tea/coffee/milk, etc., is also allowed.

However, one should avoid taking pressure therapy for up to 2 to 3 hours after taking lunch or dinner, because while rolling for stimulation the pressure points to be pressed may lie in the area which falls in the reflex zone or meridian of the stomach etc., which needs to be avoided when the stomach is full. There is no restriction for taking lunch or dinner immediately after the session is over.

Q. 16: Is the treatment through Acupressure permanent?

A. 16: This is a very commonly asked question when the patient meets the therapist for the first time. I always put a counter question to the patient before answering this question, i.e. can you name one disease, one medicine or one doctor who can claim that a particular disease can be treated for ever? The patient goes satisfied when he is informed that the treatment can't be permanent, it can be called a long term treatment instead, i.e. the disease/pain should not reappear the day the therapy is stopped, i.e. once the sittings are over. Normally, it has been seen that once the patient recovers fully, the pain/disease does not recur for years together. However, there is always a good chance of recurrence of a disease like prolapsed disc in case the patient does not choose to live cautiously, i.e. he lifts weight or indulges in strenuous exercises, bends, or jerks his body beyond a limit, etc.

As a matter of fact, certain diseases have a tendency. For example, even after surgery of kidney stone, in case certain dietary restrictions are not observed there is every possibility of its recurrence. So is the case with even high precision bypass surgery. The patient has to observe strict diet control in case a second surgery is to be avoided.

Q. 17 Is it a fact that most of the reflex points pertaining to various organs in our body are located in the soles and palms of our body? Describe.

A. 17: Yes, two charts at the end of the book exhibit the approximate, position of the reflex points pertaining to various organs/part of our body in our soles and palms. It must, however, be kept in mind that the points in respect of each individual may not be exactly on the same spot as each body differs in size. As such, as per the body structure of an individual, the location of the reflex point pertaining to an organ in a person may slightly vary. However, they will be located in the same zone. Reflex points in respect of certain parts of the body/organs overlap each other since various organs/glands fit in the body close together, overlapping each other, e.g. gall bladder, upper part of the ascending colon and liver on one hand; kidneys and small intestines on the other hand. At times they are so near or are virtually overlapping that while giving pressure, if one point hurts it becomes difficult to pin point as to which organ is actually having the problem.

To give a fairly good idea about the part(s) of palms and soles that contains, the reflex points relating to various portion of the body have been discussed below:

Part of the Sole/Palm	*Organ*
* Big toes/thumbs	Head, Neck, Part of Spine, Pituitary, Pineal
* Fingers	Head, Sinuses

* Shoulder to Diaphragm line	Armpit, Shoulders
* Upper Arch	Organs falling in upper abdominal part
* Lower Arch	Organs falling in the lower abdominal part
* Heel	Foot, Rectal area, Sciatic nerve, Sex organs
* Inner foot/hand	Spine, Bladder
* Outer foot/hand	Shoulder, Arm, Elbow, Leg, Knee, Buttock
* Wrists	Ovary, Testis, Uterus, Prostate, Penis
* Ankle	Pelvic area (Uterus, Ovary, Testis), Knee, Hip

Q. 18: It is said that zone therapy is the basis of reflexology or acupressure. Is it a fact? If yes, describe in detail.

A. 18: Acupressure/reflexology is a marvellous system of healing which is simple to understand and easy to practice. It has been found to be highly effective and totally safe with no side effects. Anyone with some basic knowledge of disease and location of the reflex points can do it sitting at home without the help of any expensive tools/machines. The whole thing becomes simpler in case one acquires some knowledge and understanding of the theory of ten invisible zones in our body. The best thing about this therapy is that it can be given to people of any age, sex, anywhere and at any time. It is a win-win situation all the way as we have nothing to lose. Because of this unique quality of acupressure, a large number of medical specialists having progressive and unbiased approach hold this therapy in high esteem and recommend acupressure treatment to many of their patients in conjunction with conventional medicine as the two can go concurrently.

It is a matter of fact that zone therapy is the basis of reflexology or acupressure. It got a new dimension and scientific recognition when Dr. William H. Fitzgerald, an American ENT specialist, undertook research during the early years of twentieth century to establish its utility. Initially, his fellow colleagues who perhaps did not have an equally progressive and unbiased approach, discouraged him. However, the continuous and dedicated approach of Dr. Fitzgerald brought to light the presence of ten energy zones in the body. These zones, which form the basis of reflexology and acupressure, are very simple to understand. According to it, there are ten invisible life force currents passing through the body from head to feet and hands, in line with all the toes and finger endings (the tips), as shown in fig-1. The specific area falling under each life force current is called a zone. In all there are five longitudinal zones on the right side of our body and five longitudinal zones on the left side of our body in equal proportions. All the ten zones run parallel over the entire body covering head, face, shoulders, arms, hands, chest, abdomen, reproductive organs, legs and feet.

Zone-1:

It extends from the top of the head to the big toes in the feet passing through the middle of the forehead, nose, palate, lips, chin, spine, abdomen and legs. This zone also goes up to the thumbs covering the shoulders and arms. Zone I thus feeds a part or entire area of the organs falling in this zone according to their actual position in the body, viz. head, brain, spine, nose, mouth, chin, the pituitary, pineal, thyroid, thymus and adrenal glands, lungs, heart (on the left side as well as on the right), esophagus, stomach, duodenum, small intestine, liver (on the right side), ureters, uterus, sex organs, prostate, urinary bladder, rectum and anus.

Zone-2:

Emanates from the top of the head and runs down to the second toe and likewise up to the tips of first finger. This zone covers certain portion of the brain, eyes, sinuses, tonsils, lungs, bronchial tubes, heart (on the left and right, both sides), stomach, liver (on right side), solar plexus, pancreas (on the left side), kidneys and small intestine.

Zone-3:

Comes from the top of the head and goes up to the third

toe in the feet and also up to second finger in hands. It includes some portion of the brain, eyes, lungs, heart (on left side), stomach (on left side), solar plexus, pancreas (on left side), liver (on right side), kidneys, appendix (on right side) and small intestine on both sides of the body.

Zone 4:

Extends from top of the head down to fourth toe in the feet and third finger in hands. This zone feeds certain areas in brain, ears, shoulders, lungs heart (on left side), stomach, spleen and pancreas (all the three on the left side), liver, gall bladder and appendix (all three on the right side), small intestine and colon on both sides.

Zone 5:

Moves from the top of the head down to little toes and little fingers in the feet and hands respectively. The fifth zone covers the outer side of the head, certain portions of the brain, ears, shoulders, upper arms, spleen (on left side), liver, gall bladder, ileocecal valve and appendix (all four on the right side) and colon on both sides.

Although all the toes, thumbs and fingers embody reflex areas for the brain and head, yet the major reflexes for the brain and head exist in the big toes and thumbs. Interestingly, each big toe and thumb contains reflexes for half portion of the brain and head on respective side. In addition each big toe and thumb sub-divides into five zones.

To facilitate quick and accurate detection of various reflex points pertaining to different organs, the founders of zone therapy have further divided hands and feet into three transverse (horizontal) zones. Thus to get maximum benefit from zone therapy, it is necessary that one must possess basic knowledge of the position of various organs in the body.

Q. 19: Does acupressure treat the cause of the disease?

A. 19: As pointed out earlier, a disease is the outcome of malfunctioning of one or more organs in our body. This occurs basically due to an imbalance in the flow of energy in the meridian(s) pertaining to these organs. In case this imbalance is somehow removed and the flow of the vital force, i.e. life energy restored in the pathways (meridians) of the affected organs, they start functioning to their optimum requirement.

It is very easy to achieve this with the help of the pressure point technique, i.e. acupressure. Once the cause is removed, the disease automatically disappears. That is why generally acupressure therapists say that they do not treat a disease but treat the organs. Once all the organs begin to function at their optimum level, the person becomes healthy and there is no place for disease.

Q. 20: Does acupressure help in chronic cases as well?

A. 20: The World Health Organization has accepted the fact that the traditional system of medicine offers valuable contribution towards the health and quality of human life. They have officially recommended the use of acupuncture for treating conditions like arthritis, bursitis, tendonitis, backache, sciatica, neck and shoulder pain, migraine, and tension headaches, etc. In acupressure, we use exactly the same points that are used in acupuncture, only difference is the methodology, i.e. the needles are not used to prick. It has been found over years of practice that very encouraging results have been obtained in all the ailments referred to above. As such it can be safely concluded that acupressure helps in both acute and chronic cases.

This pressure point therapy (acupressure) which as a matter of fact is the simplified form of acupuncture and has also been referred to as "Acupuncture without needles" has been found to be remarkably successful in treating a number of functional disorders, infertility problems, chronic fatigue, digestive disorders, asthma, insomnia, nervousness and depression.

Q. 21: What role can acupressure play as a preventive therapy?

A. 21: To prevent illness, just spend a few minutes gently massaging at certain pressure points, releasing tension; opening up the flow of energy is a wonderful way to keep your body fit. In ancient China, family physicians used to get a fee only as long as their patients remained healthy. Treating someone who has fallen sick, according to them, is like 'starting to dig a well when you start feeling thirsty'.

The aforesaid quote has been deliberately incorporated to send a word down the line, i.e. we should do everything possible to ensure pre-empting disease before it takes place. This can be achieved by eating well, exercising, learning to calm our mind and body with meditation and relaxation, etc. An additional input of pressure point therapy shall provide an extra boost to our health in keeping ourselves strong and preventing slight imbalances from turning into significant health problems.

Soon, you will realise that prevention is perhaps the most potent and practical method of health care, going by the spirit of the saying 'An ounce of prevention is worth a pound of cure', which reflects the natural law of life. Why wait till you fall sick and thereafter seek medical attention which is expensive and perhaps full of side effects.

The day you adopt acupressure, it amounts to taking charge of your own health. The more body awareness you achieve, the more quickly you will be able to notice tension in your neck, shoulders or in whatever part of the body some unusual sensation occurs. Now by yourself, you will be able to dissolve it almost there and then, before it could develop into a more serious problem. By adopting acupressure, the pressure point therapy to manage the minor ailments and imbalances before they develop into major problems, you will be able to save money, prevent pain and disability and maintain good health.

Q. 22: Can acupressure also help in overcoming habits, e.g. smoking, alcohol, drug addictions, etc?

A. 22: Generally, when you talk to addicts suffering from either of the above mentioned addictions, they tell that they resort to such habits to overcome stress. Some say that they can think better when they smoke.

Because of its deep stress releasing and stimulating effects, acupressure therapy can be very helpful for the people who have somehow become addicted to these self-destructive habits, in which they lose both money and health. Besides the destressing points on which giving pressure will help, there are specific points you can use to clear your mind, regulate your appetite, balance your digestion. The increased feeling of well being created by deep relaxation will help you overcome cravings and strengthen your resolve to quit smoking, alcohol and other negative habits.

Q. 23: Can acupressure help in improving beauty?

A. 23: Yes, acupressure therapy is being used in China for hundreds of years to increase natural beauty of women. Though it cannot be attained overnight, as can be done by a quick visit to a beauty parlour, yet the brighter side is that whereas the beauty attained at a beauty parlour is only for a few hours or days and at a big cost, the beauty uplift attained by following an acupressure schedule is sustainable and for a much longer duration and without any cost. All that you are required to do is to spare 15-20 minutes out of your busy schedule, which is again much shorter a duration as compared to your visit to a beauty parlour. The fact that one day all of us are going to have wrinkles with ageing cannot be denied, yet the important part is to feel good and healthy.

We all know that we look better when we feel relaxed, so the first tip to tone up your beauty is to feel relaxed and take care to improve your overall health and vitality. This will further help you in bringing out your natural good looks. You can also learn to relax your facial muscles and stimulate certain pressure points which increase circulation and improve complexion. There are certain pressure points which you can include in your routine and that can even help you in preventing wrinkles on your face and the body in the long run. These points shall be discussed in detail in the section dealing with the treatment of various ailments.

Q. 24: Under what circumstances should acupressure be avoided?

A. 24: Though acupressure treatment is totally harmless and can be given to anyone at any age, of any sex and any place or time, yet it is better if it is not given

(i) Over a cut or over a fractured area,

(ii) In case there is swelling in the area where pressure needs to be given,

(iii) To a pregnant woman immediately after pregnancy is

known and may be even after the very first month of conception, because giving pressure on certain pressure points may cause contractions and may result in a miscarriage. However, in such cases if it becomes essential for some ailment like cervical, migraine, insomnia or nausea, etc., related to pregnancy, pressure should be given by a professional and under no circumstances should it be given by an untrained person at home.

(iv) Pressure should not be given at least upto 2 hours after taking lunch or dinner.

(v) Pressure therapy should be avoided for a period of at least half an hour after taking bath or undergoing full body massage or physical exercise in a gym or a play ground.

Q. 25: How does acupressure give relief in the severity of pain?

A. 25: Acupressure or pressure point therapy encourages the body to relax. This has an overall positive effect on our bodily functions. It destresses our body and reduces tension which constrict our muscles thereby restricting the flow of blood in the cardiovascular system. When our muscles are relaxed, blood can circulate more easily and freely and carry oxygen and other nutrients to our body cells. This also helps to eliminate accumulated toxins in our body. This has a direct impact on the severity of pain. Moreover, when the pressure points are pressed, the body releases natural pain killers, e.g. endorphins, which again help in curtailing the sensation of pain for the patient.

Q.26: Are dietary supplements/restrictions needed with this therapy?

A.26: Diet is one of the many factors that influence our health. If we really want to look good, we must be judicious about our diets too. Whereas specifically no dietary supplements are suggested as a precursor to undergoing this therapy, it is also assumed that the individual observes the usual norms of consuming a balanced diet to keep fit and healthy.

Some basic tips are, however, offered here for those who

feel that since they are in the prime of their youth, they can digest whatever stuff they consume. When we say whatever stuff we tend to point out towards the junk food in particular as well as the trend of consuming cheese in good quantity or ice-cream and chocolates, etc. Consumption of green vegetables, an essential ingredient in our diet, is a remote possibility perhaps. But those who still consume them in good quantity as a routine and also blend them with other fibrous food are certainly better placed in so far as staying fit and healthy is concerned. Another thing that needs mention is that generally people take a lavish dinner after the day's hectic work schedule. This is somehow not the right way. The largest meal should be consumed at lunch time in a relaxed manner, since at midday our digestive system can work strongest. It takes a long time to digest a large meal late at night, unless we can ensure that we do not go to bed at least up to 2-3 hours after taking our dinner. In case we go to bed immediately after a hearty dinner, it may disturb our sleep or when we wake up in the morning, we are not fresh. Try also to restrict your fat intake and reduce it to the minimal in case you suffer from a heart ailment or are hypertensive. Consumption of fat is a major factor behind a heart attack or even in cancers. Try to consume fresh and natural food and avoid canned or frozen food to the extent possible. Take plenty of vegetables, fresh fruits (seasonal fruits in particular), and lots of whole grains and a little bit of chicken or fish. Shun red meat. In short, resort to a low fat, high fibre diet. Patients suffering from arthritis and other musculoskeletal disorders should avoid rajmah, lobia, urad sabat and curds etc., to avoid aggravation of the disease.

Q. 27: As an acupressure therapist, would you like to prescribe some guidelines for good health?

A. 27: In case you have a health problem or even otherwise, you must take a holistic approach towards your health. As a matter of fact, factors like our daily routine, diet, life style and even our job requirements influence our health and we can lead a healthy life in case we do our best in keeping our life regulated and as per the laws of the nature. Here are some guidelines which will help you in keeping fit:

(a) 'Prevention is better than cure' should be the motive of your life.

(b) Take enough rest. This is very important. You can not give your best performance when you are tired. Six to seven hours of sleep a day is essential.

(c) Half an hour of walking at a good pace gets you enough exercise to remain fit. Heart patients should not over-exert.

(d) Never try to overeat. Your diet should be balanced and contain fresh fruits, vegetables; sprouts and whole grains, etc., Fat intake should also be restricted.

(e) Learn to manage stress, practice some form of meditation for relaxation. At least 70 percent of the health problems are caused by stress. Switch over to yoga can bring in highly beneficial results.

(f) Learn to dissolve negative emotions. Anger, worry, anxiety, depression are emotional forms of stress which adversely affect your nervous system. Negative feelings generate health problems.

Q. 28: What types of diseases respond well to this therapy?

A. 28: As we have said earlier, through this therapy, we do not treat the disease but we stimulate various organs by applying pressure on the reflex points relating to the affected organs. Once the flow of energy is re-established in the affected organs, the disease gets cured. As such there is no limitation for this therapy to be able to heal a particular ailment and not the other one. Yet no doubt certain ailments like cervical/lumbar spondylosis, back pain, knee pain, heel pain, sinusitis, vertigo, migraine, headache, piles, diseases of the digestive system, bed wetting, depression, sciatica, stiff neck, asthma, solar plexus, peptic ulcers, epilepsy etc., can be cured without much problem within 12-15 sittings or so until and unless these problems have been of long standing.

However, acupressure when used as a complement to other conventional therapies has been found to yield astounding results even in most complicated cases, even involving multi organ failure, cardiovascular as well as neurological problems. The sooner this therapy is given to a patient suffering from paralysis, the better and faster results can be expected.

Q. 29: What is polio mellitus? Can acupressure play some role?

A. 29: Polio is an infection caused by a virus that enters the body through nose and mouth, attacks the nerve cells of the brain and the spinal cord. Children between the age group of 6 months to 5 years are the ones who are most effected. In its milder form, this disease is marked by fever, nausea and vomiting, headache, throat infection and body ache etc. and these symptoms disappear within 24hrs or so. However, in its other form, whereas the symptoms are more or less the same, they persist for a prolonged period. The body temperature rises, muscles grow weak, the shoulders the neck and the hip joints becomes stiff and the patient finds the movements to be difficult. Legs, neck and back becomes stiff. Cases in which the nerve cells of the brain stem are damaged, paralysis may take place. The stiffness of the joints increases with passage of time and the muscles of the limbs start shrinking due to inadequate circulation.

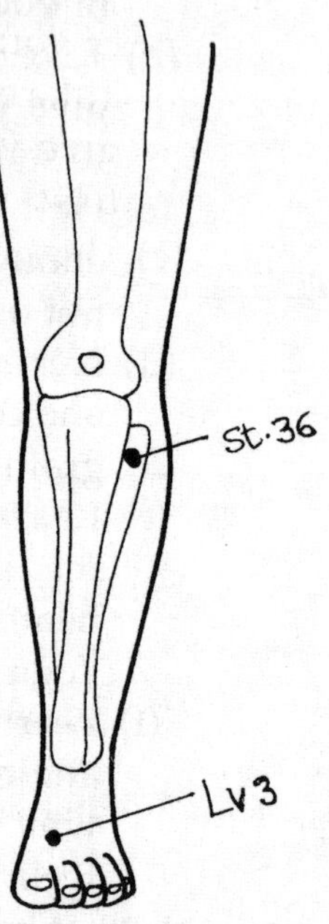

With the advent of Polio vaccines, this disease has almost been eradicated in the advanced countries. Even in India, the year 2011 has been declared Polio free year as not even a single case was reported. This could be achieved after putting in all out efforts by the Government by conducting frequent pulse polio campaigns where in people were educated through electronic and print media, as well as oral polio drops were administered to the children below the age group of 5 years. Polio injections are also given to the small children as a part of the immunization programme. This disease, once it takes place is difficult to treat, yet it has been found that acupressure therapy helps a lot in checking further deterioration and in helping the patient in overcoming the pain and stiffness in the joints and muscles.

Follow the below mentioned schedule of pressure points

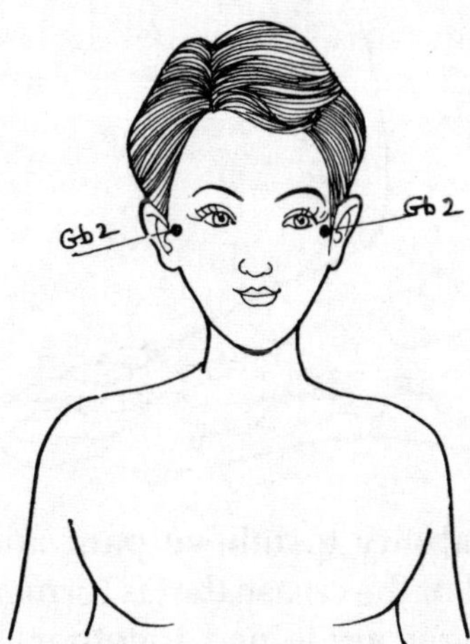

to get relief from this condition..

GB 2 is located just in front of the ear at the joint of the jaw. This point is specific to treat the Facial Paralysis.

GB 12 lies in the depression behind the ear, behind and below the mastoid bone. Is specific to treating the facial paralysis.

GB 20 is located in the hollow below the base of the skull. Steady pressure(mild to moderate) should be given on this point simultaneously on both the sides. Its effect goes well with its name i.e. 'gates of consciousness' .an extremely beneficial point to overcome stiffness in the region of the neck. It also eliminates wind and cold To restore the Bladder and Kidney meridians , stimulate B23 and B 47 points. B23 can be located in the middle of the waist, half way between the rib cage and the hip bone on the inner edge. B47 which lies in the middle of the waist four finger widths outside of the spine. These points, not only provide relief in the low back pain but also reduce muscle tension, fatigue, depression, fear and trauma . Follow it up by holding K27, 'Elegant Mansion', which is directly below your collarbone . Finally hold the 'Bigger stream', K 3, called 'Taixi'. This stimulates the 'Yin' and sedates the 'Yang' of Liver & Kidney. Hold all these points for one minute each as you breathe deep and exhale slowly.

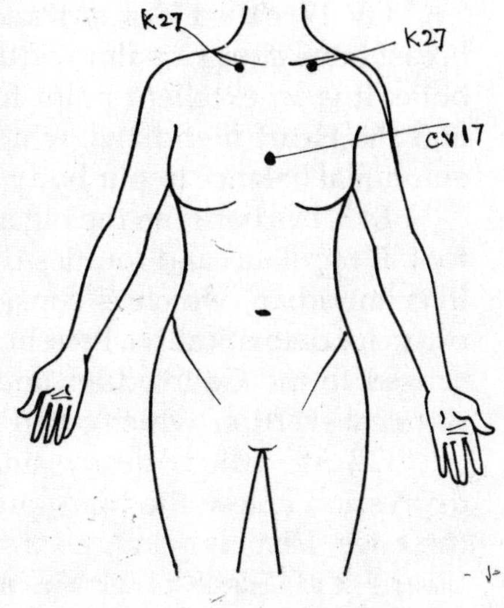

St 36, lies four finger widths below the knee cap, one finger width on the outside of the shinbone. This point strengthen thc whole body, tones the muscles and has been found to be helpful in rejuvenating the ch'i and blood. Stimulate it to benefit the Stomach and Spleen meridians.

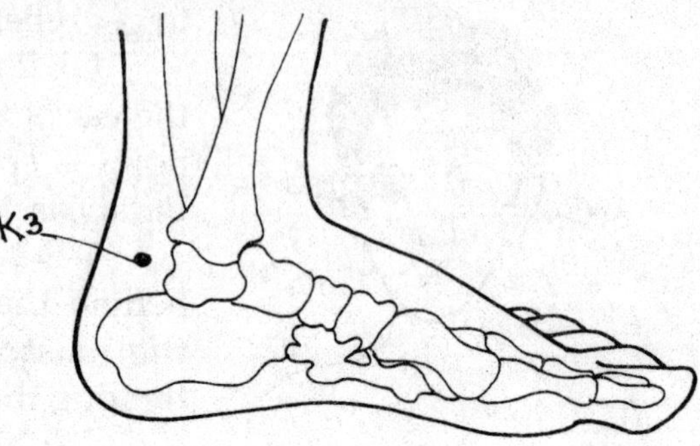

Li 4, known as adjoining valley, is known for its ability to relieve pain and circulating the Ch'i . It lies on the end of the crease that is formed when the thumb and the index finger are joined together. It stimulates elimination of toxins through bowels. It relieves stagnation of the ch,i too. Pregnant women should not use this point.

LI 11 called 'crooked pond' lies on the top outer edge of the elbow crease. It is considered to be one of the most effective points to control allergy and is also highly sensitive, as such pressure on this point should be given with utmost care lest it becomes extremely tender. Even massage like pressure can be given on this point to benefit the Large intestines and the Lung meridians.

CV 17, called 'Sea of tranquility' lies on the center of the breast bone about a palm width up from the base of the breast bone. It is an excellent point for balancing the Small intestine and the Heart meridians, which in turn result in creating the emotional balance in our body.

Lv3, lies between the big and second toes on the top of the foot. It regulates and tonifies the liver and the flow of qi in the liver meridian, which is considered to be the most powerful organ for detoxification. Pressing this point helps control damage caused to the Gallbladder and Liver meridians by excessive physical exertion, which could result into Cramps and Spasms.

GB 34, called 'sunny side of the mountain, lies in the depression below the bony prominence on the lateral side of the knee. Dispels wind, clears damp heat and stimulates the Liver's 'Yin'. Since Liver Yin nourishes the joints, mobility of the joint is improved by giving pressure to this point. Relieves excessive knee pain, muscular strain etc.

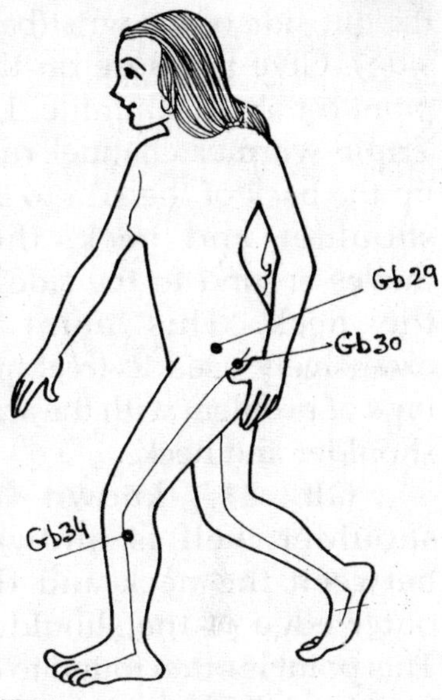

Gb 30, called the 'jumping circle', is the most important point for relieving hip pain. Stimulates circulation in the entire leg and low back. This point can be found on the buttocks about one third of distance between the hip and tail bone. Needs to be pressed with sufficient pressure, if necessary with your elbow. Pressure should be given on both sides.

B 57, 'support the mountain', is in the center of the 'V' formed between the lower border of the calf muscle, almost half way between the ankle bone and the mid point behind your knee. This pressure point helps relieve leg pain and stiffness.

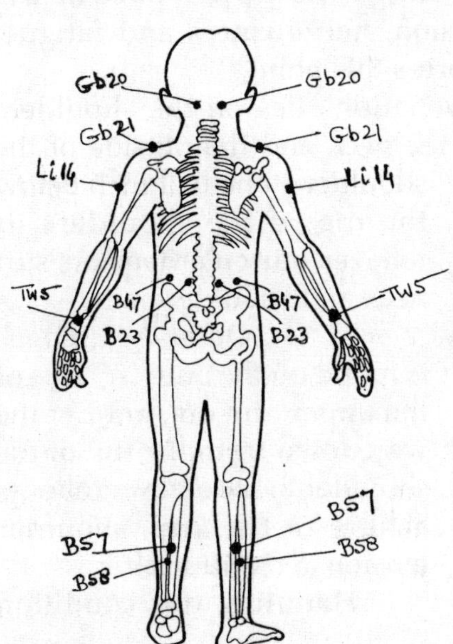

B 58, this point is about a thumb width below and a little outside of B57 point. Relieves leg pain.

Gb29, to locate this point, place your hands on both sides of your belt at the waist level. Slide down about a palm width on the hip bone. Press with the thumbs on both sides. Is a very effective point to alleviate hip pain.

TW 5, called the Outer gate is located midway between the Ulna and Radius bone about three finger widths above the wrist crease towards the elbow bone on the out side of the wrist(back side). Give pressure on this point for about a minute. The Triple warmer channel runs up the back of the arm to the shoulder and neck, then moves around to the side of the neck. This point is extensively used to treat any type of problem with the arm, shoulder and neck.

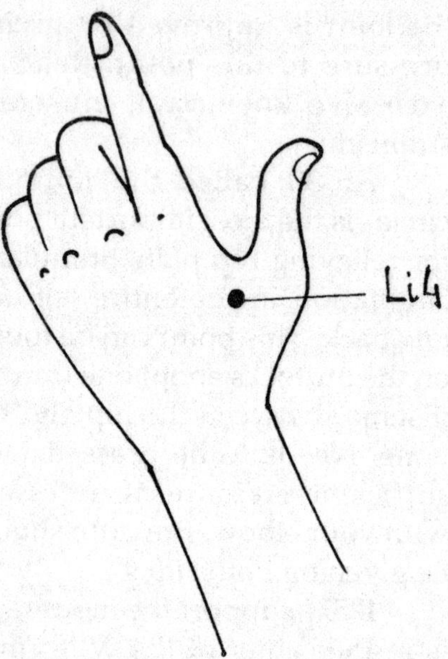

GB 21, known as shoulder well is midway between the neck and the outer edge of the shoulder. This point is often found to be very tender. This point can be pressed on both the sides of the shoulders simultaneously. It becomes even more beneficial in case the patient takes slow and deep breaths as you press various points. This points restores normal flow of ch'i in the lungs(the upper part of the body).Relieves shoulder tension, nervousness and fatigue. Pregnant women should not press this point.

TW 15, 'Heavenly Rejuvenation', lies on the shoulders midway between the base of the neck and the outside of the shoulders, one half inch below the top of the shoulders. It relieves muscular tension, stiff neck and shoulder pain.

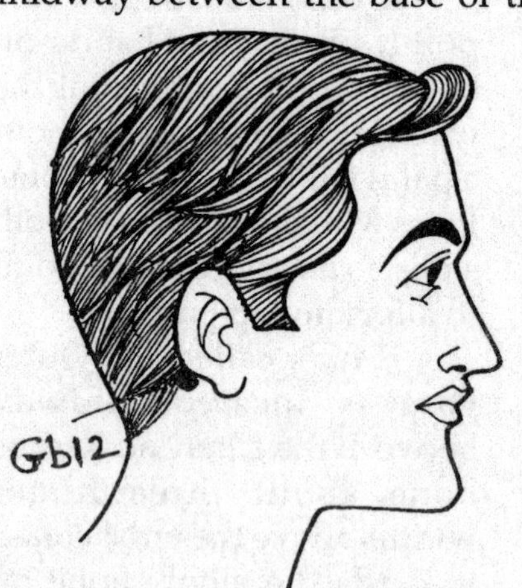

LI 14 , Outer Arm Bone', is found on the oute[illegible]rface of the upper arm one third of the way down from the top of the shoulder to the elbow. Relieves aching in the arm, shoulder tension and stiff neck.

Handling this condition

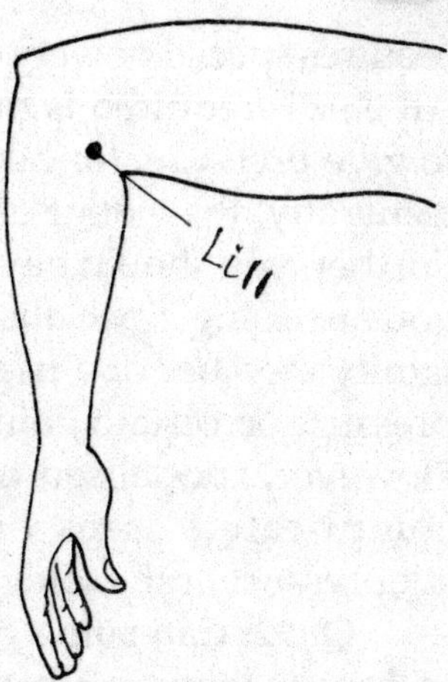

using reflexology, since this condition has a direct relationship with the brain and the nervous system, reflex points relating to brain, vertebral column, all the vital organs e.g. heart, liver, kidneys, lungs as well as endocrine glands i.e. pituitary, adrenals, thyroid and para-thyroid as well as lymph glands, scapula blades, ankles (on and around the area where the leg meets the foot), need to be thoroughly stimulated at least once a day or if possible even twice a day, in case stiffness and pain is on the high side , for about 3-4 days in the beginning and thereafter once a day for about a month and then twice or thrice a week . For location of the reflex points relating to various organs referred to above, please see the figures of the palms and the soles at the end of the book.

Q. 30: Can acupressure be of any use in stimulating the immune system and in detoxification?

A. 30: Yes, acupressure has been found to be extensively useful in detoxification and stimulation of the immune system in a large number of cases. As a matter of fact, kidneys, liver, lungs, large intestines, our lymphatic system and the skin are the major organs which help us in expelling toxins from our body. The reflex points in respect of all of them can be easily found in our palms and soles and these can be easily stimulated by giving pressure. Besides strengthening the immune system, another advantage we can derive out of it is to attain weight loss by way of throwing out of the toxins. In addition, in case we also stimulate the reflex points relating to the adrenal glands, which are located just below the ball of the foot, this regulates the stress response. Adrenals are extremely helpful in detoxification.

Q. 31: Does healing by acupressure require special powers or very extensive training?

A. 31: It is incorrect to say that healing by acupressure requires special powers or extensive training. Everyone can heal. All that is required is that it should be clear to you as to where to give pressure, for how long to press and how hard to press. Generally, the extent of pressure should be mild to moderate. Further, you should be confident and not over confident of what you are doing. Specialised training is not required for helping a family member or a friend in lending a helping hand in giving pressure on certain points which have been earmarked already. However, specialised training shall be necessary for handling complicated cases or for in-depth professional use of acupressure/reflexology independently by yourself.

Q. 32: Can some points be prescribed for daily workout to draw maximum advantage out of acupressure? Also describe their location and utility.

A. 32: To draw maximum advantage out of acupressure from certain pressure points located in very convenient locations all over our body, a daily schedule of pressing 12 Master Points can be drawn. Each point can be pressed from 30 seconds to one minute with moderate yet firm pressure. Thus, including the time to reach out to these important points, you need at best 20 minutes to complete the daily workout and see for yourself what benefit you derive! These points have been shown in the figures opposite to make it more convenient to locate them:

No. 1: Li 4, is also known by the name 'Adjoining Valley' and is located at the crease of the mound that pops up when the thumb and index finger are joined together. Pressure on the left hand can be given by the right hand and on the right hand by the left hand thumb and the index finger. This is considered to be one of the most effective acupressure and acupuncture points to relieve headache and pain in other parts of the body, to relax muscles and also balance the flow of energy in the lower and upper part of the body. It also activates the bowel movement. Pregnant women should not press

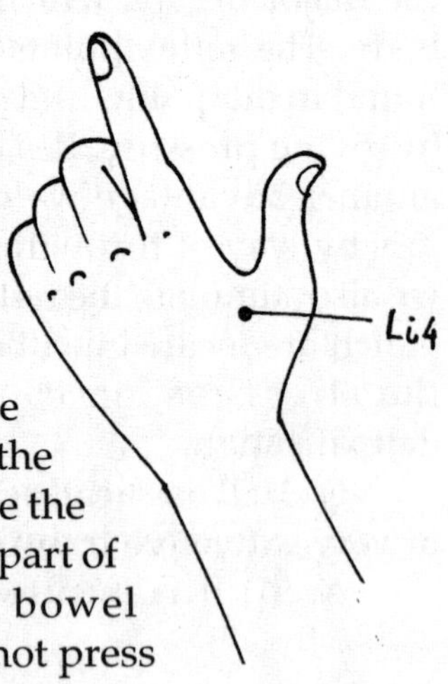

Li4

this point as it can cause miscarriage.

No. 2: Li 11, known as 'Pool at the Crook' it is located at the outside end of the crease that is formed when we bend our hand to touch our shoulder. Give pressure on both hands with the help of opposite hands. This point becomes very tender on pressing, therefore utmost caution has to be exercised. This is very useful in clearing the excess heat and dampness from the body and also pain in the elbow, arm and shoulders. It is also an important point to combat allergy and to treat tennis elbow.

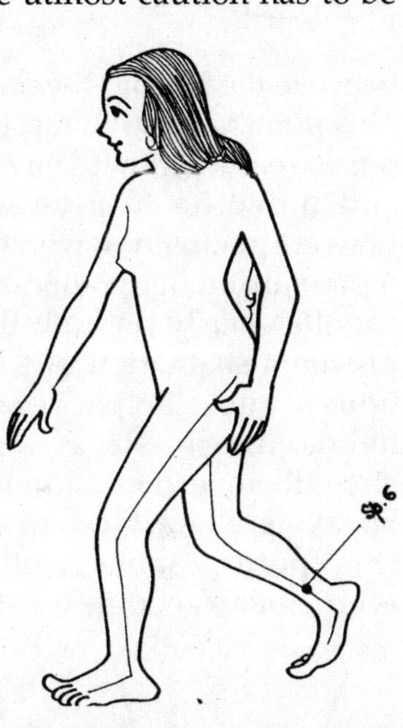

No.3: Sp 6, also called 'Three Yin Meeting Point', is located above the ankle bone towards the inside of the leg on the back side. The exact location being about four finger widths above the ankle bone. It is one of the most important pressure points as its name suggests since it strengthens the Yin of three meridians viz. spleen, liver and kidney at the same time. It is also considered master point for regulating female organs and is therefore useful in regulating periods, relieving cramps, facilitating menopause, etc. Pregnant women should not use this point.

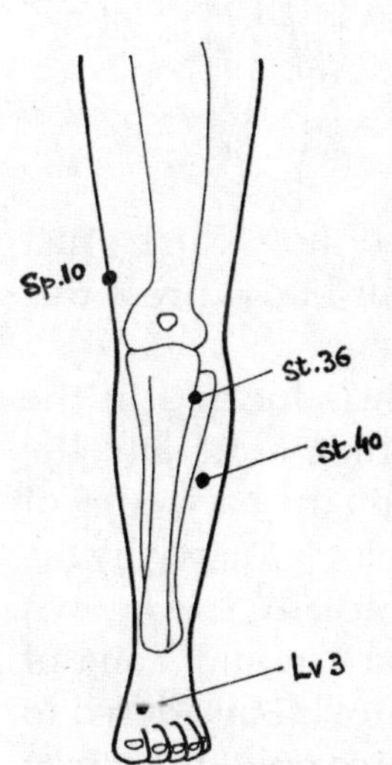

No.4: St 36, is located four, finger widths below the kneecap towards the lower

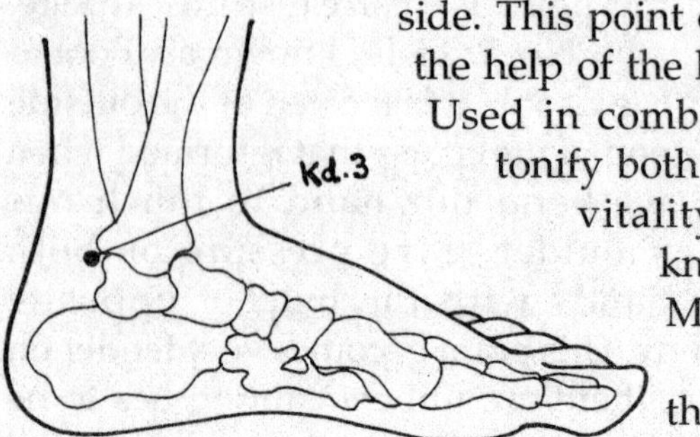

side. This point can also be pressed with the help of the heel of the opposite foot. Used in combination with Sp 6, they tonify both Ch'i and blood to bring vitality. This master point is known by the name 'Three Mile Foot'.

No.5: Lv 3, known by the name 'Bigger Rushing', is located in the web between the big and the second toes. This point is often found to be very sensitive, so start with mild pressure and move on to give moderate pressure gradually. It would be better if pressure on this point can be given simultaneously on both the feet. It prevents stagnation of Ch'i in the body and helps greatly in overcoming stress and in strengthening the immune system. Speaking about the importance of this point, some well known acupressure/acupuncture therapists at times say that in case you are given an option to press just one point on your body, press this point.

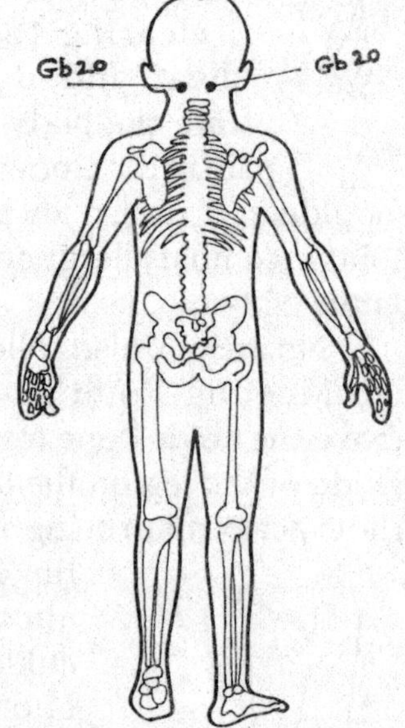

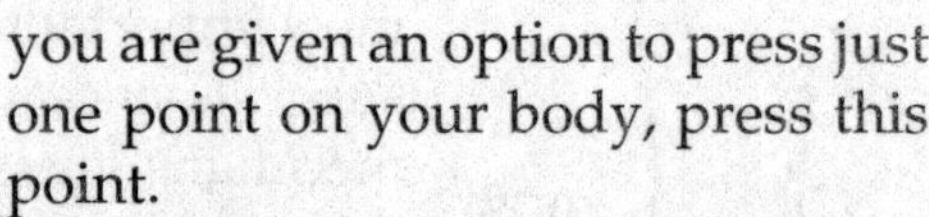

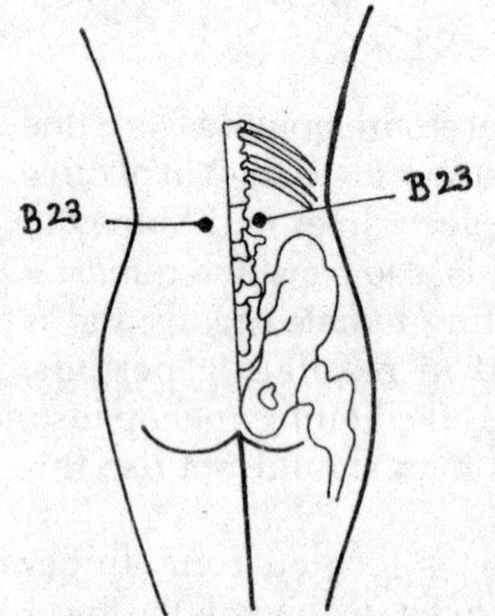

No.6: Kd 3, is located in the middle of the ankle bone and the Achilles tendon on the back edge of the ankle. This point is known by the name 'Supreme Stream'. It is known as the root of the Yin and Yang of the entire body and is considered to be the prime source point in respect

of the kidney meridian. This point has a powerful tonifying effect on the meridian and the entire body.

No.7: B 23, this point which is an associated point of kidney, is located one and a half inches on either side of the spine, above the level of your navel and below the centre of the back. These points on both sides of the spine on your back can be easily stimulated with the help of our hands. This point in combination with Kd 3 tonifies the kidney's Ch'i strongly.

No.8: Gb 20, also called the 'Wind Pool' is located in the depression on either side of the vertebra of your neck, one thumb width above the hairline of the neck, at the base of the skull. Pressure can be easily given with the help of the thumbs of both the hands simultaneously. This point is very useful in relieving neck stiffness, headache, pain in shoulders/heaviness etc., and also regulates the internal movement of energy.

No.9: Sp 10, 'Sea of Blood' is found about two thumb widths above the knee on the bulge of the thigh muscle towards the anterior side. This point prevents stagnation in the blood, particularly in the lower abdominal area. This point is also particularly useful for nourishing the skin.

No.10: St 40, is located half way between the ankle bone on the outside of the foot and centre of the kneecap. Find the tibia and go two thumb widths off the bone to the outside. It is very helpful for reducing mucus and congestion.

No.11 and 12: Extra points, as shown in figure, these lie in the middle of the forearms, between the wrist crease and the elbow crease. Whereas the point on the right arm plugs the loss of energy, the same on the left arm (also called Pc 4), about a thumb width down towards the wrist from the midpoint has been found to be very helpful in stimulating the heart.

Q.33: Can acupressure help control acidity?

A.33: Before getting on to treating this symptom, it would be better if we know a little about its cause so that by keeping out those factors to the extent possible, we can prevent acidity in the first place.

Many people suffer from one or more symptoms, e.g. gas formation, belching, flatulence, burning sensation in the region of Oesophagus. Looking at the cause we can easily say that poor diet could be the prime cause. Some people may be sensitive to a particular type of food or towards hot and spicy meals, fried food, etc. Stress could be another factor to aggravate the condition. The long term goal, should be to correct our dietary routine than to resort to an antacid or other medical remedy.

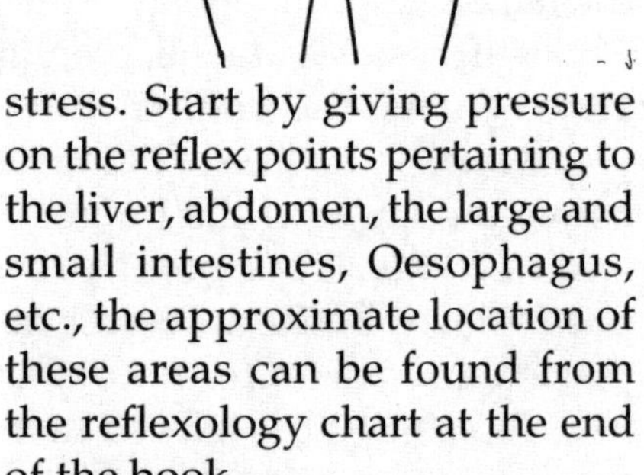

Fortunately, acupressure and reflexology have a great role to play in minimising stress. Start by giving pressure on the reflex points pertaining to the liver, abdomen, the large and small intestines, Oesophagus, etc., the approximate location of these areas can be found from the reflexology chart at the end of the book.

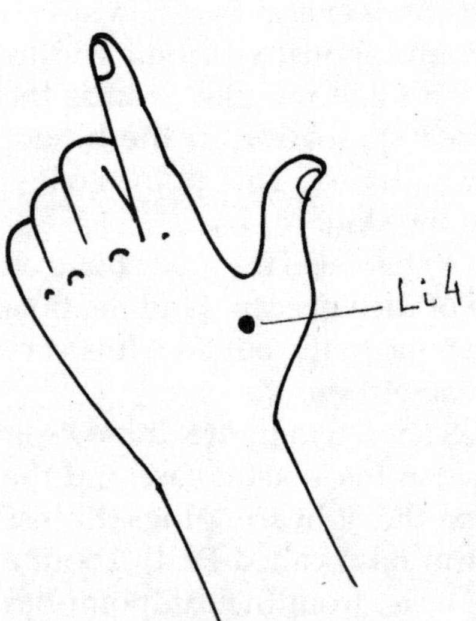

Give pressure on Li 4 point in the web where the index finger and the thumb meet. This point can be pressed on both the hands between the thumb and the index finger of the other hand one by one. It improves intestinal activity and also relieves constipation and abdominal distention.

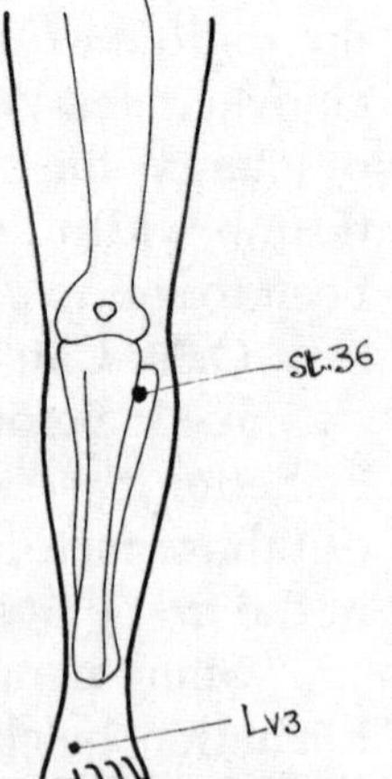

St 36, 'Three Mile Point', which can be easily found four finger widths below the lower border of the kneecap and one finger width towards the outside of the shin bone serves the purpose of a gastrointestinal tonic; it also relieves indigestion, prevents gas formation and bloating. Give pressure on this point for 30 to 60 seconds.

Then go to the Sp 6, the meeting point of spleen, liver and kidney meridians. It is located on the inside portion of your leg, above the ankle bone. Pressing this point is forbidden for pregnant women.

Lv3, is yet another pressure point which has been found to be very beneficial in overcoming stress. It is found between the big and the second toe and relieves distention, nausea, vomiting and abdominal pain.

Cv12 found midway between the breast bone and the naval helps in overcoming indigestion, heartburn, abdominal pain and constipation.

Q. 34: How acupressure can be helpful in overcoming allergies?

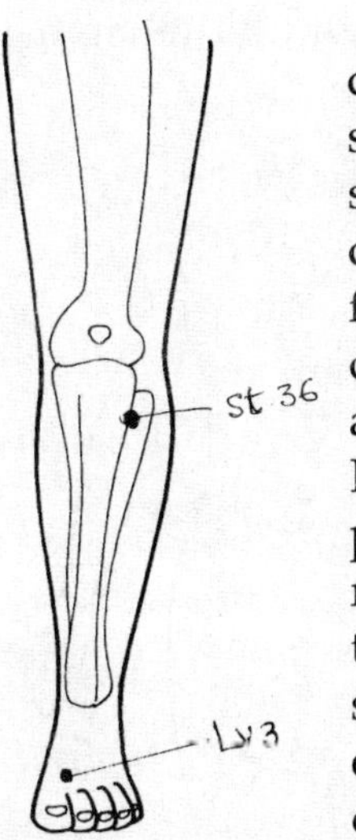

A. 34: An allergy can be termed as sensitivity towards a substance. The cause(s) could be some particular food, e.g., banana, egg, dust, pollen, pet hair or a particular type of cloth. Even a tiny particle can provoke an allergic reaction which may lead to running nose, sneezing, blood shot eyes, breathing problem, cramps and even fever.

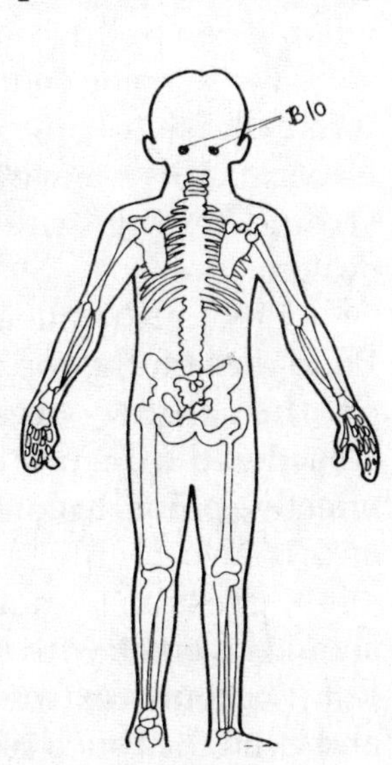

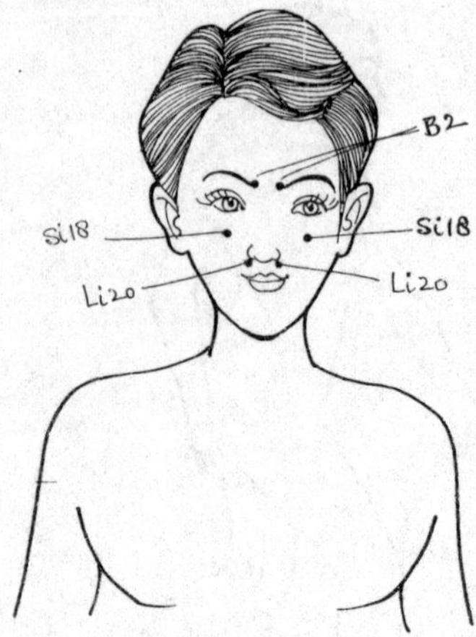

Generally, our immune system tries to take care by itself by releasing a chemical called histamine.

Acupressure is an effective method for overcoming many symptoms of allergy. This is done by balancing the flow of energy in the body. Pressure therapy can also strengthen our system to help prevent recurrence of allergic reactions. For early relief, we can use one or more than one points described below:

Lv 3 is located on the top of the foot in the valley between the big and second toe. Give pressure for about 30-45 seconds. It relieves all kinds of allergic reactions, in particular, the blood shot eyes and neuromuscular disorders.

Li 4, is considered to be an antihistamine point. It is located at the centre of the web between your thumb and the index finger. Press and release slowly, and repeat 3-4 times period 60 seconds or so on both the hands turn by turn. This point should not be used by pregnant ladies except at the time of delivery when it can be successfully used to arouse labour pain.

Tw 5 can be found two and a half finger widths above the wrist crease, on the top of the forearm. This relieves allergy by strengthening the immune system.

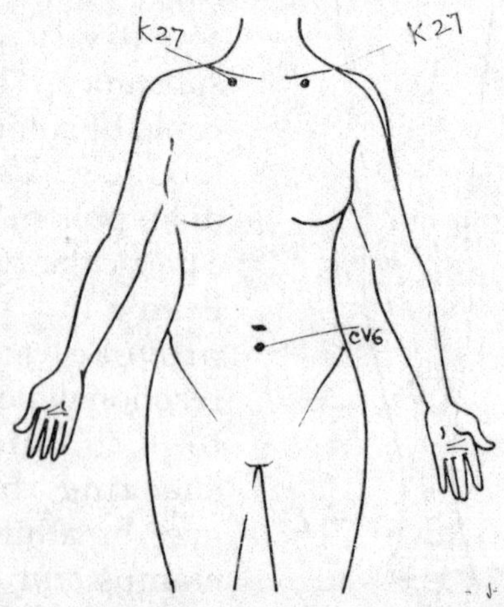

Li 11 also called 'Crooked Pond' lies on the top outer edge of the elbow crease. It is considered to be one of the most effective points to control allergy and is also highly sensitive, as such pressure on this point should be given with utmost care lest it becomes extremely tender and even the touch of cloth may hurt once it gets tender. Even massage like pressure can be given on this point.

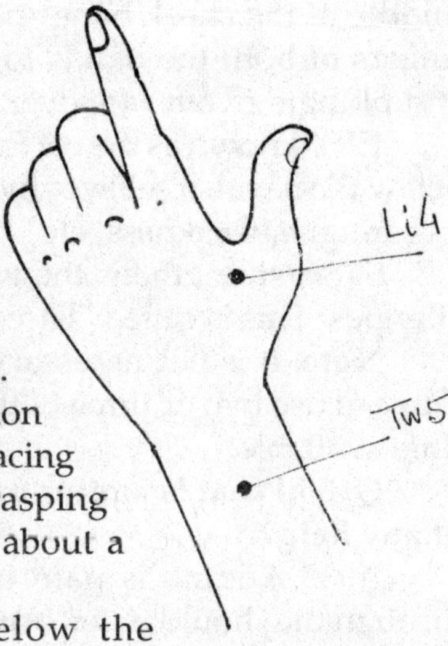

B 10 is located about one and a half inches below the base of the skull, one half an inch on either side of the spine. It has been given the name 'Heavenly Pillars' and it relieves allergic reactions, e.g. swollen eyes, headache, exhaustion etc. Pressure can be given by interlacing your fingers behind your head, grasping the neck and pressing firmly for about a minute.

K 27 is in the hollow below the collarbone next to the breastbone. Helps allergies in the shape of chest congestion, breathlessness, asthma, cough and sore throat etc. It has been given the name 'Elegant Mansion'.

B 2, known by the name 'Gathered Bamboo' is located at the inner end of the eye sockets, near the bridge of the nose, in the small indentation. It helps in relieving headache, sinus congestion and other allergy symptoms.

Li 20 is located in the groove right below the nostrils on your upper lips on both the sides. Press with the index fingers simultaneously, directing the pressure in the direction of the eyes. This point known as 'Welcome Fragrance' is highly beneficial for nasal allergies particularly stuffy nose and sinus. Pressure can be given for up to a minute.

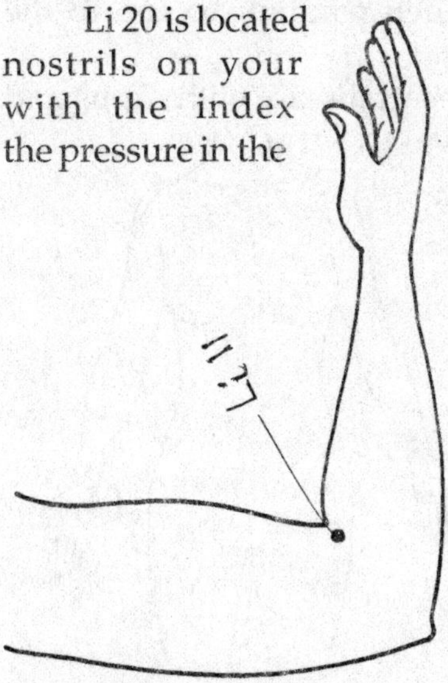

Si 18 is yet another important point from which maximum benefit can be derived in getting relief from sinus congestion in particular. This point called 'Check bone Crevice' as the name suggests is in the middle of the cheek bone and can be pressed by placing three fingers of both the hands together just below the cheek bone and plunging your face over these fingers for a minute.

CV 6 known as 'Sea of Energy' is located two finger widths below the naval. It relieves the allergies that follow constipation, gas, fatigue, weakness, etc.

St 36, strengthens the whole body to prevent and relieve allergies. This is called 'Three Mile Point'.

Note: It is not necessary to press all the points at a time. You can use two or three of them at a time depending upon the time available.

Q. 35: What is angina and its cause? Can acupressure be of any help?

A. 35: Angina is pain in the chest area which radiates through the shoulder, left arm and at times to the tip of the little finger. It is caused by insufficient supply of oxygen reaching the heart muscle owing to some blockage or spasm in the arteries leading to the heart.

Short temper, laziness (no exercise), smoking (increases the level of carbon monoxide in the blood) may be one of the causes. The prime culprit is, however, a fatty diet, as it leads to narrowing down of the blood vessels that restricts the supply of blood and consequently the much wanted oxygen to the heart.

Conventional medicines treat heart disease with strong and powerful medicines that reduce cholesterol level and control high blood pressure. Options like angioplasty and bypass surgery are also available. However, besides being risky and full of side effects, the cost of surgical procedures and medicines is on a very high side and the common man can ill afford it. Research has shown that risk of a heart attack can be substantially decreased by

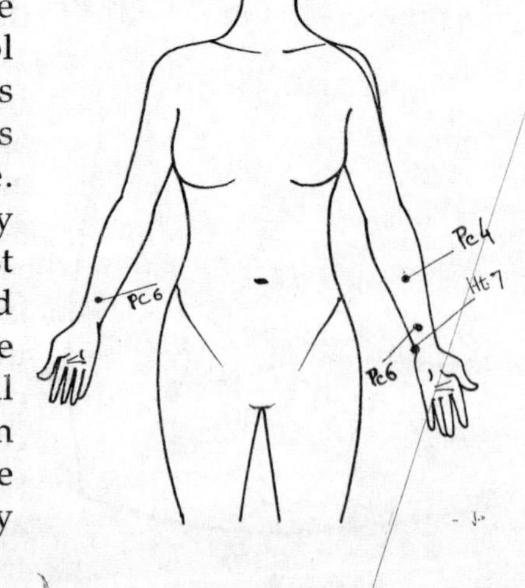

natural means, e.g. acupressure. However, a word of caution, in case the angina attack or heart condition is severe, medical aid must be taken without loss of time. Acupressure is advisable only as a preventive and first aid. There is, however, no harm in continuing with acupressure, in addition to treatment under conventional medicine, as it has been found to increase the pace of recovery of the patient(s) and looking into the results, many highly qualified cardiologists in well reputed hospitals have started combining this technique successfully.

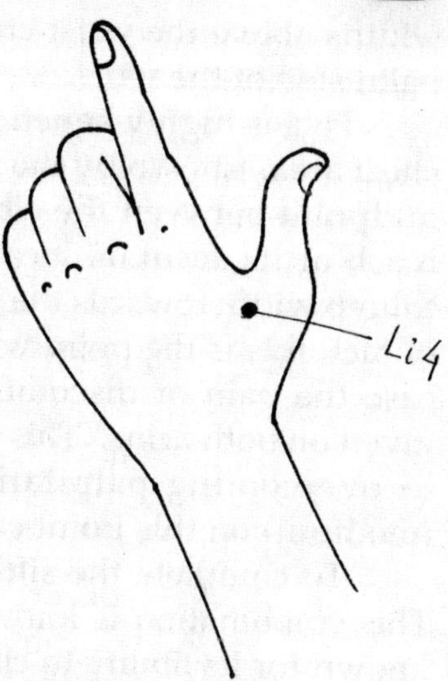

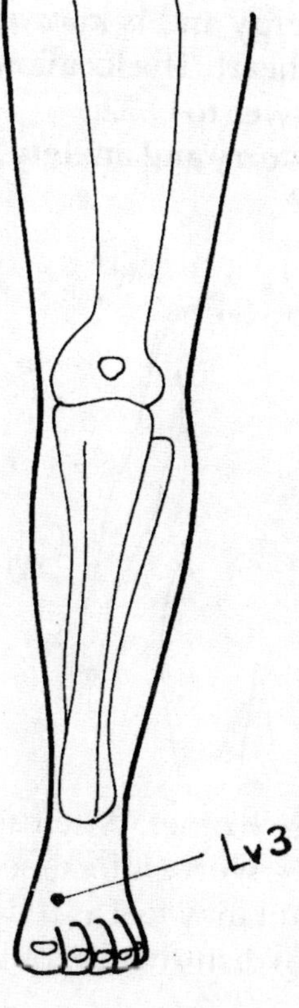

Ht 7 also called the 'Mind Door' needs to be pressed to begin with. This point is located next to the bone on the outside of your left wrist. Precisely the area where the palm and the wrist meet. This is the source point in respect of the heart meridian and is highly effective. It not only nourishes the heart but is also helpful in soothing the emotions by calming the mind.

Pc 6 is also known by the name 'Heart Protector'. As the name itself suggests, pressing this important point strengthens the heart. It also relieves pain and discomfort in the heart region. Further it restores the Ch'i and blood flow in the heart region. Give firm yet moderate pressure on this point in both the hands, particularly the left hand and for up to 30 seconds at a time. Build up slowly and release gradually. Pressure can be repeated 2-3 times. The exact location of this point is two thumb widths above the wrist crease in the centre of the arm on the palm side of the wrist.

Pc 4 is highly beneficial for any sort of discomfort in the chest area. Known by the name 'Cleft Gate', it is located at the midpoint between the elbow crease and the wrist crease. To reach at its accurate location, you have to go down about a thumb width towards the wrist from this midpoint. As a matter of fact, this is the point which should be pressed first of all in case the pain or discomfort is intense. Pressure needs to be given on both arms. This point can also be found to be helpful in overcoming palpitation. If the pain is acute, pressure (medium) on this point can be repeated even 3-4 times.

To complete the sitting, give pressure on Li 4 and Lv 3. This combination is known by the name 'Four Gates', and is known for its ability to circulate Ch'i through the entire range of meridians in our body. This helps both physically and emotionally, by breaking up the blocked energy and is known for its beneficial effect for keeping a healthy heart. The location of these points has been described in the answer to Q.32.

Q. 36: What is the difference between worry and anxiety? Can acupressure help in overcoming them?

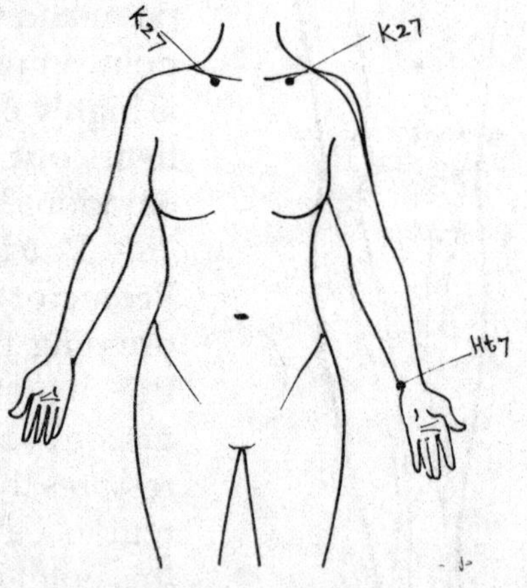

A. 36: It is a well established fact the mental stress consumes more energy than physical stress. It is believed that excessive thinking consumes much of the energy in our body and deprives the rest of the body of the vital Ch'i. On the other hand, it cannot be denied that worry is a natural part of living and it prompts us to get ready for the upcoming challenges in our life. Anxiety and worry are, as a matter of fact, related to each other. Whereas, anxiety is more focussed on the current events, worry is focussed on the future. During an attack of anxiety, you may feel as if the heart is sinking, breathlessness and emotional disturbance could

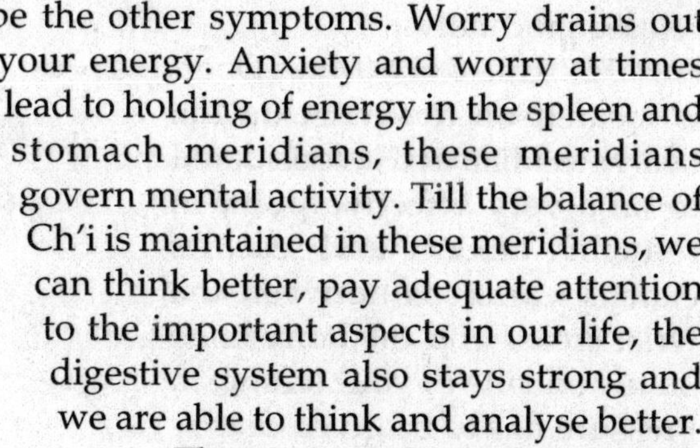

be the other symptoms. Worry drains out your energy. Anxiety and worry at times lead to holding of energy in the spleen and stomach meridians, these meridians govern mental activity. Till the balance of Ch'i is maintained in these meridians, we can think better, pay adequate attention to the important aspects in our life, the digestive system also stays strong and we are able to think and analyse better. The moment this balance is lost, we face great hardship with our reasoning and that leads to worry. Imbalance of Ch'i in the stomach and spleen meridians also causes deficiency in the heart meridian.

Interviews, exams, first public speech, etc. are a few instances, which are potential causes of anxiety in our life. Once the event is over, the worry and the anxiety automatically come to an end. However, in case the anxiety continues for long and starts interfering with our normal day to day functions, or is associated with panic attacks, phobias, then without loss of time a doctor's help should be sought. Most of our routine worries and anxiety can be managed easily using acupressure as discussed below:

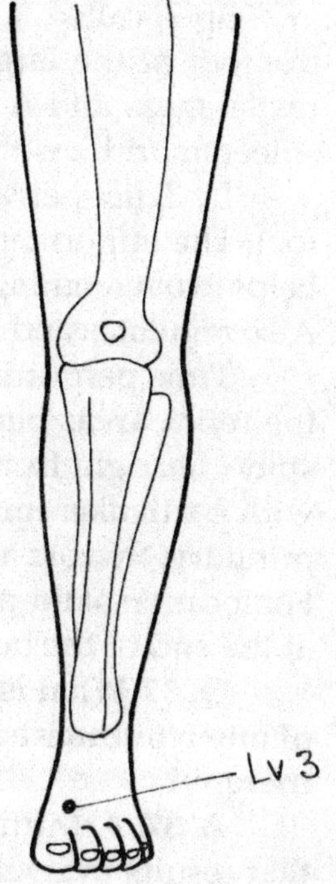

Gb 13, go to the outer edge of the eyebrow and move up one palm width to the point just on the hair line. This point calms the mind and relieves anxiety. This point is known by the name 'Mind Root'.

Gv 24, known as 'Mind Courtyard', this point falls just inside the hairline of the forehead. This also gives a calming effect on the mind. Give moderate yet firm pressure for about a minute and then release gradually.

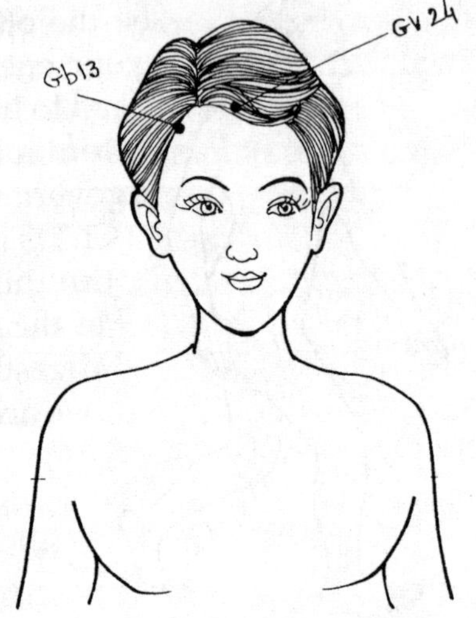

H 7, called the 'Mind Door' is located on the wrist on the heart meridian and is considered to be a very effective point in reducing anxiety and fear. Its exact location is between the wrist crease and the bony knob on the outside of your left wrist. Pressure has to be given one by one on both the hands for a period of 30 seconds on each by pressing firmly and releasing gradually.

K 27 is located under the collarbone in the depression next to the breastbone. It is a very potent point and helps overcome headache, mental strain, disorientation, anxiety and palpitation.

Sp 2, called 'Great Metropolis' in located on the inside of the foot at the large joint at the base of the big toe. It calms restlessness and it also regulates the Ch'i in the stomach and spleen meridians thereby helping the heart meridian as well.

Lv 3, lies between the big and second toes on the top of the foot. The importance of this point cannot be overemphasised. It helps in overcoming worry and stress related to decision making. Also regulates and tonifies the liver and smooth flow of Ch'i.

Time permitting, also spend some time giving pressure on the reflex areas pertaining to the stomach, liver, spleen, entire spine, i.e. right from the top of the big toe to the heel, chest area with particular emphasis to heart and lungs. Give pressure on pituitary, thyroid and adrenals and around the diaphragm also. For location of the areas corresponding to them, refer to the chart at the end of the book.

Q. 37: What is arthritis? Can it be managed with the help of much publicised daily exercise programme and acupressure therapy?

A. 37: Arthritis means inflammation in or around the joints that results in swelling, pain and stiffness. Though as many as

100 + types of arthritis are known, yet most of them can be grouped into two categories :

(a) Osteoarthritis (OA) and

(b) Inflammatory type of arthritis includes rheumatoid arthritis (RA), while bursitis and tendonitis, which are caused by the changes due to wear and tear are not considered as an arthritic condition.

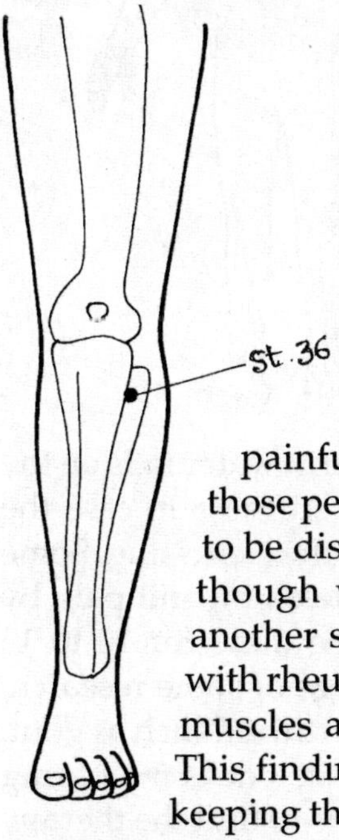

St. 36

The results of a study published in July, 2002 in the journal '*Arthritis and Rheumatism*' confirm that if you do-not move around and keep your muscles strong and joints flexible, your arthritic symptoms will worsen. Following the findings of the study conducted over 107 people with osteoarthritis of the knee, the researchers asked the participants to what degree they avoided activity during a painful arthritic flare up; they concluded that those people who avoided activity were more likely to be disabled than people who continued activity though with some amount of modifications. In another study researchers have found that women with rheumatoid arthritis, who had the thickest thigh muscles also had denser and stronger femur bone. This finding supports the importance of exercise for keeping the muscles and bones strong for preventing painful fractures caused by osteoporosis. Exercise may also be the most effective treatment for those with fibromyalgia, as it helps to relieve deep muscle pain, chronic fatigue and other exasperating symptoms.

There are many more benefits of exercise for the people suffering from arthritis. Regular exercise produces alpha waves in the brain that brings a feeling of relaxation, reduces anxiety and stress, and improves mood. Moreover, body releases endorphins during exercise; these brain chemicals are natural mood elevators and natural pain-killers. However, in case you are on medication and want to start an exercise programme, consult your doctor whether or not some medicine in your prescription interferes with the heart rate or the blood pressure. Also seek his advice as to how rigorous an exercise you can undertake safely to begin with. The following three steps will be found to be highly beneficial by the arthritic patients:

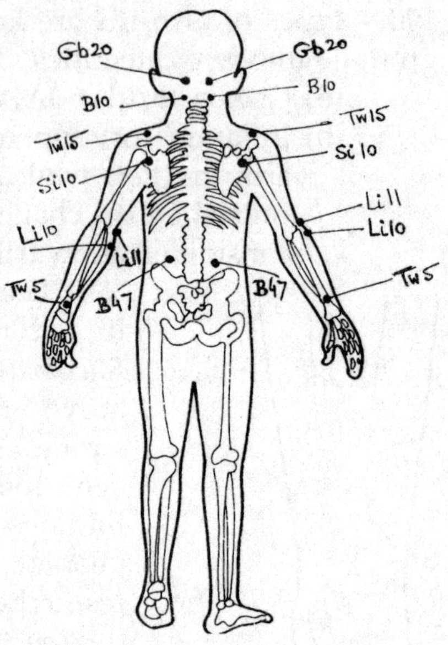

Step 1 : Use Moist heat or ice application on the arthritic joints or painful muscle for 15 minutes before exercise. Moist heat dilates blood vessels and increases the flow of blood and oxygen to the painful site. You may use a moist heating pad or a warm damp towel. You can even sit or stand under a shower so that warm water falls on the painful area. It will help overcoming the stiffness in case the process is repeated for a few minutes after the exercising. Some patients prefer ice packs, which reduces swelling and pain by constricting the blood vessels. This can be done for 10 to 15 minutes at a time. According to the findings of some research, ice packs may be of help in some kinds of arthritis such as gout. Alternating moist heat applications with ice packs may bring optimum relief. The most important thing is to find the therapy that brings relief from pain and that works best for you. Make it a habit before and after your exercise.

Step. 2: Balance exercise with rest periods, since after a workout, most of the arthritic patients feel some discomfort. In case your pain or discomfort does not reduce even after moist heat or ice pack, give yourself more rest. Restart the exercise after a break of 24 hrs at best and after a moist heat or ice pack as it suits you; make sure that you begin again with fewer repetitions this time and follow up again with moist heat or an ice pack. Increase gradually.

Step. 3: If your pain becomes severe during an exercise, stop until you check with your doctor. In case, however, there is

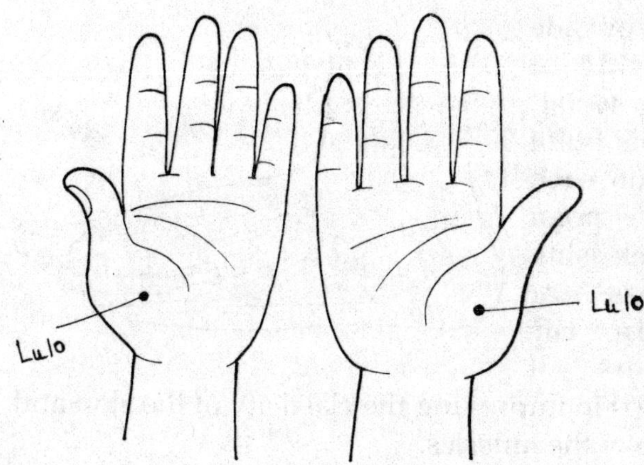

little discomfort but you can continue exercise, try only with a fewer repetitions and try to build up gradually. Remember, if your joints are swollen and inflamed some types of exercises may not be helpful. So first speak to your doctor before continuing with the exercise programme. Make it a point to balance exercise with rest in between in case of aggravations.

There are acupressure points that strengthen specific joints and relieve arthritic symptoms and rheumatism. By stimulating those points daily with finger pressure and hot and cold compresses, you can improve your overall condition and manage your arthritis.

1. Li 4 is located at the highest spot of the muscle where the thumb and index finger are held together. Press in the web between them directing towards the bone that attaches to the index finger. This anti-inflammatory point is beneficial in relieving pain caused by arthritis in all parts of the body, specifically in the hands, wrists, elbows and shoulders.
2. Lu 10 is located on the palm side of the hand in the centre of the big mount at the base of the thumb. Apply firm pressure to the centre of the pad where the thumb joins the palm of the hand. This point relieves arthritis in the hand.
3. Tw 5 can be located by flexing your hand backwards. This point is on the outer side of the forearm about one and a half inches from the wrist crease. Press firmly between the ulna and radius. To give firm pressure, wrap your hand around the wrist to clamp

onto the outside and inside of your wrist. Hold this point firmly on each arm. This point helps releasing tightness or pain in the shoulders. It also helps in improving the elasticity of the skin and the tone of the muscles.

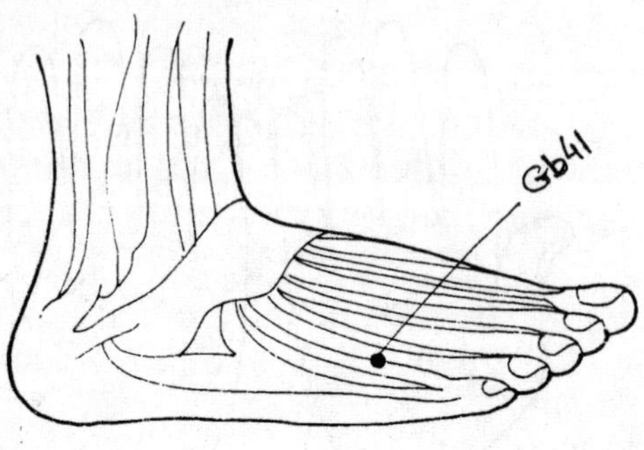

4. LI 10 can be located by bending your arm to form a crease at the elbow joint. This point is located about an inch towards your hand from the end of this crease, on a muscle. Apply gradual pressure in the centre of the forearm muscle. This anti-inflammatory point relieves arthritis in the upper portion of the body particularly in the hand, wrist and elbow joints. This point is of great value for relieving aching, tired muscles and joints. Arthritic patients should make it a habit to stimulate this point on both the arms when they get up in the morning.
5. LI 11 is located in the elbow joint at the outer end of the crease when you bend your arm. Give steady but mild to moderate pressure on this point with your arm partially flexed. It relieves joint inflammation specially in the elbow and the shoulder joints.
6. SI 10 is located where the arm joins the back between the top of the shoulder bone and the back crease of the armpit. Press on the muscular cord on the shoulder joint. This point relieves arthritis, bursitis and rheumatism. Also releases shoulder and upper back pain.
7. TW 15 is found on the top of the shoulder, i.e. midway between the outside of the base of your neck and the outside of your shoulder, about one-half inch below

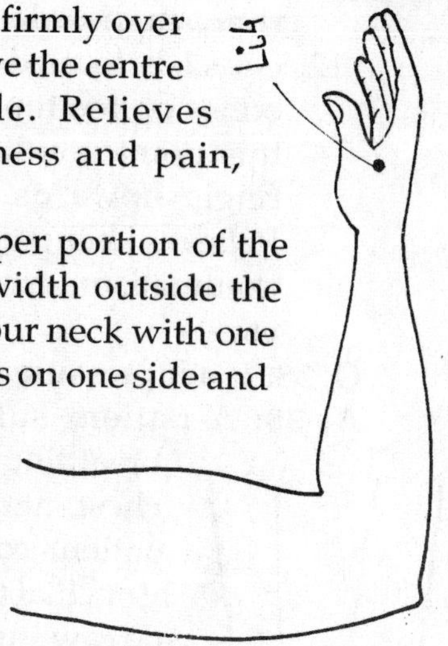

the spot. Press gently but firmly over the shoulder muscles above the centre of each shoulder blade. Relieves shoulder and neck stiffness and pain, including rheumatism.

8. B 10 is located on the upper portion of the neck, about one thumb width outside the spine. Hold the back of your neck with one hand using all your fingers on one side and the thumb on the other to squeeze the neck muscle. Is considered as a key point for overcoming stiffness, rigidity and arthritic pain in the neck and back. It is specially beneficial to combat stress and trauma.
9. GB 20 is located in the hollow below the base of the skull. Steady pressure (mild to moderate) should be given on this point simultaneously on both the sides. It relieves arthritic pain, headache, back pain and stiff neck.
10. B 47 is located on the lower back between the 2nd and 3rd lumbar vertebrae about one and a half inches away from the spine. Pressure can be given by making fists and rubbing the lower back portion briskly. It relieves lower backaches, fatigue, etc.
11. St 36, is located about four finger widths below your kneecap and one finger width outside of your shin bone. This point can be best stimulated by the patient himself by using his own heel to rub this point (use right heel to stimulate left foot and vice versa). Helps in overcoming arthritic pain all over the body, particularly pain in the knee joints. Is also considered to be the most effective acupressure point for alleviating sore, tired muscles and general fatigue. Pressure on this point strengthens the whole body, tones up the muscles, aids digestion and relieves

stomach disorders.

12. GB 41 is located between the 4th and 5th metatarsal bones on the top of the foot. For giving pressure on this point you have to slide your index or middle finger upwards, pressing just below the juncture. Relieves knee pain and also hip and shoulder tension, rheumatism, excessive water retention and sciatica, etc.

Q. 38: Is acupressure effective in asthma?

A. 38: A patient suffering from asthma experiences breathing problem, tightness in the region of chest, and wheezing. Most of the times, the patient coughs up mucus. The walls of the bronchial tubes spasm, the air passage becomes narrow, and the patient finds it difficult to exhale. Majority of asthmatic conditions are a result of allergies, and pollutants, e.g. pollens from grass, flowers, animal fur, dust, etc. Climate change is yet another important cause for this condition. Breathing difficulties can cause the body to become toxic. For their proper functioning, all the cells, organs and systems of our body need proper supply of oxygen, which it does not get when the patient is having breathing problems. We keep on breathing throughout the day but never think about it. Severe asthma is one of the most dreadful health conditions in which the patient struggles to get just a little air, this reminds us of the importance of air in our lives.

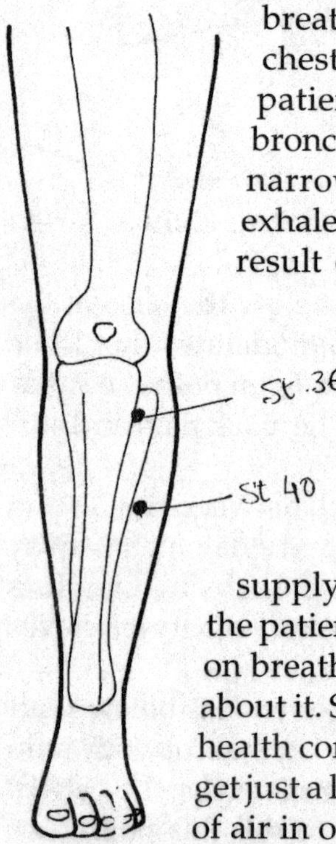

St.36

St 40

Modern medicine can easily take care of asthma with the help of bronchodilators which relax the bronchial muscles and make breathing easier. However, such drugs can have negative side effects, e.g. rapid heart rate, which itself could be life threatening. Pressure point therapy can offer much relief from asthma. Combined with changes in your diet and some exercise, this therapy can help control asthma and allow reduction or elimination of medications you might be taking, with due approval of the physician under whose care you are. In a preliminary research study conducted by the Acupressure Institute in Berkeley, California, it was found that four out of five of the adult asthmatic patients tested had a 20 percent increase in their vital lung capacity immediately after receiving twenty minutes of acupressure.

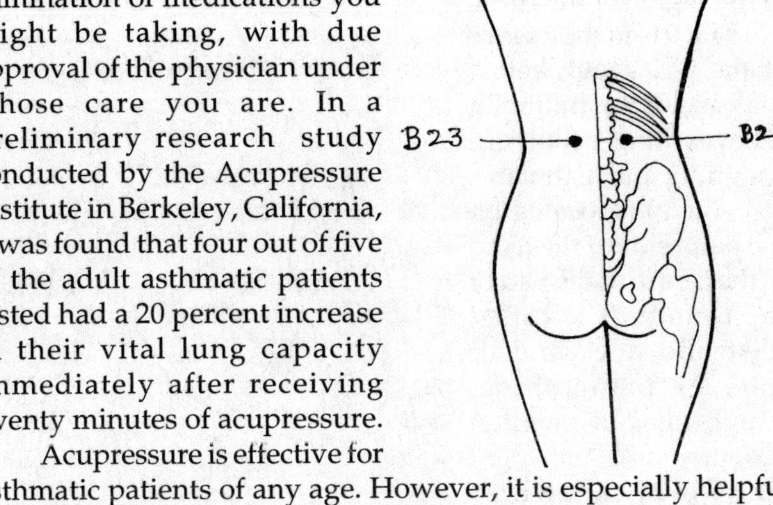

Acupressure is effective for asthmatic patients of any age. However, it is especially helpful for children and young adults. Acupressure has no conflict with the use of inhalers. You can continue to use it while taking acupressure therapy, what we suggest is to monitor and curtail using inhaler in consultation with your physician. Very soon you will find that within five sittings or so you can do without an inhaler or you have to use it only once in a while (i.e. SOS.). The pressure points to be used are:

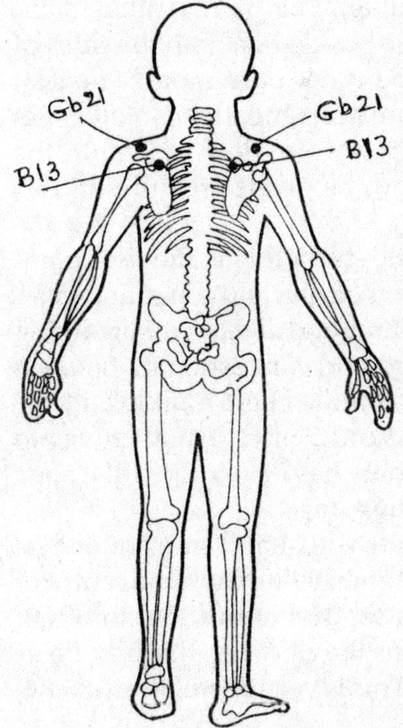

B 13 is located between the spine and the scapula bone, just one finger width below the upper tip of the shoulder blade. This is known as 'Lung Associated Point'. It relieves asthma, coughing, sneezing, etc.

K 27 is located in the hollow below the collarbone next to the breastbone. This point relieves breathing difficulty, chest congestion, coughing and stress in the region of the chest.

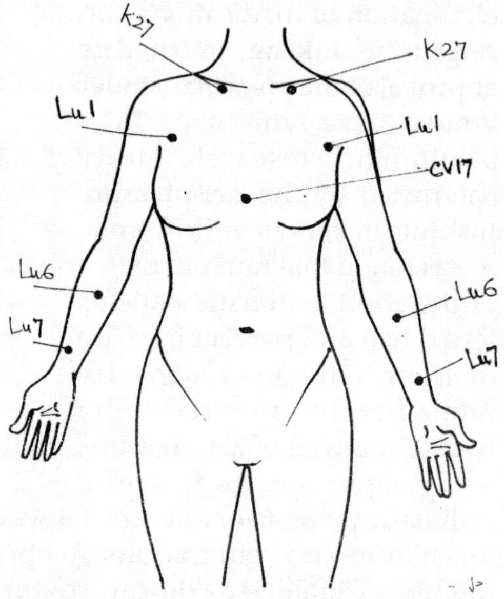

Lu 9 is in the groove at the wrist fold, below the base of the thumb. It relieves lung problems, coughing and asthma.

Lu 10 is located on the palm side of the hand in the centre of the pad of the thumb. It is called 'Fish Border' and it relieves breathing, coughing and swollen throat.

GB 21, known as 'Shoulder Well', is midway between the neck and the outer edge of the shoulder. This point is often found to be very tender. This point can be pressed on both the sides of the shoulders simultaneously. It becomes even more beneficial in case the patient takes slow and deep breaths as you press various points. This point restores normal flow of Ch'i in the lungs. Pregnant women should not be given pressure on this point.

Lu 1, known as 'Central Residence', this is the first point on the lung meridian. It helps stop wheezing and coughing, tones the lungs, is helpful in relieving asthma and all kinds of breathing difficulties. It also alleviates tension and congestion in the chest region. This point is located between the chest muscle and the deltoid in the space between the 1st and 2nd ribs. Another way to locate this point is to go about two inches below the collarbone or about one inch inwards from the armpit.

Lu 6, to locate this point, hold your hand in front of you with palm facing up. Draw an imaginary line from the centre of the elbow crease to the wrist crease, divide this line into half and move one thumb width towards the elbow on this line. Press this point with medium pressure. This is very useful in any acute condition involving the lungs.

Lu 7 is located about one and a half inches above the Lu 9 point above the wrist crease on the thumb side. It has been named 'Broken Sequence' and is used for its tonifying effect on the lungs.

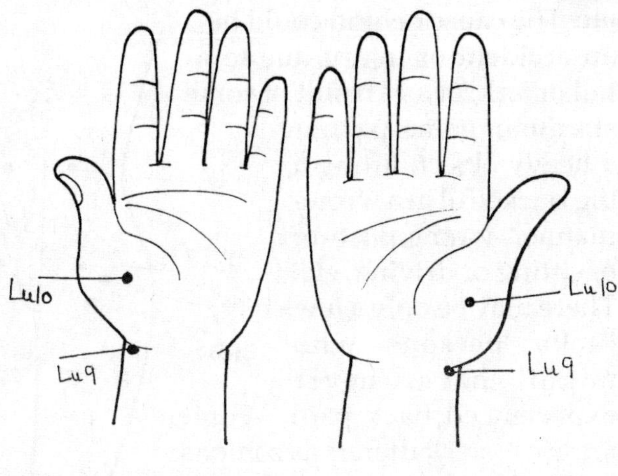

CV 17 is directly on the breastbone, between the 4th and 5th ribs. For men, this is at the level of the nipples. For women, you can easily find it about three finger widths up from the bottom of the breastbone. Use the tips of three fingers to press. It would be more beneficial in case the points CV17 and B13 are pressed one after the other. This point has been found to be beneficial in chronic cases of asthma.

Following points may also be of use in case situation demands and time permits: B23; St 36 and St 40.

It is not necessary to press all the aforesaid points in one session, you can omit some of them in one session and add them in the other session omitting some of the points attended to in the previous session.

In case you also wish to add pressure points used in reflexology, the important areas you cannot afford to miss shall be the lung and the bronchial reflexes on the top and bottom of the feet; solar plexus/diaphragm point; the adrenals, the sinus reflexes on the toes and the fingers.

Q. 39: A large number of patients suffer from back pain. Can acupressure help? What are the causes?

A. 39: Usually, back pain is a temporary ailment that comes and goes and is caused because of some strenuous activity or overexertion. It gives a feel of pain, discomfort, tenderness in the lower back, in the region of the spine, hips, etc. The cause behind could be an accident or injury due to a fall or jerk, or as a result of some strenuous game, pushing a heavy object, lifting a big bucketful in a wrong manner, wrong posture of sitting or driving, etc. There may be only a few lucky persons who might have never experienced back pain. Women are the worst sufferers as compared to men because of certain biological factors (e.g. childbearing) and probably due to the lumbar curve in their back. The only redeeming feature is that in most of the cases generally the pain is bearable and only in few cases is it disabling or excruciating. Other reasons could be overweight, weak muscles, lack of movement, etc.

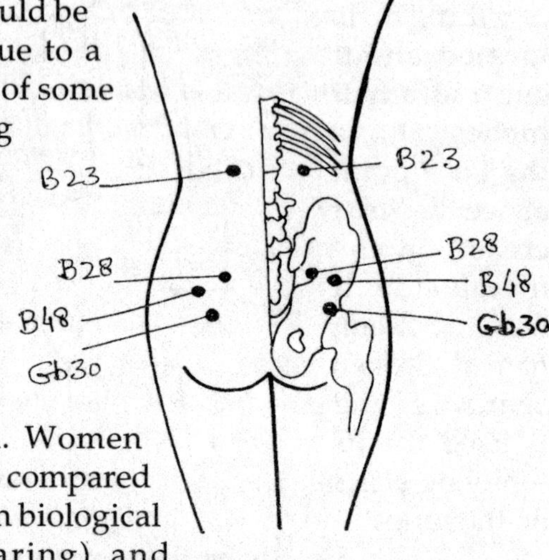

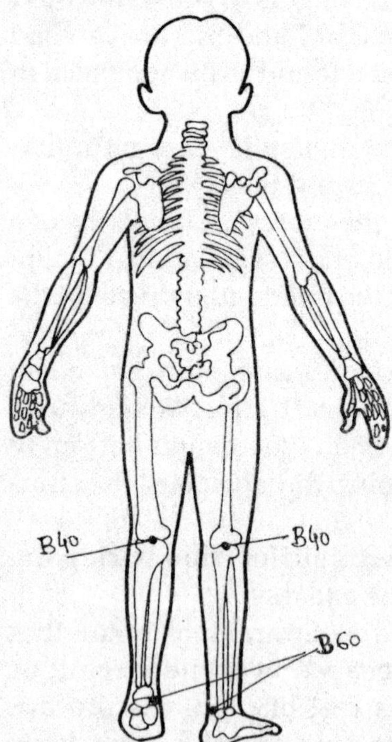

One can, however, adopt to undertaking certain exercises to strengthen the muscles and make them more flexible; poor or improper posture can also be corrected. Acupressure can prove to be a boon in tackling this problem. In case you suffer from back pain, the first thing that should come to your mind is to correct the energy flow in your bladder meridian, as this is the meridian passing through your entire back starting from the eye, going through the top of your head and down to the little toe in the foot. Backache is considered to be caused by the blockage of the Ch'i in the bladder meridian.

To begin with, give pressure on B 23 which can be located in the middle of the waist, half way between the rib cage and the hip bone on the inner edge, and B 47 which lies in the middle of the waist on the outside of the erector muscle. These points, not only provide relief in low back pain but also reduce muscle tension.

Next points to be pressed are B 28 and B 48, which lie on the inner bladder line, halfway between the top and bottom of the sacrum and half way between the inner and outer edge and on the outer bladder line as shown in the figure. These points are highly beneficial for lower back, buttock and pain in the sacral region. They also help in relieving sciatica pain.

B 40, lies in the middle of the crease in the back of the knee. This point is highly beneficial in relieving lower back pain, stiffness and tension, etc., by moving the Ch'I through the knee, thereby reducing knee pain, spasms and stiffness in the lower back area.

GB 30 is located on the buttocks, about a third of the distance between the hip bone and the tail bone. Press this point strongly, using your thumb or even elbow if the buttock muscles are too heavy. It helps reduce hip joint inflammation, relieve muscle sprains, spasms and pain in the low back. This point is also useful in alleviating sciatica pain.

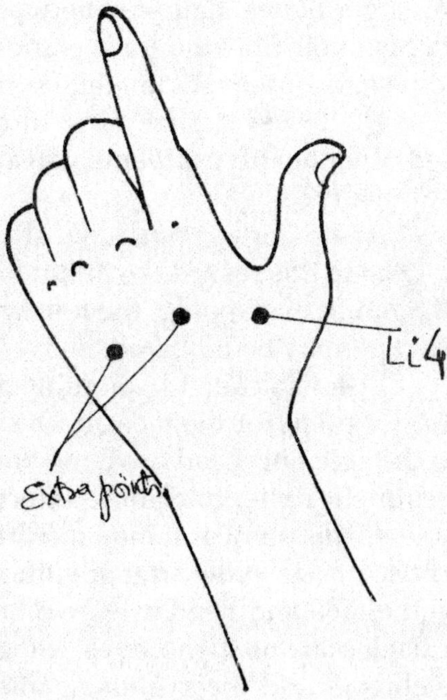

B 60, lies half way between the Achilles tendon and the outer ankle bone. It relieves back pain in the lower and upper back and the legs. Also give pressure on

GV 4, which can be found at the waistline 2-3 finger widths below the B 23 point, to get relief from pain.

Since one may find it difficult to give pressure on the points which are on the back, pressure on the following points on the back of the hand may be given which have been found to be extremely beneficial.

Li 4, known as 'Adjoining Valley', is known for its ability to relieve pain and circulating the Ch'i. It lies on the end of the crease that is formed when the thumb and the index finger are joined together. Pregnant women should not use this point. Just half inch above and below this point, there are two more points which are highly beneficial in relieving back pain. Apply sufficiently strong pressure on these points with the help of the thumb of the other hand. Repeat the process on the other hand. Interestingly, it has been found that in case of pain on the left side, pressure works better if given on the right hand, and if on the right side then pressure should be given on the left hand. Two more extra points lie on the back of the hands. First between the 2nd and 3rd finger bones and the second between the 4th and 5th finger bones, half way between the knuckles and the wrist. In case you find the pain comes back, repeat the process for some sessions, as it may take some time to get fully cured.

Q. 40: Besides helping in overcoming all sorts of pains and other health problems, can acupressure also help in toning up beauty?

A. 40: Certain tips have already been provided in answer to Q.23 in this regard. To attain long term natural beauty sitting at home at no expense, the following schedule of pressure point therapy may be followed:

Li 4 also called 'Adjoining Valley' is considered to be the master point for the face and head. It opens the flow of energy to the face and head area and thus helps in making rest of the treatment easier and more effective. Pregnant women should not use this point as it may result in premature contractions and a miscarriage. Now after opening the gate for the flow of energy to the face and head area, we have to focus on toning up the muscles around the eyes for getting a better look for the eyebrows and the eyelids as also to provide a better lustrous look to our skin.

Si 17 can be found in the indentation directly behind the ear lobe. It stimulates the thyroid gland to improve the luster of the skin. Perhaps that is why it has been given the name Heavenly appearance.

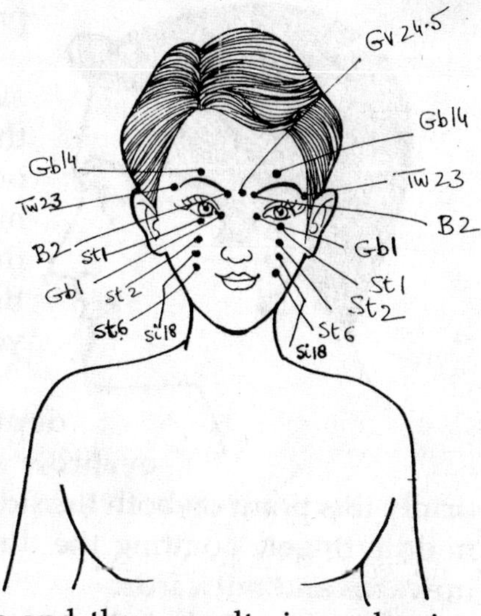

Gv 24.5 is located between the eyebrows, in the indentation where the bridge of the nose meets the forehead. This tones up the endocrine system, particularly the pituitary gland. This tones up the entire body, reduces stress and thus results in a glowing facial look bubbling with energy.

Gv 16 can be found at the top of the spinal column in the hollow under the base of the skull. Pressure on this point should be mild and should be given with caution. It helps in overall toning up of the eye, ear, nose and throat which in turn results in better looks.

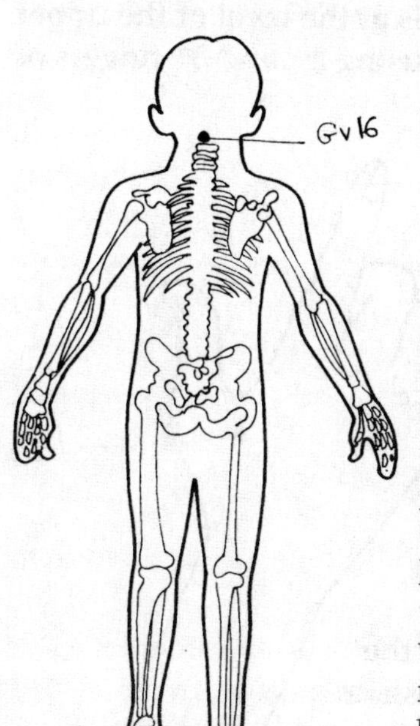

B 2 is located at the inner edge of the eyebrow, next to the bridge of our nose, in the small indentation. Press here with the middle finger of both the hands together on both sides for 30 to 60 seconds, starting with mild pressure, hold and then release gradually. Keep the eyes closed and breathe deeply while applying pressure.

Gb 14 is located one thumb width above your eyebrows in the middle of the eyebrow. Pressure can be applied with the index or middle finger for about a minute, directing the

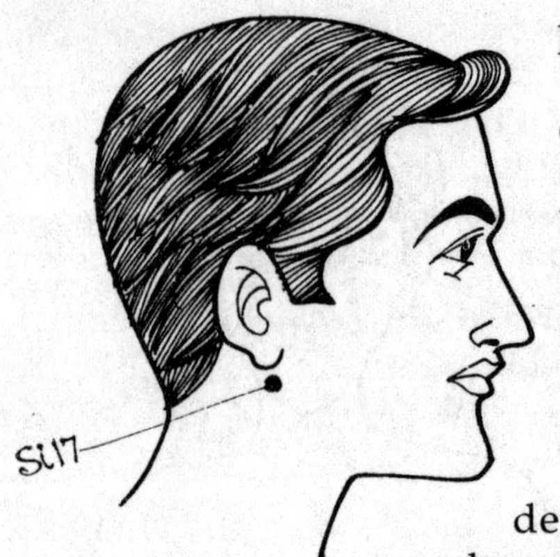

pressure towards the hairline.

TW 23 is located on the eyebrow line at the outer edge of the eyebrow. Apply pressure on both the sides for about one minute in the depression, with the help of the index or middle finger as may be convenient to you.

Gb 1 try to feel the depression in the outside of the eyebrow as shown in the figure. Press firmly this point on both the sides with the help of the index or middle finger, pointing the direction of the pressure slightly upwards and outwards.

St 1 is just below the eye socket in line with the centre of the pupils. Feel the ridge of the bone of the eye socket. Give mild but direct pressure towards the bone for about 30 seconds. Follow it up by giving pressure on St 2 beneath St 1 on the same line below the pupils. This points falls at the level of the upper border of the nostrils. Give pressure using 2nd and 3rd fingers of both the hands simultaneously.

St 4 falls just outside the corners of the lips in the dimples that are formed when you smile. Press for 30 seconds with your index fingers.

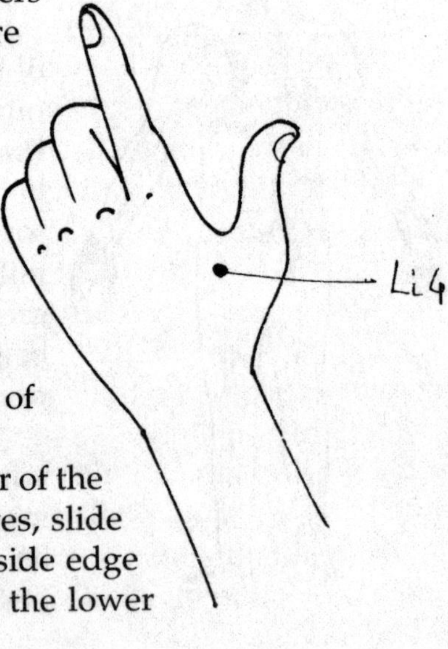

St 6 can be located easily by clenching your teeth and looking for the point where the endpoints of the jaws meet. Press slowly at the point of the bulge for about one minute with the help of middle and index fingers.

Li 4

Si 18 starting from the corner of the eye on the sides of both your eyes, slide down your fingers from the outside edge of the eye sockets till you reach the lower border of the cheek bones. Put your three fingers below the cheek bone on both the sides of the cheeks and plunge your head on these three fingers giving medium pressure for about a minute or less.

Points St 2, St 4, St 6 and Si 18 help in tightening and lifting the cheeks.

In case you also wish to add pressure points used in reflexology, the important areas you cannot afford to miss shall be the lung points on the bottom of the feet to open the chest and facilitate deeper breathing with a view to get more of Oxygen which is vital for a healthy skin as it is for energy and metabolism. To promote digestion and throw the toxins out of our body, work on the solar plexus/diaphragm point, the adrenals, the abdomen and liver, kidneys, large and small intestines. Pressure should also be given on the webbing between the toes and the lymph area where the foot meets the lower leg, to throw out the toxins. Also give pressure on the sinus points to improve circulation which will result in a healthy glow on the skin of the entire body. For the reflex areas of various organs mentioned here refer to the diagrams of soles and the palms at the end of the book.

Q. 41: What is bed wetting? Can acupressure help in this condition?

A. 41: Bed wetting is a condition seen as lack of control over urine due to deficiency in water element which means that the kidney and urinary bladder meridians need to be strengthened. Generally, children in the lower age group suffer from this problem and no major cause is attached to it and this condition is controlled by itself in the natural way. However, in case this

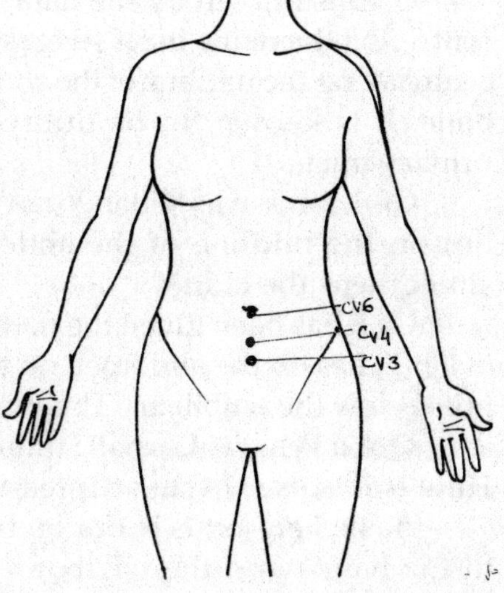

problem persists even after the age of three years or so or at times when even the elderly people wet their beds, it calls for attention. Generally, people say that it can be controlled by reducing the intake of water/fluids particularly in the night after 8 pm, however, there seems to be not much truth in all this. Following the acupressure schedule discussed below would be found to be useful in overcoming and controlling this condition:

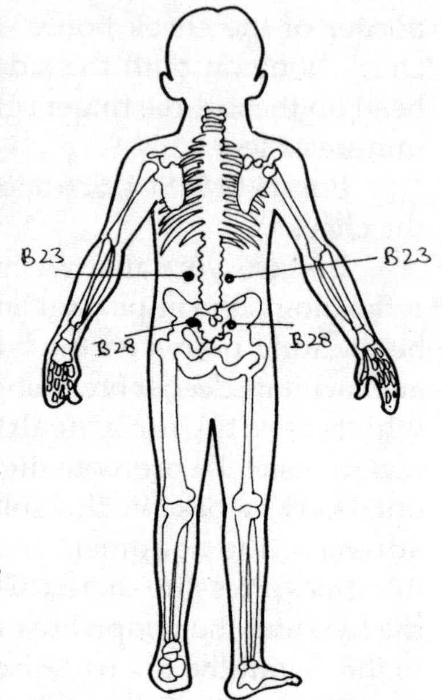

B 23 is located on the sides of the spine, at the level of the waist. This strengthens the Ch'i of the kidney. This is considered to be a major point for treating disorders of the urogenital system and has a direct effect on kidneys.

B 28 is located in the sacral region, i.e. the lowest part of the spine, on the side, and this point strengthens the Ch'i of the bladder.

Cv 3 is known by the name 'Zhongji' which means exact centre. As the name itself suggests, this point lies exactly at the centre along the midline of the abdomen, slightly above the pubic bone. It is known for its utility for treating disorders of the urinary tract.

Cv 4, known as 'Guan Yuan' meaning Storage Place of Ch'i lies on the midline of the abdomen, a little above Ren 3. It strengthens the kidney.

Cv 6 has been given the name 'Ch'i Hai' which means 'Sea of Ch'i', lies on the abdomen on the midline, above Ren 4 and a little below the umbilicus. This point also strengthens the kidney.

Q. 42: What is Carpal Tunnel Syndrome and Tendonitis? How is it caused? Can acupressure help?

A. 42: Few joints in our body are as important as the joints in the hands and the wrists for carrying out our day-to-day

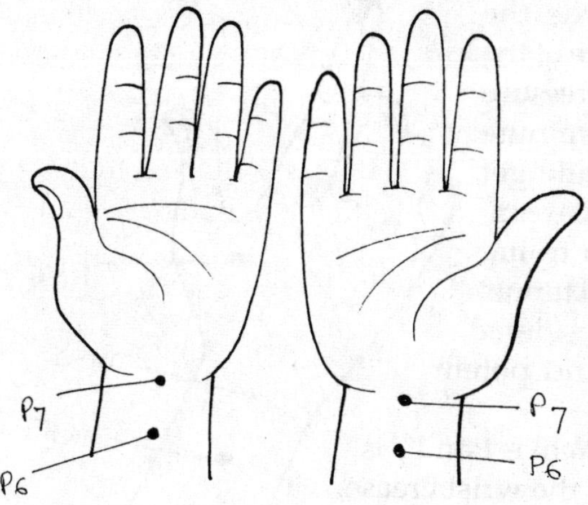

activity. Acupressure has been found to be effective for healing from a sprained wrist to carpal tunnel syndrome and tendonitis. Dr. Keith Kenyon found that acupressure relieved wrist arthritis also. Carpal tunnel syndrome can be a very painful condition. The carpal tunnel is a tunnel through your wrist in which tendons, arteries, veins, and nerves travel to the hands. It is caused by the swelling that creates pressure on the medial nerve and is caused from overuse in activities, e.g. working on computers for long hours, playing video games and sending SMS on mobile phone very frequently. Likewise, tendonitis is an inflammation of the tendons due to their overuse. When the tendons inflame, they compress the median nerve going into your hand. Pressure points discussed below are capable of relaxing the tendons and muscles attached to the wrist which results in less pain and discomfort in using the fingers:

Li 4, known as 'Adjoining Valley', is known for its ability to relieve pain and inflammation and circulating the Ch'i. It lies on the end of the crease that is formed when the thumb and the index finger are joined together. Pregnant women should not use this point.

P 6, known as the 'Inner Gate' is located in the middle of the inner side of the forearm, two and a half finger widths above the wrist crease towards the elbow. It relieves wrist pain.

P 7, the big mound is in the centre of the wrist on the palm side. Giving moderate pressure on this point with the thumb for about a minute helps overcome wrist pain (carpal tunnel syndrome), rheumatism and tendonitis to a great extent.

Tw 5, called the 'Outer Gate' is located midway between the ulna and radius about two and a half finger widths above the wrist crease towards the elbow bone on the outside of the wrist (back side). Give pressure on this point for about a minute to strengthen the wrist and get relief from pain, rheumatism, sensation of pain when trying to hold something, carpal tunnel syndrome, etc. This is considered to be a very effective and potent point in acupressure.

Tw 4, known as 'Active Pond', is located in the hollow of the wrist crease, at the centre, on the outer wrist. Pressure on this point can be given by placing the thumb on the centre of the outer wrist crease, with the fingers supporting from the inside of the wrist. Apply firm pressure and ask the patient to take deep, long breaths. Continue for a minute or two till the pain in the wrist subsides. Release gradually. Throughout the process, ask the patient to continue with deep slow breathing. Repeat the process on the other wrist.

Q. 43: A large number of people suffer from cervical spondylosis. Can acupressure be of any help to such patients?

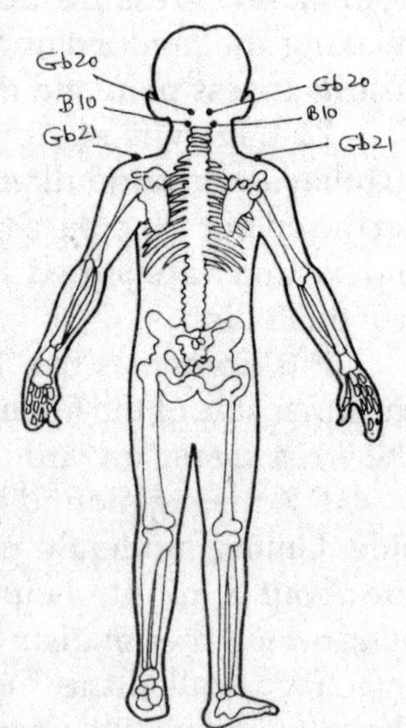

A. 43: Today, cervical spondylosis is perhaps the most common disease from which over 50 percent of the population is suffering. The interesting part is that of these 50 percent, at least 70 percent are not aware that they are suffering from this ailment. Basically, poor or faulty posture can be attributed as a major cause of this ailment. Watching TV for long hours in lying position or half lying posture with head resting on the palm, working on

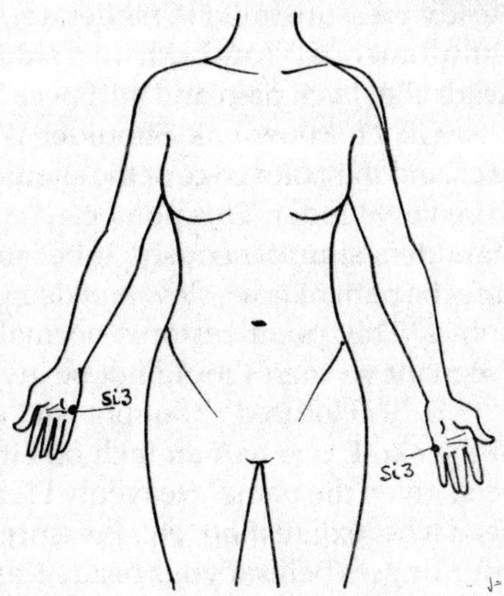

computers for long hours, driving long distances every day, sitting in a wrong posture on a scooter, motor cycle or in the car can also be an underlying cause of this disease.

In medical terms, it can be termed as a chronic degeneration of the cervical vertebrae. Generally, the disease occurs in men and women over 30 years of age. But there is no age bar as such and even youngsters and elderly people have been seen to be suffering from this ailment. The symptoms that draw attention about the onset of this disease are stiffness or uneasiness or pain in the neck that radiates through shoulders towards lower arm. A sensation of numbness in the hand or even up to the fingers is also at times experienced. It may be accompanied with headache and vertigo at times, and in advanced cases the patient may have a feeling as if he/she would fall down even while sitting or lying in the bed because of the intensity of the vertigo. The symptoms of cervical spondylosis, at times are so much similar to that of angina that people are misled. The major difference is that in case of a cervical attack, sweating is missing and the extent of discomfort in the region of the chest is also much less comparatively.

This condition can be easily overcome by pressure point technique and reflexology. Most of the times, you do not even require an x-ray to identify the vertebrae where the problem has occurred. An experienced acupressure therapist will be able to identify the exact location by the touch of the big toe or the first knuckle of the thumb. Moreover, until and unless the problem has been existing for years, this condition can be controlled within 8-10 sittings.

GB 20 is located in the hollow below the base of the skull.

Steady pressure (mild to moderate) should be given on this point simultaneously on both the sides. Relieves arthritic pain, headache, back pain and stiff neck.

GB 21, known as 'Shoulder Well' is midway between the neck and the outer edge of the shoulder. This point is often found to be very tender. This point can be pressed on both sides of the shoulders simultaneously. It becomes even more beneficial in case the patient takes slow and deep breaths as you press various points. This point restores normal flow of Ch'i in the lungs. Pregnant women should not be given pressure on this point.

B 10 is located about one and a half inches below the base of the skull, one half an inch on either side of the spine. It has been given the name 'Heavenly Pillars'; it relieves swollen eyes, headache, exhaustion, etc. Pressure can be given by interlacing your fingers behind your head, grasping the neck and pressing firmly for about a minute.

Si-3, make a fist and twist, then twist your wrist to view the side of your little finger. Using your thumb, apply pressure on the side of your palm just below the knuckle of the little finger, between the bone and the muscle. Press firmly for about a minute.

For overcoming this condition using reflexology, work on the reflex areas of the cervical vertebrae on the big toes and the thumbs up to the first knuckle on both feet and hands. Also work on the pads below the big toes and the thumbs with a view to stimulate the areas between the shoulder blades. See figure at the end of the book for locating specific areas.

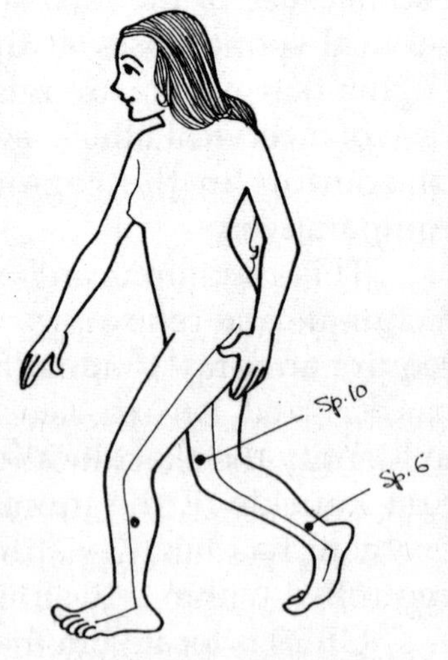

Q. 44: Can acupressure help overcome blood circulation problems?

A. 44: Stagnation in any form of life is not considered to be good. Water in a river remains fresh as long as the flow is at a good pace. It starts stinking the moment the flow is stopped/obstructed. Even in a work situation, the moment stagnation starts taking place, there comes a feeling of discontentment amongst the workers and the output reflects a negative impact. Similarly, in the context of our physical health, stagnation in the flow of the life force Ch'i is the cause behind most of the ailments. Blocked flow of this vital life force in various meridians in our body leads to disease.

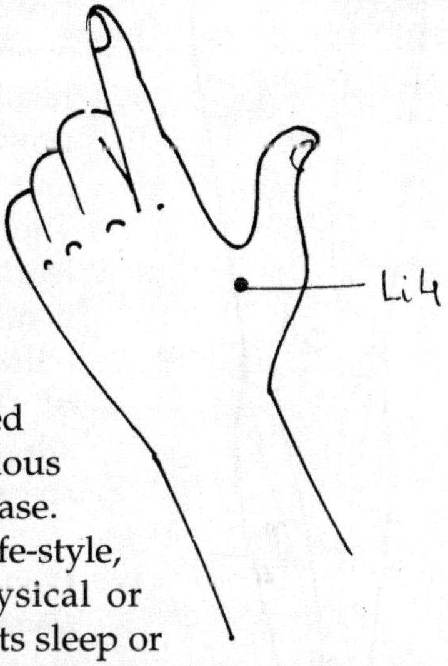

Li4

Wrong food habits, sedentary life-style, stress in any form, i.e. either physical or emotional, which also directly effects sleep or even inadequate sleep, can be the cause behind the disruption in the smooth flow of Ch'i in our body. Ch'i being primarily responsible for blood circulation. Therefore, it is of prime importance to get rid of any sort of obstruction with a view to allow unobstructed flow of Ch'i and in turn better circulation. Once this is achieved, it results in restoration of the entire system to a state of better health and balance.

Acupressure can help you break the stagnation in the flow of blood circulation with the help of following few pressure points:

Li 4 is located at the highest spot of the muscle when the thumb and the index finger are held together. Press in the web between them directing towards the bone that attaches to the index finger. Li 4 also called 'Adjoining Valley' is considered to be the master point in removing stagnation in the flow of Ch'i, and thus helps in making rest of the treatment easier and more effective. Pregnant women should not use this point as it may result in premature contractions and miscarriage.

Now after opening the gate for the flow of energy we touch upon yet another vital point known by the name 'Bigger Rush' Lv 3 is known to be the most effective point for regulating the flow of Ch'i throughout our body and in the Liver meridian in particular, which in turn keeps the Ch'i throughout our body

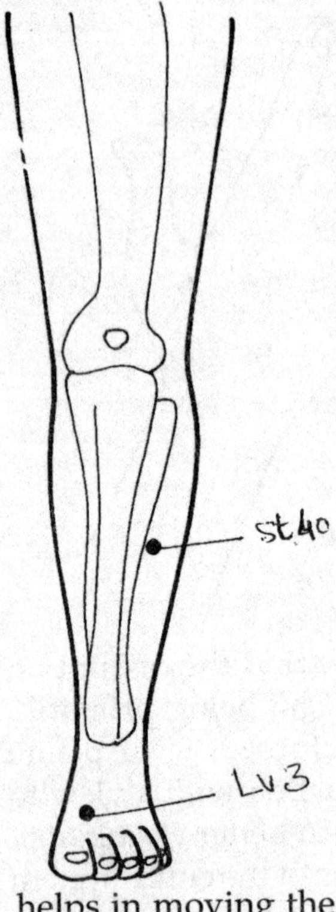

flowing smoothly. Once the flow of energy in the liver goes out of balance, it results in stagnation and imbalance in the flow of Ch'i and blood in every meridian and the result is discomfort and disease. Though this point is found to be extremely tender generally, looking into its utility, it needs to be included in the workout without fail and as a routine, since a touch of this point can tell us about the stagnation of any type in the body anywhere.

Sp 6, also called 'Three Yin Meeting Point', is located above the ankle bone towards the inside of the leg on the back side. The exact location being about four finger widths above the ankle bone. It is one of the most important pressure points as its name suggests since it strengthens the Yin of three meridians, viz. spleen, liver and kidney at the same time. It also helps in moving the liver Ch'i throughout the body. Pregnant women should not use this point.

Sp 10, is yet another important point that can be used with success for removing stagnation in the flow of blood.

St 40, is located half way between the ankle bone on the outside of the foot and centre of the kneecap. Find the tibia and go two thumb widths off the bone to the outside. Is very helpful for reducing congestion.

Q. 45: Can acupressure be of any help in alleviating discomfort caused by cold?

A. 45: When the resistance of your body is low, you are exhausted, and your system is not able to get attuned to the climatic changes quickly. This is the time when you are prone to catching a cold. Your mucus membrane becomes a breeding ground for the virus. These viruses keep breeding in our nose and throat and attack when the conditions in the body suit them best, e.g. when the temperature and moisture is congenial.

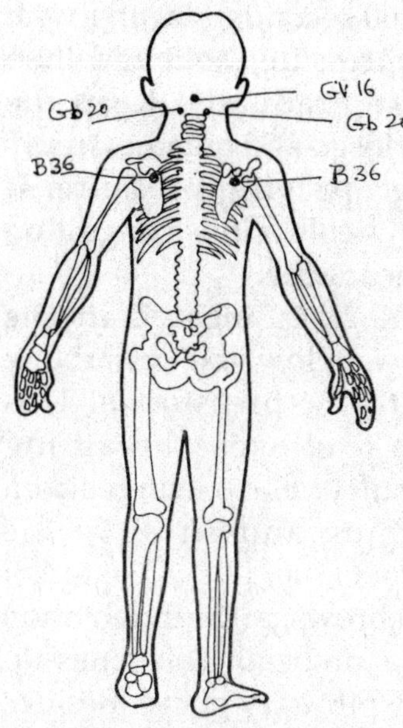

Cold is a symptom and the body's attempt to protect itself from viruses, and in doing so, it secretes more mucus to flush them away.

Interestingly, it is said that cold cannot be treated by any means, i.e. if you take medicine, it takes seven days to cure and if you do not take any medicine it will get cured within a week. On the same analogy acupressure also cannot cure cold yet it can certainly help you in alleviating the amount of discomfort one feels otherwise. It can help the body to expel the viruses that have entered the body and is capable of increasing the body's resistance to protect it from cold in future.

B 36 called 'Bearing Support' is good for building up the body's resistance to combat colds. Located near the spine, on the shoulder blades as shown in the figure, it is said that wind and cold enter the pores of the skin at this point. Pressure can be given on this point easily by holding your shoulders with your hands. Even a good massage on this area, i.e. upper back, shoulders and neck helps a lot in decongesting.

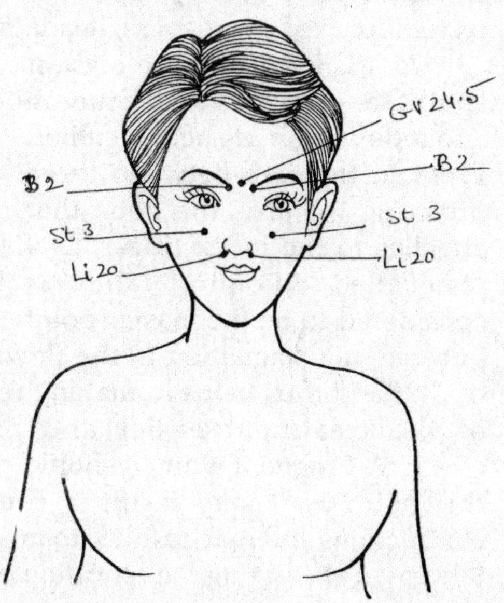

B 2 is located at the inner edge of the eyebrow, next to the bridge of our nose, in the small indentation. Press here with the middle finger of both the hands together on both sides for

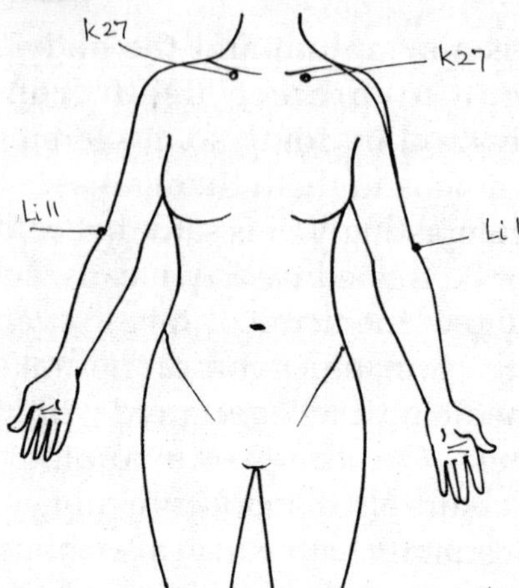

30 to 60 seconds, starting with mild pressure, hold and then release gradually. Keep the eyes closed and breathe deeply while applying pressure. It relieves cold, sinus congestion and headache.

K 27 is located in the hollow below the collarbone next to the breastbone. This point relieves breathing difficulty, chest congestion, coughing and stress in the region of the chest and sore throat.

GV 24.5 is located between the eyebrows, in the indentation where the bridge of the nose meets the forehead. This tones-up the endocrine system, particularly the pituitary gland. Besides it tones up the entire body, reduces stress and relieves head congestion, stuffy nose and headache.

GV 16 can be found at the top of the spinal column in the hollow under the base of the skull. Pressure on this point should be mild and be given with caution. It helps in relieving head congestion, red eyes, stress, headache and stiff neck.

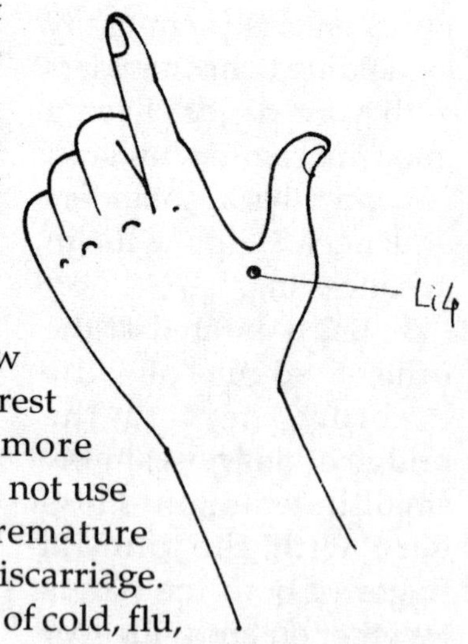

Li 4 is located at the highest spot of the muscle when the thumb and index finger are held together. Press in the web between them directing towards the bone that attaches to the index finger. Li 4 also called 'adjoining valley' is considered to be the master point in removing stagnation in the flow of Ch'i and thus helps in making rest of the treatment easier and more effective. Pregnant women should not use this point as it may result in premature contractions and may result into miscarriage. It helps in alleviating the condition of cold, flu, congestion in the head and headache.

GB 20 is located in the hollow below the base of the skull. Steady pressure (mild to moderate) should be given on this point simultaneously on both the sides. Relieves head congestion, headache, neck pain, stiff neck and irritability.

LI 11 is located at the outer end of the elbow crease. This point is very effective in relieving symptoms of cold, fever and in strengthening the immune system to help develop resistance from future colds. As this point gets very tender on touching, mild or massage-like pressure only should be given on this point.

St 3 can be found at the bottom of the cheek bone in line with the pupil. It relieves stuffy nose, head congestion, discomfort in the eyes, e.g. burning and swelling.

LI 20 is located outside each nostril on the cheeks. Nasal congestion, sinus and facial swelling is overcome by giving pressure on these points.

Q. 46: What are the causes behind constipation? Can it be cured by acupressure treatment?

A. 46: Faulty diet without enough fruits, green vegetables, insufficient fibre rich food/grains, many types of items at a time in one meal, white flour which does not contain enough roughage as the husk is thrown out as also lack of exercise lead to constipation. Occasional constipation does not pose a serious problem, but chronic constipation may lead to serious consequences and cause the waste matter to block the colon. The colon muscle that throws out the waste can become too relaxed or too tense to move. It is believed that one can take care of this condition by eating a properly balanced diet and doing regular exercise or even brisk walk, jogging, etc. Enough quantity of water/fluids

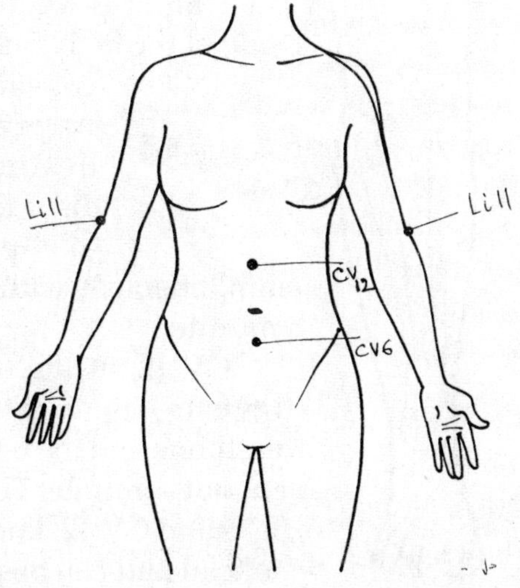

should also be consumed.

Acupressure treatment can also be given to overcome this condition by following the schedule outlined below:

CV 6 known by the name 'Sea of Energy' is located three finger widths below the navel. Pressure on this point can be given in lying position (empty bladder). It relieves abdominal pain, constipation, colitis and gas formation.

St 36 is located about four finger widths below your kneecap and one finger width outside off your shin bone. This point can be best stimulated by the patient himself by using his own heel to rub this point (use right heel to stimulate left foot and vice versa). Helps in alleviating sore, tired muscles and general fatigue. Pressure on this point strengthens the whole body, tones up the muscles, and aids digestion and relieves stomach disorders, e.g. constipation, by overcoming intestinal disorders.

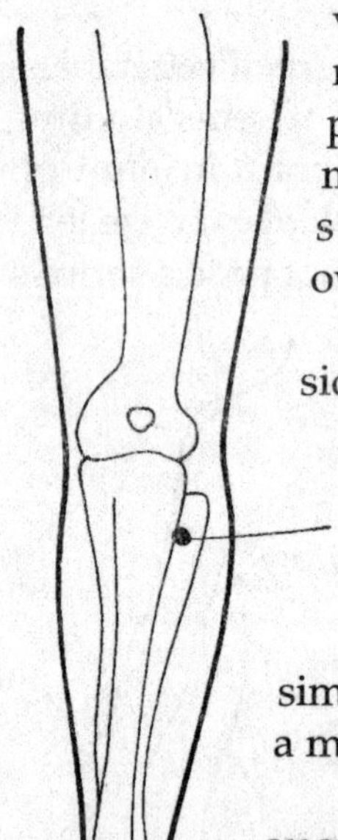

St 25 is located two thumb widths to the side of the belly button on both the sides This is considered to be one of the most important pressure points for treating a wide range of intestinal disorders as well as constipation. Try to press both the sides simultaneously with medium yet firm pressure for a minute.

CV 12, as the name 'Middle Stomach' itself suggests, is located midway between the breastbone and the belly button. Give firm pressure for about a minute. This famous combination of CV 6, St 25 and CV 12, known as 'Four Doors', is highly beneficial and can be used to overcome any type of

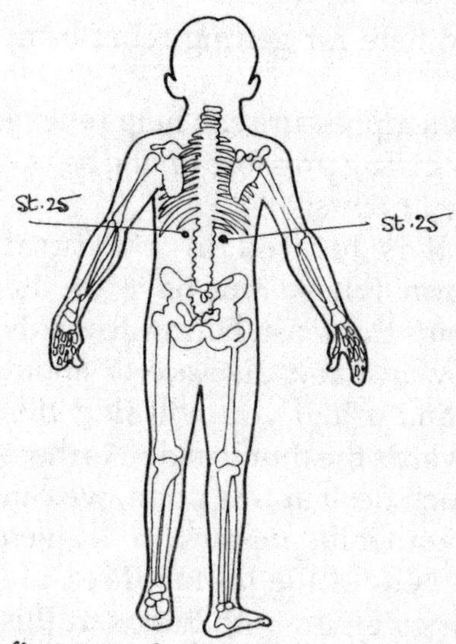

stomach or gastrointestinal disorder including constipation and diarrhoea.

One of the causes of constipation is excess internal heat. This dries up the stool which makes it too hard to pass. Give pressure on Tw 6 which is located three finger widths from the wrist crease on the back of your forehand, in the centre between the ulna and radius bones. This helps in clearing the excess heat when pressed in conjunction with Li 4 and Li 11 as shown in the figure to help cure constipation in case the stool being passed by the patient is very hard and black. Whereas one of the functions of Li 4 is to clear excess heat, Li 11 clears heat in general from the body and helps regulate the activity of colon to soothe bowel movement.

Q. 47: What makes us cough and what is the cause? Can acupressure help?

A. 47: The flow of Ch'i in the lungs usually flows downwards. For whatever reason if the lung Ch'i starts moving in the upward direction, we suffer from cough. Generally, cough accompanies cold and in case you suffer from both at the same time, also give pressure on the points discussed above for getting relief from cold in addition to the points that are being

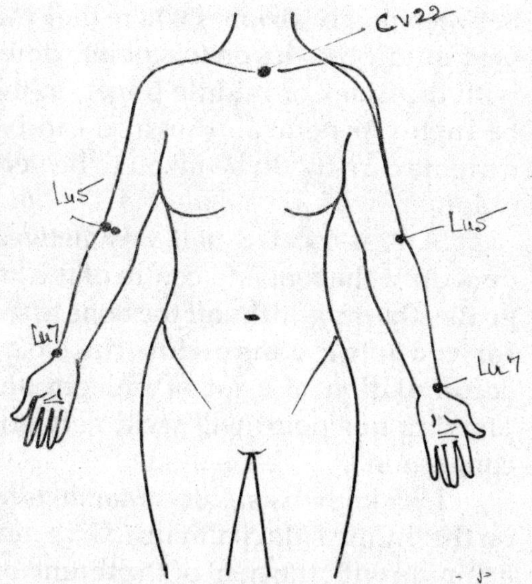

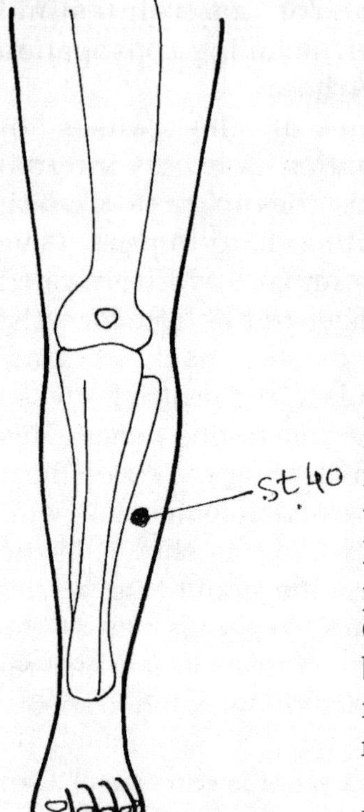

discussed here for getting relief from cough.

Yes, acupressure can help relieve cough by giving pressure on the below mentioned points:

Lu 7 is located in a natural depression where the base of the thumb joins the wrist. Follow towards the elbow and at a distance of about an inch and a half you will find this point towards the thumb side. As there is not much flesh at this point, we can manage with mild pressure to be given with the help of the thumb. Pressure has to be given on both hands at this point. This point reverses the flow of Ch'i in the downward direction to bring relief. Can also be used to get relief from cold, sneezing and running nose.

Cv 22 known as 'Heaven Projection' is in the depression between the collarbones where they meet the breastbone. Giving very mild pressure on this point, downwards and not inwards, with the index or middle finger, to the count of 10, is found to be highly beneficial. Pressure can be repeated 2-3 times but extreme care has to be taken to be very gentle and mild on this point.

St 40 is located half way between the ankle bone on the outside of the foot and centre of the kneecap. Find the tibia and go two thumb widths off the bone to the outside.It is very helpful for reducing congestion. In case you feel that there is accumulation of a lot of phlegm and mucus in your lungs, pressing this point will yield very good results in clearing the congestion.

Lu 5 known as 'Cubit Marsh' is located in the elbow crease on the thumb side (palm up). Give moderate pressure for about a minute with the help of the thumb of the other hand. This will clear heat and moisten the throat. Repeat pressure on the other hand also.

To overcome this condition using reflexology, warm up the reflex areas of the palms and soles and give pressure on the reflex areas of chest, lungs, bronchial area, sinus points, area pertaining to throat and neck, etc. Refer to the figures of palms and soles at the end of the book to know the approximate location of reflex areas pertaining to various organs.

Q. 48: What causes cramps? Can acupressure/reflex-ology provide any relief in this condition?

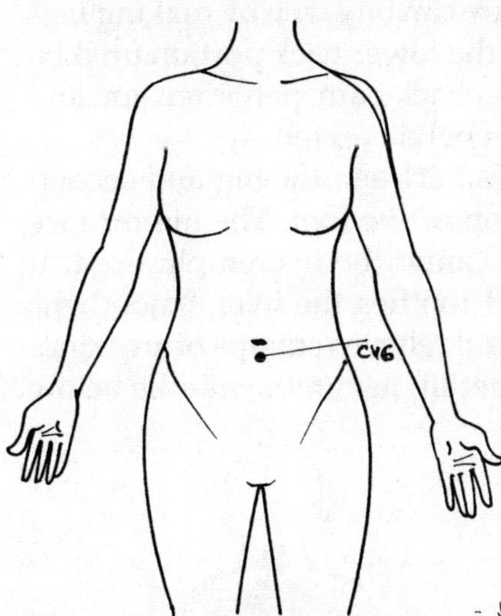

A. 48: Cramps are generally caused by muscular tension. They can develop anywhere in the body, however, they usually occur in the muscle(s) which have been overused. During a cramp, the nerves of the affected muscle become hyperactive that causes an extreme contraction of the muscle involved. Runners get cramps in their legs. They are often felt in the calves and generally occur during or after an exercise or other physical exertion. At times even if you stretch your legs with a little force, cramp occurs. Dehydration may also be the cause responsible for cramps in the legs, as such sportspersons must ensure that they stay properly hydrated during the period they are on the field.

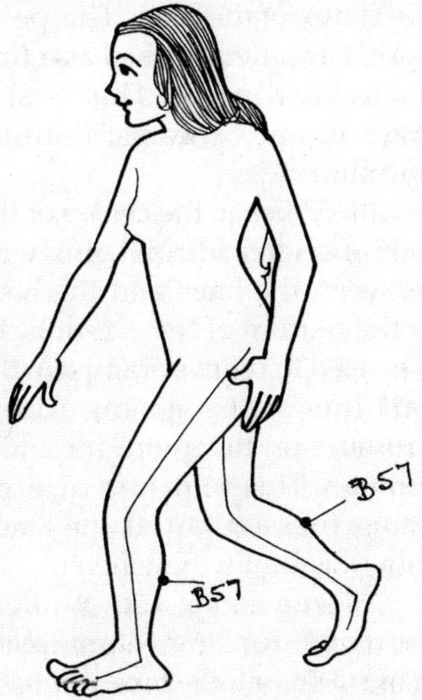

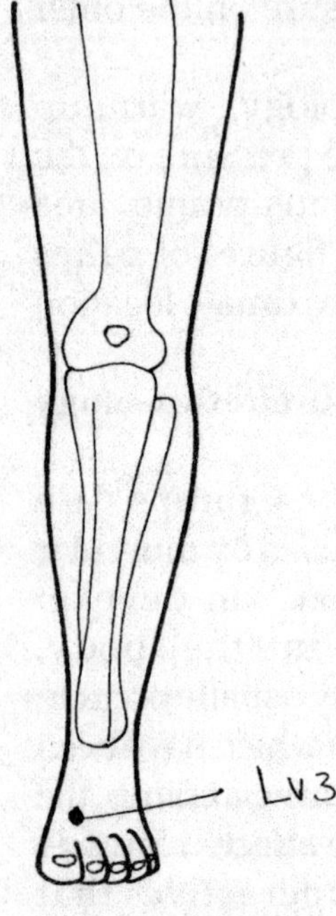

The following pressure points in acupressure can be of much relief to patient suffering from this highly painful condition.

CV 6 known as 'Sea of Energy' is located three finger widths below the navel on the midline of the body. It helps relieve menstrual cramps.

B 47 is located on the lower back between the 2nd and 3rd lumbar vertebrae about one and a half inches outside from the spine. Pressure can be given by making fists and rubbing the lower back portion briskly. Relieves lower back pain, pelvic tension and cramps in the pelvic region.

Lv 3, lies between the big and second toes on the top of the foot. The importance of this point cannot be overemphasised. It regulates and tonifies the liver, smoothens flow of Ch'i and relieves cramps of any kind.

GV 26 is located on the upper lip just in the middle below the centre of the nose. This point is very frequently used as a first aid revival point. This is also used to cure cramps, fainting and dizziness.

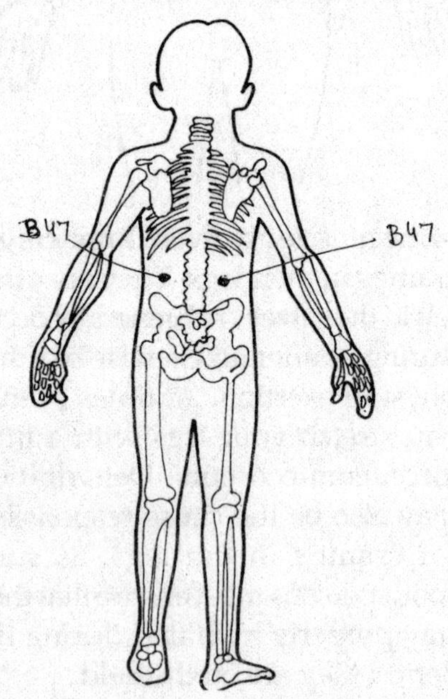

B 57 lies in the centre of the calf muscle, almost midway between the knee and the heel, at the bottom of the calf muscle. It is used to relieve cramps in the calf muscle by giving direct pressure on this point for 2 to 3 minutes. This point hurts a lot on being pressed but at the same time it is highly beneficial.

Using reflexology to help this condition, give stimulation around the ankle bone on both

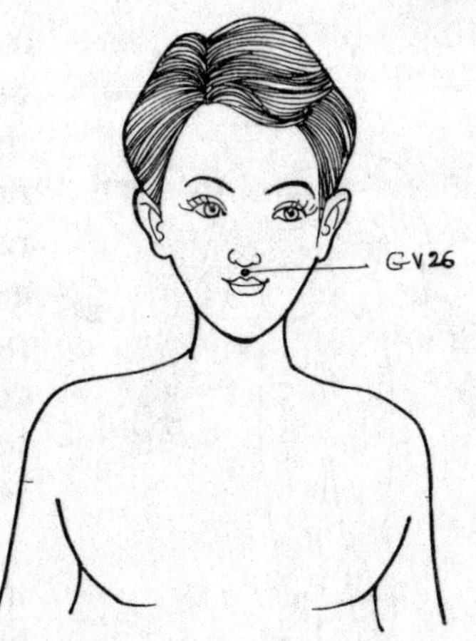

sides of the feet (anterior and posterior) on both feet in massage like semicircular motion, to and fro. Stimulation of these areas helps a lot. Also give pressure with the help of thumb and index figure over the area of the Achilles tendon about four to five inches height above the base of the heel on the back side of the foot, on both feet. Let it be followed by giving pressure with the help of your thumb on the calf muscle, the point between the crease of the knee on the back side and the base of the ankles. This point hurts a lot but is equally effective. Hold your thumb on this point for about 30 seconds with moderate pressure, breathe deep and gradually release the pressure. Repeat 2-3 times. Massage the area with the pad of your palm to remove the tenderness over this spot.

Q. 49: What is depression and how is it caused? Can acupressure help in overcoming depression?

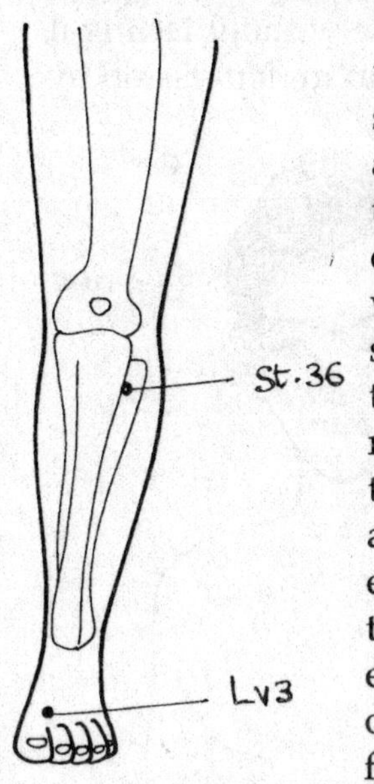

A. 49: Depression is a signal to notify that something is lacking. In every one's life sooner or later a time comes when things are not happening the way one would-like them to or have planned. It seems as if everything is going out of hands. Any one would feel bad in such a situation. However, some people who have learnt to live with time and take things the way they come do not feel the pinch too much and are thus able to bear the brunt without much trouble. Yet another set of people who are used to taking every petty thing to their heart, are not able to sustain the situation and they become extremely sad as and when they suffer a loss or in case someone close to them in the family or even nearby relation dies. In such

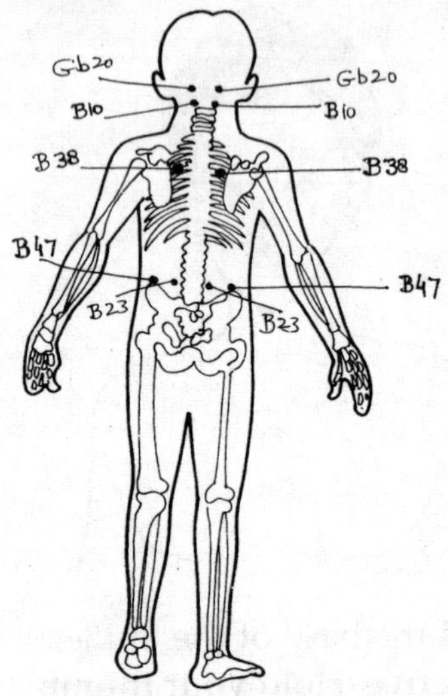

a situation these people tend to focus only on the negative side of life. Every thing seems to have been lost. In short, no charm is left in their life and they feel low energy levels. At times it assumes alarming proportions and the patient does not want to even talk or confide with anyone. He does not like to talk, and starts crying bitterly without an apparent cause.

At this juncture, it becomes important to distinguish between a short term depression, which is caused by what we call 'blues', the short term circumstances that appear and disappear vis-à-vis a chronic or acute depression which requires intervention of a professional for counselling or treatment, as the case may be.

The causes of depression could be external as discussed above, biological as caused by chemical imbalances in the system and psychological, that are caused in case you keep on controlling your anger for a pretty long time without letting it out or expressing the same. This may end up in depression by turning the inward anger against yourself. Depression can thus be the result of repressed emotions and stagnant energy, i.e. the flow of Ch'i particularly in the liver meridian. At times it could also be caused by the deficiency of Vit. C and E, which can be made good by the use of salad of parsley and cucumber, dressed with fresh lemon juice. Deep breathing is also useful in overcoming emotional

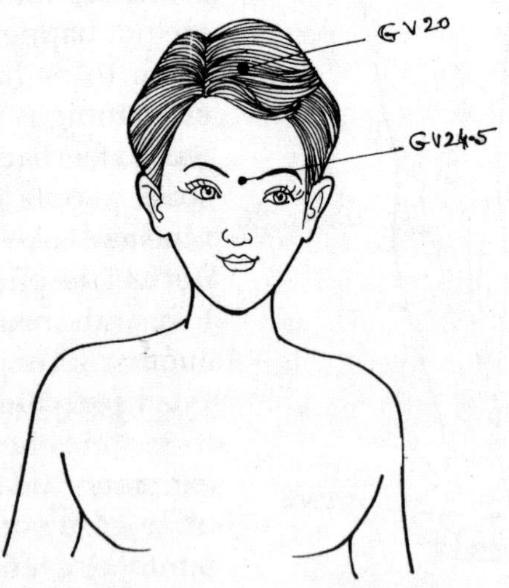

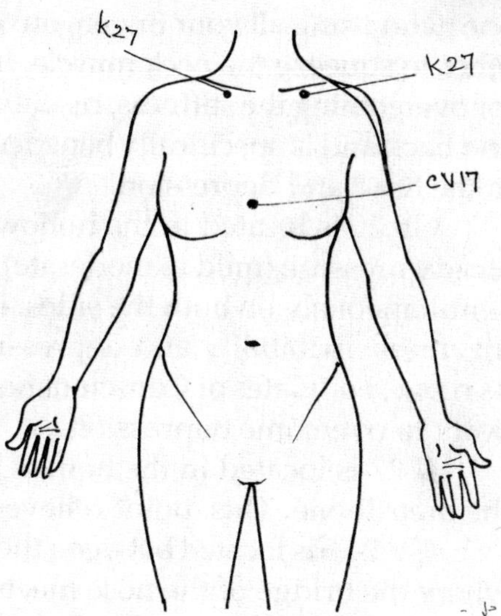

imbalance which is at times caused by inadequate supply of oxygen in our blood due to shallow breathing.

Acupressure can successfully treat this condition by unblocking the stagnation and rejuvenating the flow of Ch'i in the meridians which adversely impact the emotions. Following schedules would be helpful:

Li 4, known as 'Adjoining Valley', is known for its ability to relieve pain and circulating Ch'i. It lies on the end of the crease that is formed when the thumb and the index finger are joined together. Pregnant women should not use this point.

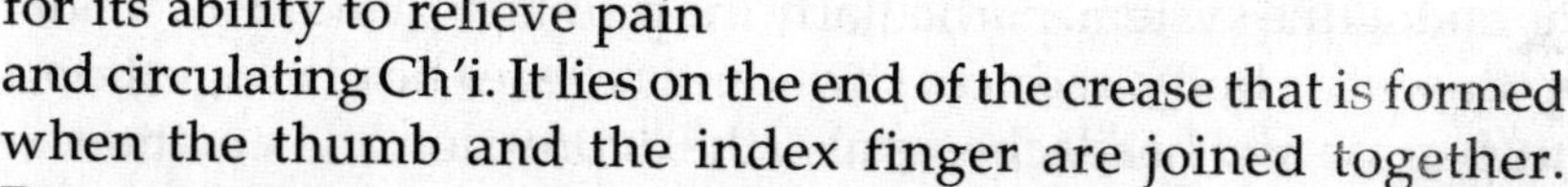

Lv 3, lies between the big and second toes on the top of the foot. The importance of this point cannot be overemphasised. It regulates and tonifies the liver and the flow of Ch'i in the liver meridian. These two points in combination are capable of 'lifting the spirits' and healing emotional upsets which cause depression.

Tw 3 is located on the back of the hand in the channel between the little and 4th finger, in the depression almost half way between the knuckles and the wrist. Press for about one minute on both the hands.

Gv 20 known as 'Hundred Meetings' is so called because all the Yang channels of the body meet at this point. It is located at the vertex. Use medium pressure for about a minute.

B 38 called 'Vital Diaphragm' is located between the shoulder blades and the spine at the level of the heart. It helps relieve anxiety, grief and emotional disturbances and is very helpful in overcoming depression.

B 10 is located on the upper portion of the neck, about one thumb width outside the spine. Hold the back of your neck with one hand using all your fingers on one side and the thumb on the other to squeeze the neck muscle. It is considered as a key point for overcoming the stiffness, rigidity and arthritic pain in the neck and back and is specifically beneficial to combat stress, heaviness in the head and depression.

GB 20 is located in the hollow below the base of the skull. Steady pressure (mild to moderate) should be given on this point simultaneously on both the sides. Relieves headache, stiff neck, dizziness, irritability and depression. Its effect goes well with its name, i.e. 'Gates of Consciousness'. Is an extremely beneficial point to overcome depression.

K 27 is located in the hollow below the collarbone next to the breastbone. This point relieves anxiety, and depression.

GV 24.5 is located between the eyebrows, in the indentation where the bridge of the nose meets the forehead. This tones up the endocrine system, particularly the pituitary gland. This tones up the entire body, reduces stress and relieves head congestion, stuffy nose and headache, as also the depression and emotional imbalances.

CV 17 known as 'Sea of Tranquility' is located in the centre of the breastbone, four finger widths above the base of the breastbone. It helps relieve nervousness, grief, depression, hysteria and other emotional imbalances.

B 23 can be located in the middle of the waist, half way between the rib cage and the hip bone on the inner edge. It relieves depression, fear and trauma.

B 47 lies in the middle of the waist four finger widths outside of the spine. This point, not only provides relief to lower back pain but also reduces muscle tension, fatigue, depression, fear and trauma.

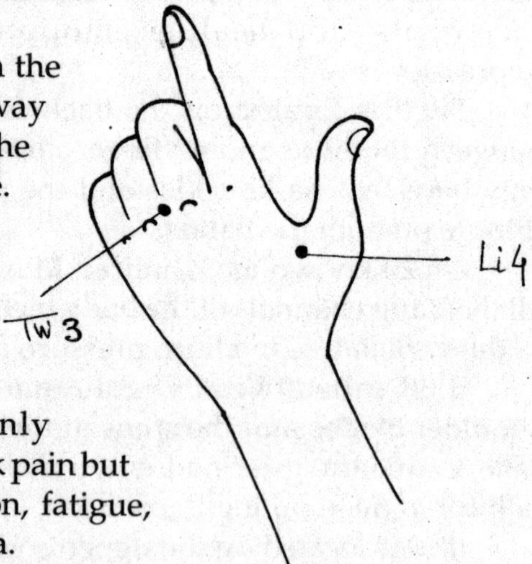

St 36 (Three Mile Point), which can

Li4

Tw 3

be easily found four finger widths below the lower border of the kneecap and one finger width towards the outside off the shin bone, serves the purpose of a gastrointestinal tonic. It also relieves indigestion, tones up the muscles of the whole body, balances the emotions and helps in overcoming depression. Give pressure on this point for 30 to 60 seconds.

Q. 50: What are the symptoms of diabetes? Can it be cured by acupressure/reflexology?

A. 50: The major symptoms of diabetes are :

(i) excessive thirst,
(ii) frequent urination,
(iii) increased appetite,
(iv) craving for sweets,
(v) loss of weight, etc.

Diabetes is caused by insufficient or non-production of 'insulin' by the pancreas. Lack of insulin results in an increase in the blood sugar level. The blood sugar level (fasting) in non-diabetics should be something between 80-100 and the same after taking breakfast (PP) should be something between 120-140. Long term complications of diabetes include damage to the retina at the back of the eye, cataracts, kidney damage, ulcers, high blood pressure and heart disorders.

Diabetes is a disease that cannot be cured but it can certainly be kept under control. Acupressure/reflexology can play a vital role in keeping it under control. However, an interesting feature about this disease is that medicine plays only a partial role in its control. It would not be incorrect to say that no medicine or even insulin injections can keep blood sugar level under check unless the patient helps himself by keeping a good control on his diet, is extremely calorie conscious, does a good amount of exercise or morning and evening walk (4 to 6 Kms per day put together), at a sufficiently good pace. In case, however, owing to some other health problems one is not able to move at a quick pace or undertake a brisk walk, walking at a normal pace would be fine.

Handling this condition using acupressure technique has to be in combination with the conventional medicine and while doing so our main target should be to stimulate the circulatory

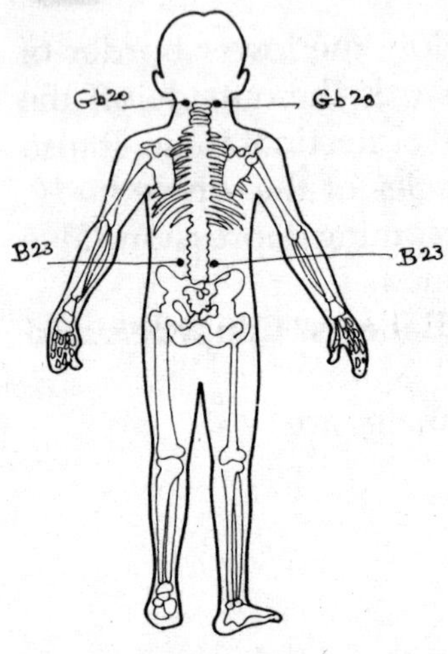

system and the immune system, for which the following schedule can be followed:

LI 4 is located at the highest spot of the muscle when the thumb and the index finger are held together. Press in the web between them directing towards the bone that attaches to the index finger. Li 4 also called 'adjoining valley' is considered to be the master-point in removing stagnation in the flow of Ch'i. Pregnant women should not use this point as it may result in premature contractions and miscarriage.

Now after opening the gate for the flow of energy we touch upon yet another vital point known by the name 'Bigger Rush' Lv 3 is known to be the most effective point for regulating the flow of Ch'i throughout our body and in the liver meridian in particular, which in turn keeps the Ch'i throughout our body flowing smoothly. Once the flow of energy in the liver goes out of balance, it results into stagnation and imbalance in the flow of Ch'i and blood in every meridian and the result is discomfort and disease. Though this point is found to be extremely tender generally, looking into its utility, it needs to be included in the workout without fail and as a routine. As far as possible this point should be stimulated simultaneously on both the feet. Speaking about the importance of this point, some well known acupressure/acupuncture therapists at times say that in case you are given an option to press just one point on your body press this point.

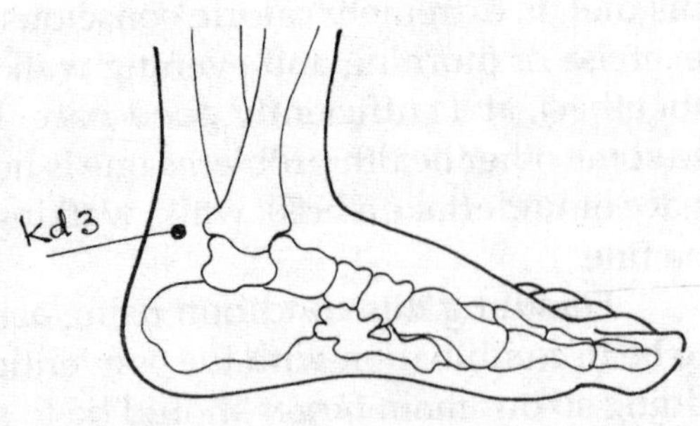

Sp 6, called 'Three Yin Meeting Point', is located above the ankle bone towards the inside of the leg on the back side. The exact location being about four finger widths above the ankle bone. It is one of the most important pressure points as its name itself suggests since it strengthens the Yin of three meridians viz. spleen, liver and kidney at a time. It also helps in moving the liver Ch'i throughout the body. Pregnant women should not use this point.

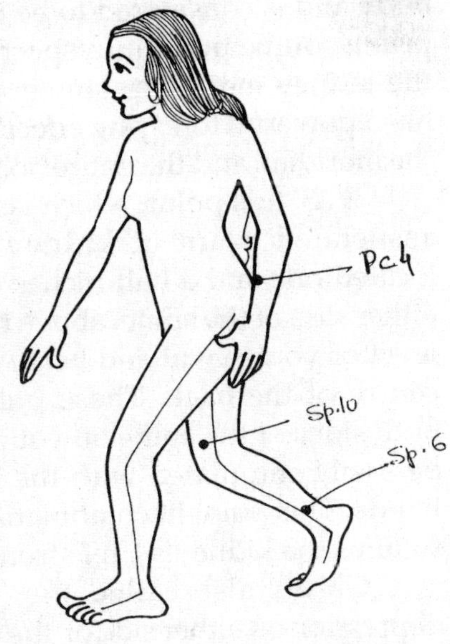

Sp 10 is yet another important point that can be used with success for removing stagnation in the flow of blood.

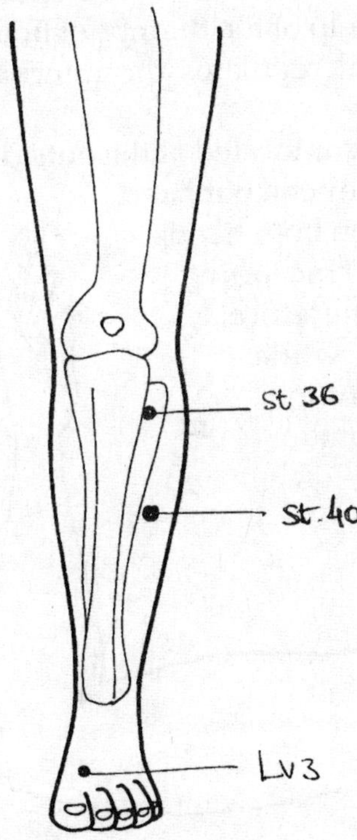

St 40 is located half way between the ankle bone on the outside of the foot and centre of the kneecap. Find the tibia and go two thumb widths off the bone to the outside. It is very helpful for reducing congestion

St 36, is located four finger widths below the kneecap towards the lower side. This point can also be pressed with the help of the heel of the opposite foot. Used in combination with Sp 6, they tonify both Ch'i and blood to bring vitality. This master point is known by the name 'Three Mile Foot'.

Kd 3, is located in the middle of the ankle bone and the Achilles tendon on the back edge of the ankle. This point is known by the name 'Supreme Stream'. It is known as the root of the Yin and Yang of the entire body and is considered to be the prime source point in respect of the kidney meridian. This point has a powerful tonifying effect on the meridian and the entire body.

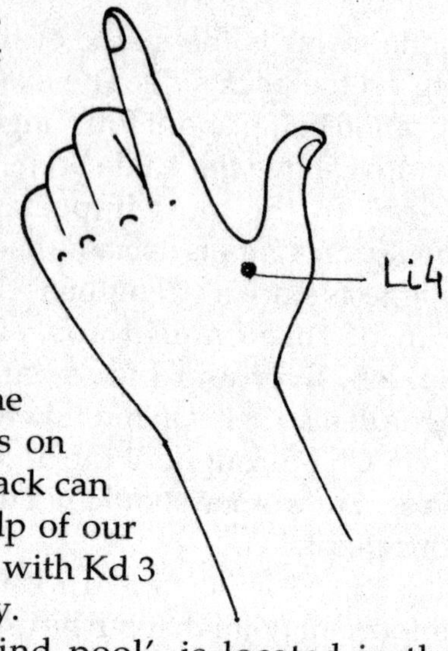

B 23, this point, which is an associated point of kidney is located one and a half inches on either side of the spine, above the level of your naval and below the centre of the back. These points on both sides of the spine on your back can be easily stimulated with the help of our hands. This point in combination with Kd 3 tonifies the kidney's Ch'i strongly.

Gb 20, also called the 'Wind pool', is located in the depression on either side of the vertebra of your neck, one thumb width above the hairline of the neck, at the base of the skull. Pressure can be easily given with the help of the thumbs of both the hands simultaneously. This point regulates the internal movement of energy.

Li 11, known as 'Pool at the Crook' is located at the outside end of the crease that is formed when we bend our hand to touch our shoulder. Give pressure on both hands with the help of opposite hands. This point becomes very tender on pressing therefore, utmost caution has to be exercised while pressing this point which is very useful in clearing excess heat and dampness from the body

Extra points, as shown in figure, these points lie in the middle of the fore arms, between the wrist crease and the elbow crease. Whereas the point on the right arm plugs the loss of energy and the same on the left arm (also called Pc 4), about a thumb width down towards the wrist from the midpoint, has been found to be very helpful in stimulating the heart.

Based on our experience, we feel that stimulating on the reflex areas of the following organs by giving pressure on their trigger points on a regular basis for at least 5 times a week would be of great help in keeping the blood sugar level under good control so that the patient is saved from the complications arising from this disease which are dreadful. Care has to be taken to give only gentle pressure when treating a diabetic patient because the skin of diabetics gets thinner and may bruise easily. Pressure on the reflexes of the pancreas has to be given with utmost care and ensured that it is gentle/mild.

The important areas to be stimulated are:

(i) the pancreas;
(ii) the pituitary gland
(iii) the adrenal gland
(iv) the thyroid gland
(v) the heart
(vi) the eyes
(vii) the kidneys and bladder
(viii) the liver and
(ix) the intestines.

The position of the reflex areas of the aforesaid organs has been shown in the figure (s) at the end of the book for the sake of convenience. Whereas, the reflex points indicated at (v) to (ix) have nothing to do with the control of diabetes as such, yet it is of utmost importance to stimulate these organs with a view to avoid complications/side effects of this disease. Each reflex zone needs to be properly stimulated and thereafter mild to moderate pressure given on each area (thirty seconds to one minute).

Q. 51: How is diarrhoea caused? Discuss how it can be cured using pressure point therapy.

A. 51: Diarrhoea is a natural way adopted by our body to throw toxins out from our system. It is detected by the abnormal watery bowel movements which are very frequent. Poor digestion, eating unhealthy and unhygienic food can cause bacterial infection which can lead to diarrhoea. At times it occurs

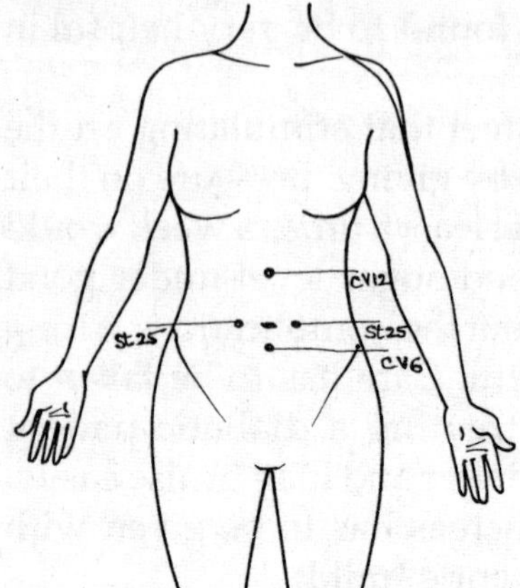

because of food poisoning or as a side effect of some strong antibiotic drug. Normally it should subside within a few hours but in case it takes more than 24 hours, you must increase the intake of fluids and must take all possible precautions to avoid dehydration. The symptoms of dehydration are dry lips, sunken eyes, dizziness etc., and it needs immediate attention.

By giving pressure on the following pressure points, we can conveniently control this condition:

CV 6 lies two finger widths below the naval, it relieves diarrhoea, and strengthens the abdominal muscles.

St 36 lies four finger widths below the kneecap, one finger width on the outside of the shin bone. This point strengthens the whole body, tones the muscles, aids digestion and helps overcome other stomach disorders.

Sp 4 is located on the arch of the foot, one thumb width in the back of the ball of the foot. It relieves indigestion, diarrhoea, stomach-ache and nausea, etc.

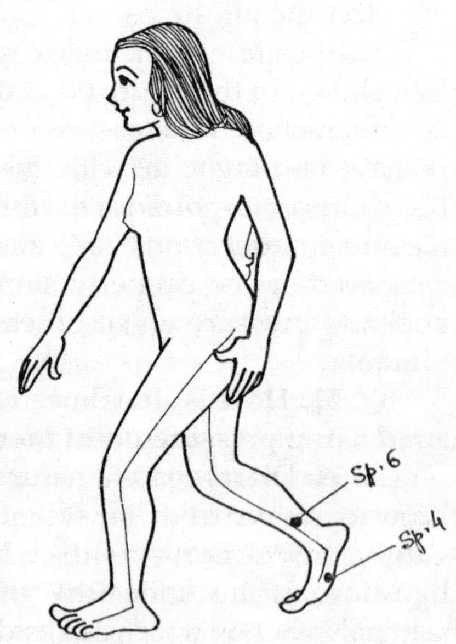

Lv 2 lies at the junction of the big and the second toes. Relieves diarrhoea, stomach-aches and nausea.

Sp 6, also called 'Three Yin Meeting Point', is located above the ankle bone towards the inside of the leg on the back side. The exact location being about four finger widths above the ankle bone. It is one of the most important pressure points as its name itself suggests since it strengthens the Yin of three meridians viz. spleen, liver and kidney at the same time. It is also considered master point for regulating female organs and is therefore useful in regulating periods, relieving cramps, facilitating menopause, etc. It is also considered to be very helpful in combination with St 36 for restoring the normal function of the gastro-intestinal tract. The two help to nourish the Ch'i and increase vitality. Pregnant women should not use this point.

St 25 is one of the most important points in the body for treating a wide range of intestinal disorders. It can be used to heal both diarrhoea and constipation. The point is located at a distance of three finger widths on both sides of the naval. Points on both sides should be given pressure simultaneously.

Cv 12 is midway between the notch at the bottom of the breastbone and the naval. Give moderate yet firm pressure on this point for relief from diarrhoea.

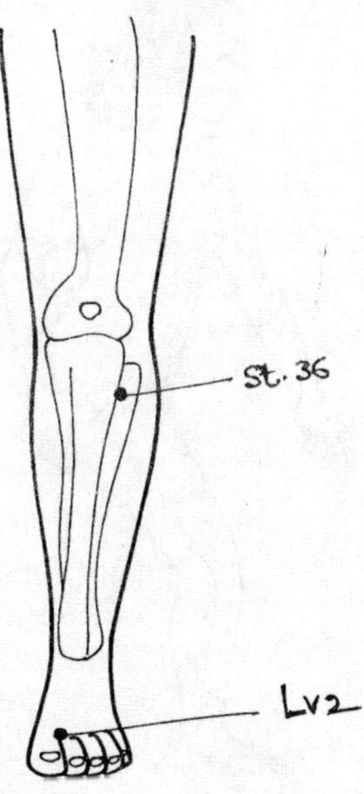

St 44 is located in the web on the top of the foot in the margin between the 2nd and the 3rd toes. This point is very effective in case diarrhoea is caused due to bad food or food poisoning.

Q. 52: What is dizziness, how is it caused? Can acupressure help this condition?

A. 52: Dizziness could be caused due to menopause, motion sickness or migraine where the patient feels as if either he is spinning or the things around him are spinning. He has a feeling of light headedness. It is also said to be a

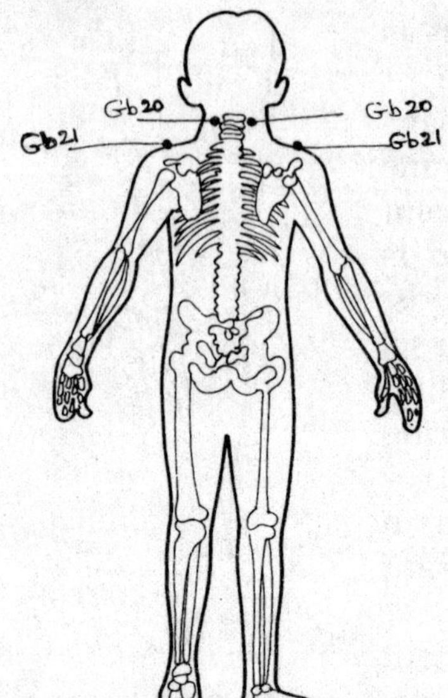

symptom of the inner ear condition known as Meniere's disease. In case the dizziness is accompanied with numbness, difficulty in speech, blurred vision or chest pain or much discomfort in the region of the heart, you must seek medical help immediately as this may be a symptom of an ensuing heart attack or a stroke.

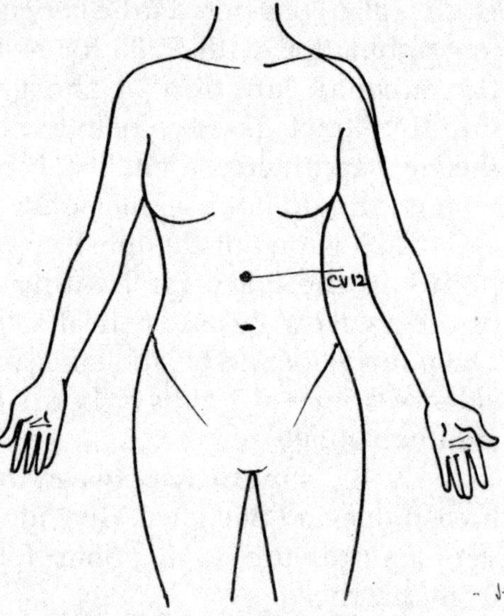

Sometimes in cases of mild dizziness, loss of appetite or constant tiredness is reported. In such cases we can overcome the condition by simply boosting the overall vitality by strengthening the Ch'i and nourishing the blood.

The following pressure points will bring relief to simple dizziness:

Sp 6, also called 'Three Yin Meeting Point', is located above the ankle bone towards the inside of the leg on the back side. The exact location being about four finger widths above the ankle bone. It is one of the most important pressure points as its name itself suggests since it strengthens the Yin of three meridians viz. spleen, liver and kidney at the same time. It is also considered to be a master point for female organs and is therefore useful in regulating periods, relieving cramps, facilitating menopause, etc. It is also considered to be very helpful in combination with St 36 for restoring normal function of the gastro-intestinal tract. It helps to nourish the Ch'i and increase vitality. Pregnant women should not use this point

St 36 lies four finger widths below the kneecap, one finger width on the outside of the shin bone. This point strengthens the whole body, tones the muscles, aids digestion and helps overcome other stomach disorders.

Cv 12 is midway between the notch at the bottom of the breastbone and the naval. Give moderate yet firm pressure on this point for relief from diarrhoea.

Lv 2 lies at the junction of the big and the second toes. This point is useful in balancing the excess Ch'i created by strong emotions.

GB 21, known as 'Shoulder Well' is midway between the neck and the outer edge of the shoulder. This point is often found to be very tender. This point can be pressed on both the sides of the shoulders simultaneously. It becomes even more beneficial in case the patient takes slow and deep breaths as you press various point. This points restores normal flow of Ch'i in the lungs (the upper part of the body). Pregnant women should not be given pressure on this point.

GB 20 is located in the hollow below the base of the skull. Steady pressure (mild to moderate) should be given on this point simultaneously on both the sides. It relieves headache, stiff neck, dizziness, irritability and depression. Its effect goes well with its name, i.e. 'Gates of Consciousness'. Is an extremely beneficial point to overcome depression.

Q. 53: Can acupressure help earache? What could be the causes of an earache?

A. 53: Ear ache is a very common condition and can be easily taken care of by acupressure. Generally, this condition is

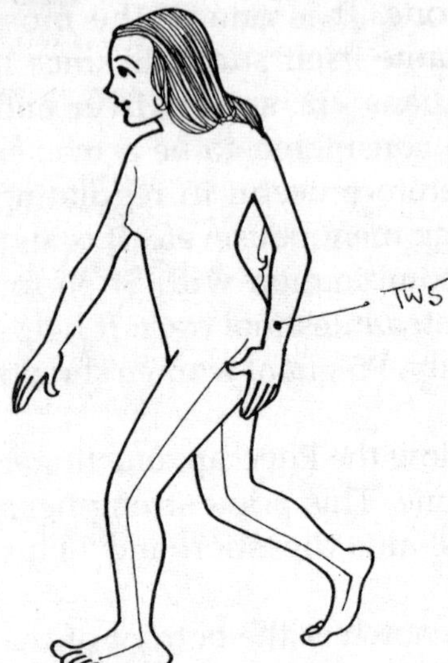

rarely serious, yet in case the discomfort does not subside in a couple of days, it would be better to seek medical advice to avoid complications from ear infections, if any. Otherwise it could be caused by an infection in the outer ear canal or in the inner ear. It may occur during an air journey owing to the change in cabin pressure which may cause unequal pressure in the inner and outer eardrum.

Li 4, known as 'Adjoining Valley', is known for its ability to relieve pain and circulating the Ch'i . It lies on the end of the crease that is formed when the thumb and the index finger are joined together. Pregnant women should not use this point.

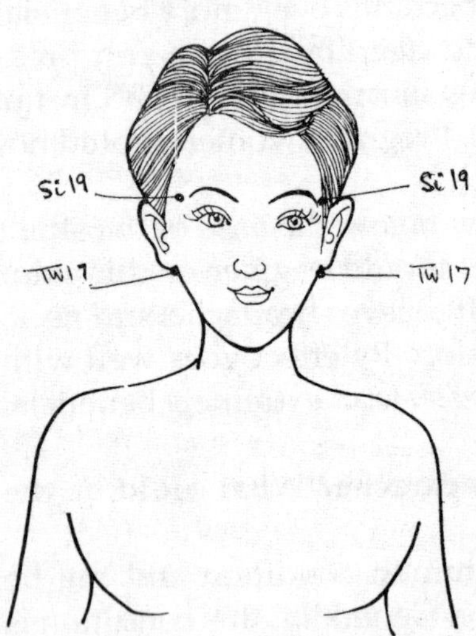

Tw 5, called the 'Outer Gate' is located midway between the ulna and radius about three fingers width above the wrist crease towards the elbow bone on the outside of the wrist (back side). Give pressure on this point for about a minute. Stimulating this point in conjunction with Tw 17 has been found to be beneficial for any type of ear problems. This is considered to be a very effective and potent point in acupressure

Tw 17 is located in the natural depression behind the earlobe. Apply mild pressure, as this point may be tender.

Si 19 known as 'Listening Palace', is located in the depression that forms when the mouth opens. Try to feel this point with your index fingers on the side of your face near the ears, as shown in the figure. Use your second, third and fourth fingers together to give pressure on this point to stimulate the entire area and to get maximum benefit.

Q. 54: Can acupressure help in keeping our eyes healthy and provide some relief to tired eyes?

A. 54: Acupressure can provide much relief in keeping the eyes healthy and also keeping our vision strong. As a matter of fact, all of us and particularly the people in the elderly age group, who have to work as typists/ stenographers or those who work on computers for long hours or those who are in the habit of watching television for a better part of the day or those of us who drive above 50 Kms or more on a day, strain their eyes.

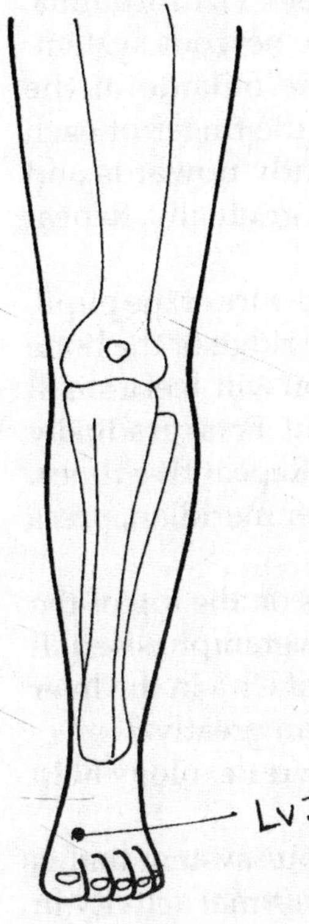

Acupressure points if used as a routine can help a lot in maintaining good eyesight and better and clear vision without any strain on the eyes whatsoever. We should not wait for the eyes to be strained or infected and then start giving or taking pressure.

A good number of pressure points which are capable of keeping the eyes fit are located close to them on the face itself. They are:

B 1, known as 'Eye Clarity', is located between the eyebrow and the eye, where the socket of the eye touches the nose. Press gently towards the nose (upwards).

Hold to the count of five and release gradually. Repeat five times.

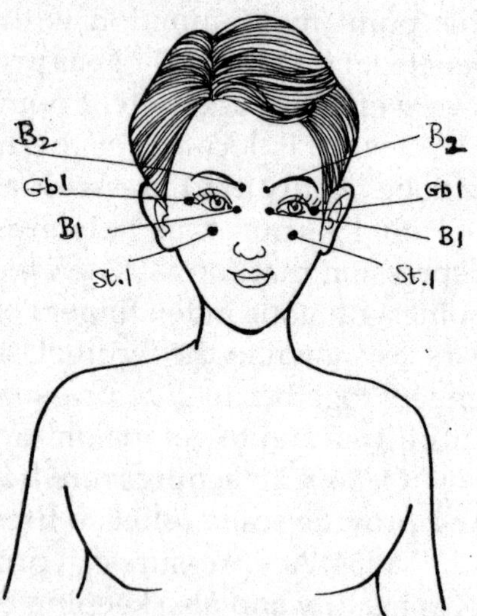

B 2, called 'Collecting Bamboo', is located just above B 1 just where the eyebrows start near the bridge of the nose. Give pressure as given at B 1.

Thereafter, hold your eyebrows with thumb under the eyebrow and index finger over the eyebrow. Pinch the eyebrow commencing from the inner side and going towards the outside. Repeat pinching on the entire area of the eyebrow at least three times. Pressure on these points is also given in handling diseases viz. insomnia, depression, etc., as it soothes the eyes and the nervous system.

Gb 1,'Pupil Crevice', is located on the outside of the eyebrow. Press firmly with the index or middle finger of each hand, with the direction of the pressure slightly upwards and outwards. Hold to the count of five and release gradually. Repeat five times.

St 1, 'Contain Tears', is located below the centre of the pupil, in the middle of the eye socket. Try to feel the ridge of the bone on the eye socket, gently moving sideways, you will feel a small notch in the bone. St 1 is located here at this point. Press gradually upto the count of five and release gradually. Repeat five times.

As the vision area is connected to the liver meridian, press Lv 3.

Lv3 lies between the big and second toes on the top of the foot. The importance of this point cannot be overemphasised. It regulates and tonifies the liver and the flow of Ch'i in the liver meridian. Stimulating this point benefits vision greatly.

Q. 55: What is epilepsy? Can acupressure/reflexology help this condition?

A. 55: Epilepsy is a disorder of the nervous system that is characterised by seizure or fainting due to abnormal activity in

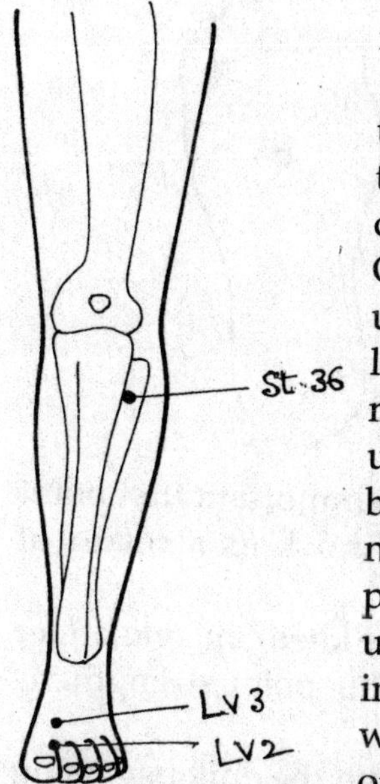

the brain. This disorder usually appears in childhood or adolescence.

In acupressure, pressure points are used to rebalance and rejuvenate the body that bring out the patient from this condition. Of many revival potent points, GV26 is most useful. It is located in the middle of the upper lip right below the nose. This point can be used in itself or in conjunction with certain other points to revive the patient instantly. The point also stimulates the body's natural mechanism for restoring health. The most important thing to be done in this context is to strengthen the

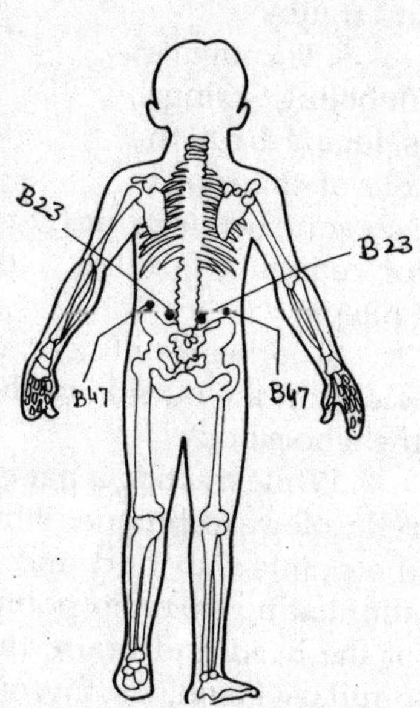

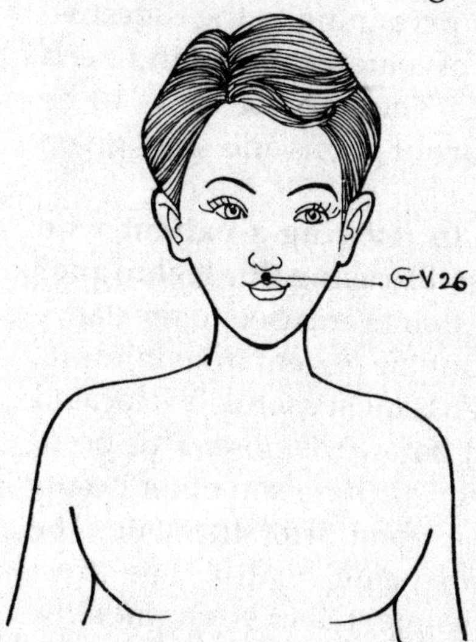

nervous system. In the event of recurrence of the condition, it is advisable to seek medical assistance and continue to give acupressure treatment, adding the following pressure points:

B 23 can be located in the middle of the waist, half way between the rib cage and the hip bone on the inner edge. It relieves depression, fear and trauma.

B 47 lies in the middle of the waist four finger widths outside of the spine. This point, not only provides relief in the lower back pain but also reduces muscle tension, fatigue, depression, fear and trauma.

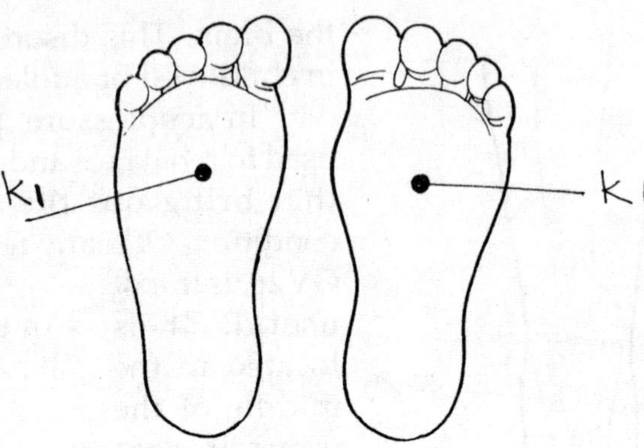

K 1, known as 'Bubbling Springs', is located on the sole of the foot in the centre between the two pads. This is an important first point for relieving fainting, convulsions or shock as a result of Epilepsy.

St 36, lies four finger widths below the knee cap, one finger width on the outside of the shin bone. This point strengthens the whole body

While treating a patient suffering from the epilepsy using reflexology technique, stimulate both the soles and look for all the points that hurt and stimulate them repeatedly besides stimulating the reflex points falling in the reflex zones in respect of the head and brain; the solar plexus, adrenal glands, the pituitary gland, the thyroid gland. The spine particularly, the area of the neck and all the reflexes pertaining to the digestive system, with emphasis on the area of parathyroid gland need to be stimulated to treat epilepsy. The specific areas to be stimulated can be seen from the figure of palms and soles given at the end of the book.

Q. 56: Can acupressure help in reviving a patient who has fainted? Is a long term cure possible using this technique?

A. 56: In acupressure, pressure points are used to rebalance and rejuvenate the body that bring out the patient from fainting. Of many revival potent points, GV 26 is most useful. It is located in the middle of the upper lip right below the nose. This point can be used by itself or in conjunction with certain other points to revive the patient instantly. The point also stimulates the body's natural mechanism for restoring health. The most important thing to be done in this context is to strengthen the

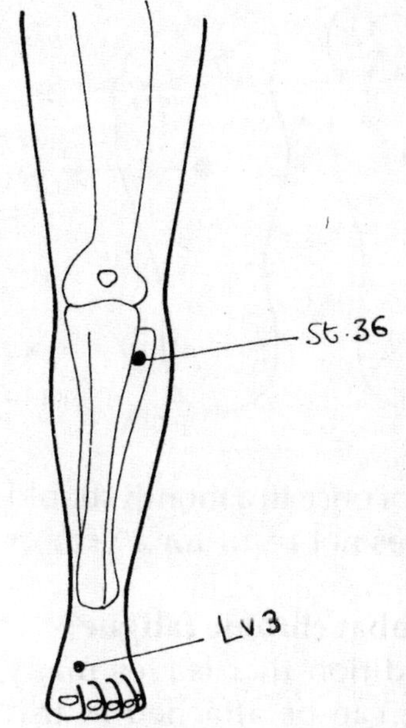

nervous system. In the event of recurrence of the condition, it is advisable to seek medical assistance and continue to give acupressure treatment, adding the following pressure points:

B 23 can be located in the middle of the waist, half way between the rib cage and the hip bone on the inner edge. Relieves depression, fear and trauma.

B 47 which lies in the middle of the waist four finger widths outside of the spine, not only provides relief in the lower back pain but also reduces muscle tension, fatigue, depression, fear and trauma.

K 1, known as 'Bubbling Springs', is located on the sole of the foot in the centre between the two pads. This is an important first point for relieving fainting convulsions or shock as a result of epilepsy.

St 36, lies four finger widths below the kneecap, one finger width on the outside of the shin bone. This point strengthens the whole body, and tones the muscles. It also helps in regaining consciousness.

Lv 3 lies between the big and second toes on the top of the foot. The importance of this point cannot be overemphasised. It regulates and tonifies the liver and the flow of Ch'i in the liver meridian. These two points, viz. St 36 and Lv3, in combination are capable of 'lifting the spirits' and healing emotional upsets. It

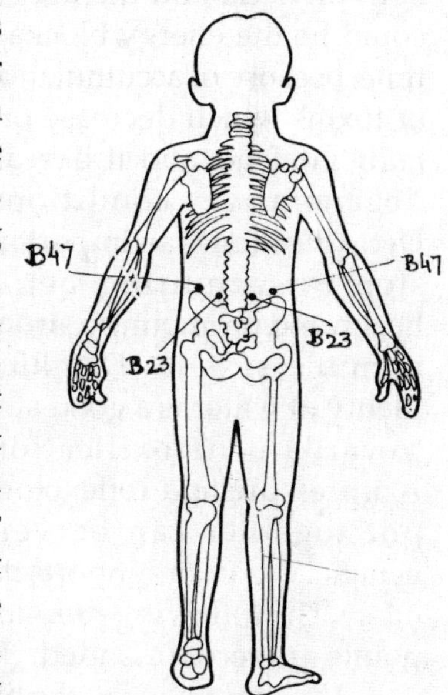

relieves fainting, dizziness, exhaustion, nervous disorders and hangovers.

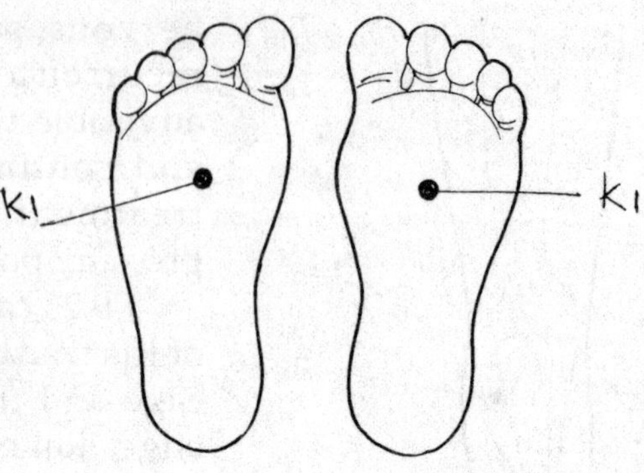

For getting long term relief, the aforesaid pressure points should be pressed initially for 10 days or so and thereafter once a week for 2-3 months and once the incidents of fainting stop, a follow-up of once in a month should be sufficient. In case the condition does not recur for a year or so, even follow-up can be stopped.

Q. 57: Can acupressure help combat chronic fatigue?

A. 57: Chronic fatigue is a condition that leaves many people exhausted. No specific cause can be attached to this condition in which the person remains tired all the time. The only cause one can perhaps think of is that it may be caused because everyone is engaged in hectic activity which results in both physical and mental exhaustion. Another probable cause could be the energy blockage that makes you feel tired all the time, because of accumulation of toxins which decrease our body's defence and also create degenerative conditions. Detoxification is an important step for acquiring better health and promoting a strong immune system. Drinking plenty of water is a good step towards detoxification. Acupressure and reflexology put together can be very beneficial as each supports the other. The following pressure points are recommended:

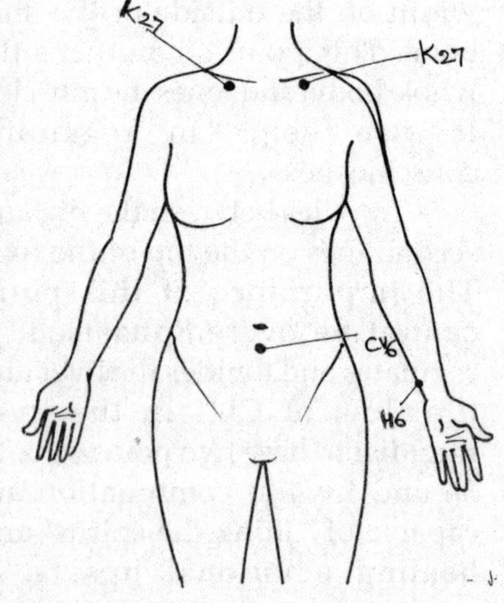

Lv 3 lies between the big

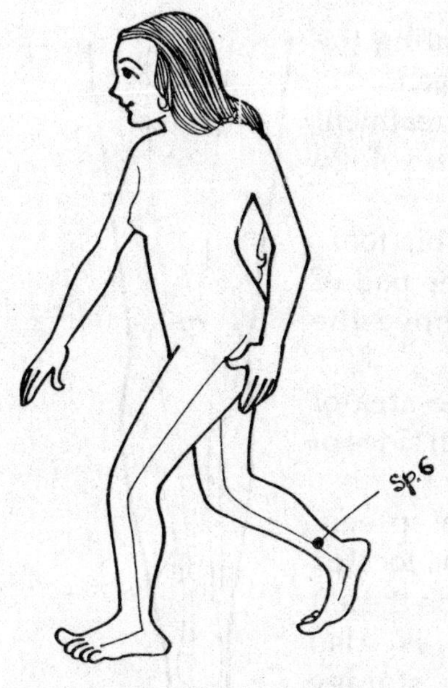

and second toes on the top of the foot. It regulates and tonifies the liver and the flow of Ch'i in the liver meridian, which is considered to be the most powerful organ for detoxification.

Sp 6, also called 'Three Yin Meeting Point', is located above the ankle bone towards the inside of the leg on the back side. The exact location being about four finger widths above the ankle bone. It is one of the most important pressure points as its name itself suggests since it strengthens the Yin of three meridians viz. spleen, liver and kidney at a time. It helps flush Ch'i and blood through the body.

Li 4, known as 'Adjoining Valley', is known for its ability to relieve pain and circulating the Ch'i . It lies on the end of the crease that is formed when the thumb and the index finger are joined together. It stimulates elimination of toxins through bowels. Pregnant women should not use this point.

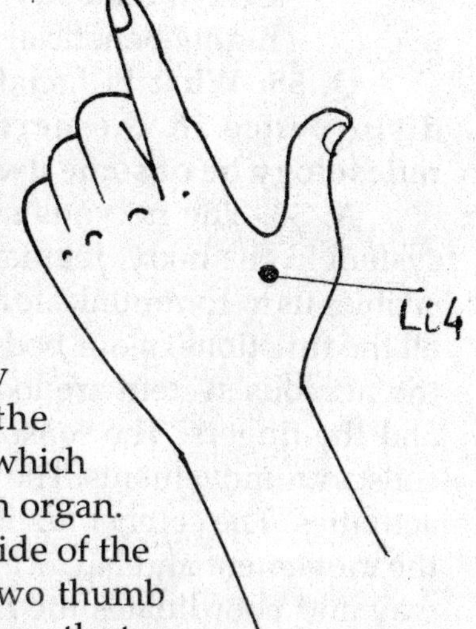

CV 6 known by the name 'Sea of energy' is located three finger widths below the naval. Pressure on this point can be given in lying position (empty bladder). Relieves general fatigue and fortifies the immune system.

K 27 is located in the hollow below the collarbone next to the breastbone. It tonifies the kidneys, which are considered a key detoxification organ.

HP 6 is located on the palm side of the hand, in the middle of the arm, two thumb widths above the wrist crease between the two tendons. It is effective in regulating the Ch'i of liver, heart and the stomach.

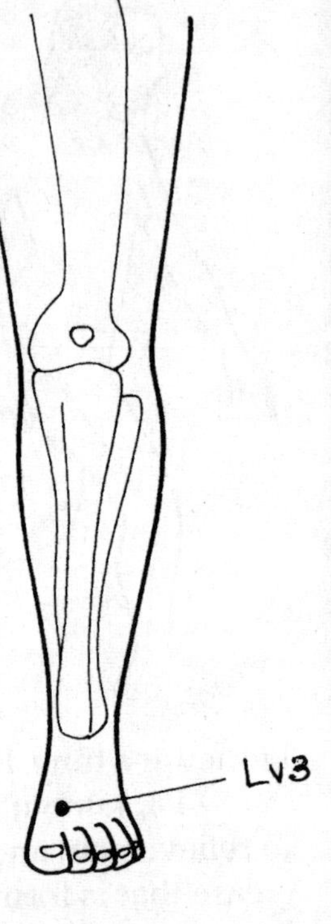

Besides giving acupressure treatment as discussed above, giving reflexology workout on the areas of:

(i) Pituitary gland on the big toes
(ii) The adrenals below the pad of the soles and just above the kidney point
(iii) Sex glands around the area of the ankle bones on both sides of the foot
(iv) Conditioning of the spleen, reflex point of which is located below the heart point on the left foot as this organ is also considered to be the storage container of life force in the body and also responsible for production of red blood cells and
(v) Liver, which is known for toning up the circulation of Ch'i in the body, in conjunction shall be found to be highly beneficial in combating chronic fatigue.

Q. 58: What is facial paralysis? Is it caused by some disturbance in the nervous system? Can acupressure/ reflexology be of some use?

A. 58: The nervous system, which is the most complex system in the body, regulates numerous activities at a time. It enables us to communicate and feel. It also monitors and controls all the functions of our body. The reflex areas corresponding to the nervous system are located in the big toe and the thumbs and the fingers. The sensory motor cortex detects and directs conscious movements. The master gland pituitary directs all the activities. The cerebellum is responsible for the coordination of the movement and balance. The brain stem is the common path way and coordinates the flow of information to and from the brain. Lack of stimulation affects the overall nervous system.

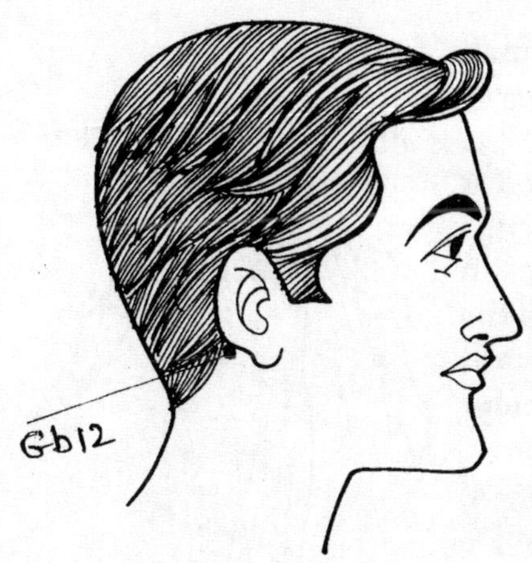

Facial paralysis, also known by the name 'Bell's palsy' is the paralysis of one side of the face due to impingement on the facial nerve. It is devastating because of its visibility. This is usually accompanied with paralysis of at least one side of the body. For paralysis resulting in rigidity, the technique of reflexology is applied especially to the brain area. We have to target the spine area for paralysis resulting in loss of control. Besides working on the big toe and the thumb areas, it would be beneficial if we work on the reflex areas of the eye and ear too as these regions also reflect the cranial nerves. Whereas in cerebral palsy we have to apply the technique on both the sides, i.e. right and left, the technique has to be focussed on the side opposite to the paralysed side.

Follow the below mentioned schedule of pressure points to get relief from this condition. At times the patient recovers within a fortnight or a month, but at times total recovery may take up to 6 to 9 months. However, the patient recovers fully. All that is required of him is willingness to recover and patience.

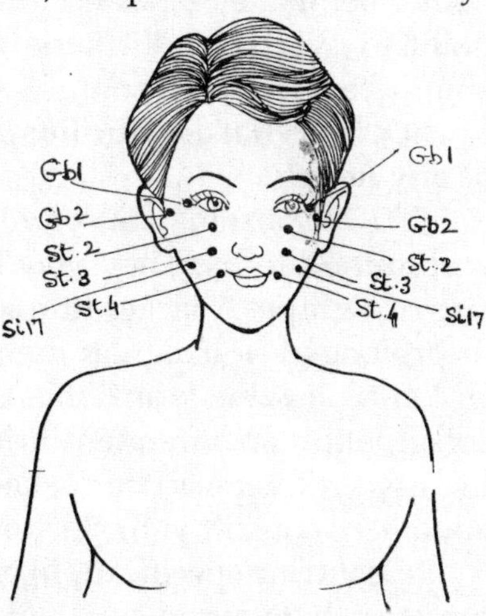

St 2 known by the name 'Four Whites' is located one finger below the lower ridge of the eye socket in line with the centre of the iris in an indentation of the cheek. Eliminates wind and improves eyesight in all the four directions.

St 3 known as 'Facial Beauty' is found at the bottom

of the cheekbone, below the pupil. It helps sagging cheeks and improves facial circulation.

St 4 is a local point specific for the treatment of the disease specific.

Sj 17 known as 'Yi feng' lies in the depression behind the bone of the ear. It is considered an important point for treating problems of the face and head. Expels wind.

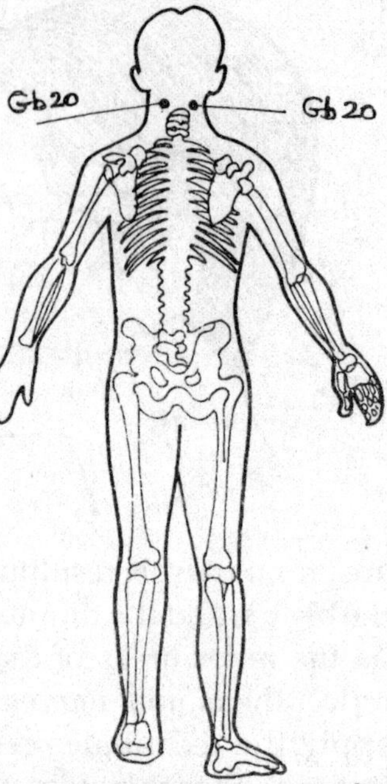

GB 1 is found in the depression next to the outer angle of the eye. Eliminates wind.

GB 2 is located just in front of the ear at the joint of the jaw. This point is specific to treat facial paralysis.

GB 12 lies in the depression behind the ear, behind and below the mastoid bone. Is specific to treating facial paralysis.

GB 20 is located in the hollow below the base of the skull. Steady pressure (mild to moderate) should be given on this point simultaneously on both the sides. Its effect goes well with its name, i.e. 'Gates of Consciousness'. An extremely beneficial point to overcome stiffness in the region of the neck. It also eliminates wind and cold.

Q. 59: What are fibroids? Can acupressure/reflexology be of any help?

A. 59: Fibroids are common, harmless tumours that grow within the uterus. They may be small or may grow up to the size of a grape. A larger fibroid may cause symptoms as heavy or prolonged or irregular menstruation with pain in the lower abdomen, leading to anaemia. Other problems include back pain, constipation and frequent urination or difficulty in urinating. In case you experience a sharp or chronic pain in the lower abdomen, consult your doctor immediately.

Occurring specifically in or on the uterus, fibroids are benign tumours that vary in size, and usually grow slowly. They occur

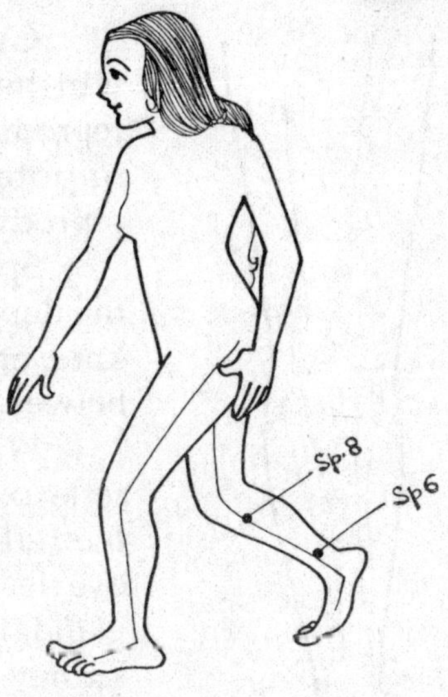

in more than 20 per cent of women above the age of 35. Though they are not problematic, fibroids may cause enlargement and distortion of the uterus and may cause hindrance in pregnancy. Generally, a female comes to know about having fibroids only when her physician feels them during the course of a routine pelvic examination. Their presence can be confirmed by ultrasound scan. At times, to prevent further fibroid growth, your physician may ask you not to take oral contraceptives or to stop taking any hormone replacement therapy.

Alternative therapies, e.g. acupressure and reflexology can ease the symptoms of this sort of uterine disorder, particularly the pain part, but it would be better if they are used as a complement to conventional medicine to get better results.

Lv 3 lies between the big and second toes on the top of the foot. It regulates and tonifies the liver and the flow of Ch'i in the liver meridian, which is considered to be the most powerful organ for detoxification.

Sp 6, also called 'Three Yin Meeting Point', is located above the ankle bone towards the inside of the leg on the back side. The exact location being about four finger widths above the ankle bone. It is one of the most important pressure points as its name itself suggests since it strengthens the Yin of three meridians, viz. spleen, liver and kidney at the same time. It helps flush Ch'i and blood through the body.

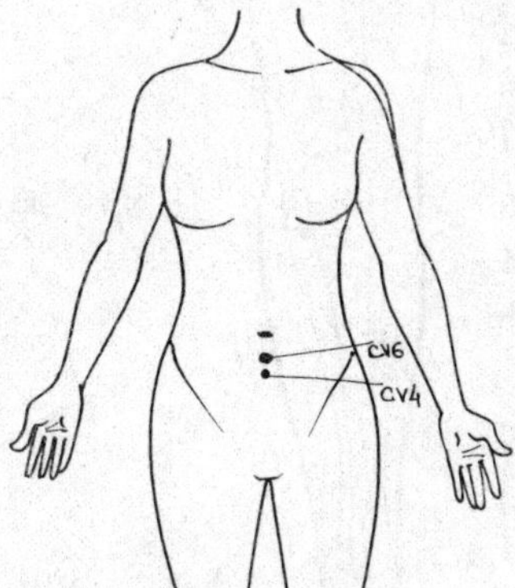

CV 4 'Gate Origin', is located four finger widths below the belly button or the naval. Helps relieve impotency and irregular menstrual periods.

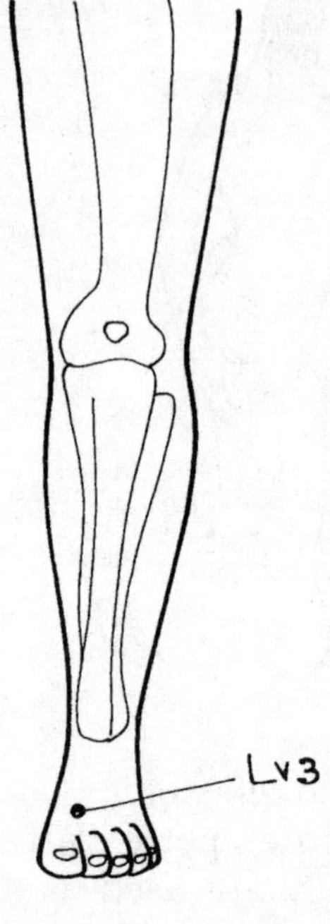

CV 6, 'Sea of energy', lies three finger widths below the naval. It relieves reproductive problems, irregular periods and impotency. Strengthens the overall reproductive system.

Sp 8 is located inside of the lower leg in the depression four finger widths below the knee on the inside of the leg. Press firmly between the calf muscle and the leg bone.

When treating fibroids using reflexology technique, we have to focus on the reflex points relating to the uterus, the ovaries, the fallopian tubes, the pituitary gland, the lymphatic system, the spine, the kidney and bladder area and all the areas connected with the digestive system by handling each reflex area for about 2-3 minutes or so. A good number of sessions will bring much relief.

Q. 60: What is meant by flatulence, and what are its causes? Can acupressure/reflexology be of any help?

A. 60: Gas formation is a normal part of the digestive process. People pass gas more than 10 times a day or even more but can still be perfectly healthy. The passing out of gas through the anus is called flatulence and at times foul smelling emissions take place which is very unpleasant and embarrassing. Gas passed from upper abdominal tract is given the name 'belching'.

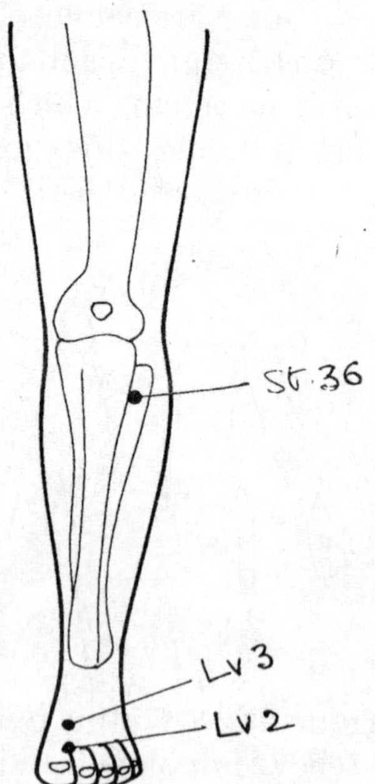

The causes of this condition may be poor diet, incorrect combinations of food and eating food very quickly without chewing it properly. We take in air when we eat or drink, particularly through a straw, or by drinking carbonated beverages, etc. Symptoms include bloating, abdominal cramps, belching and emission of gas through anus.

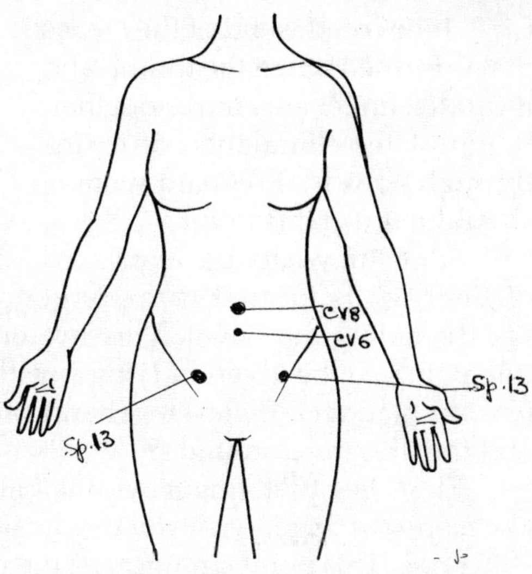

In case you eat high fibre food, e.g. beans, vegetables, fruit, grains, etc., the partially digested cell walls of these will pass into your intestines, where bacteria begins the fermentation process that produces gas. In certain cases, consumption of dairy foods, viz. milk and curds also result in the formation of gas.

This condition can be treated without active involvement of a healthcare professional by yourself, using acupressure schedule and reflexology as discussed below:

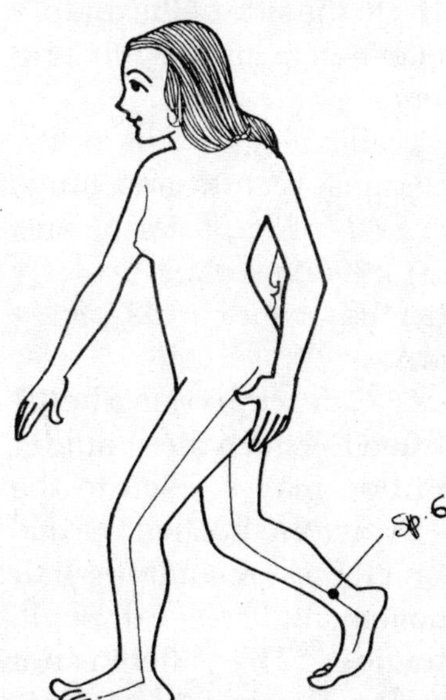

Sp 6, also called by 'Three Yin Meeting Point', is located above the ankle bone towards the inside of the leg on the back side. The exact location being about four finger widths above the ankle bone. It is one of the most important pressure points as its name by itself suggests since it strengthens the Yin of three meridians, viz. spleen, liver and kidney at the same time. It helps flush Ch'i and blood through the body.

Li 4, known as 'Adjoining Valley', is known for its ability to relieve pain and circulating the

Ch'i. It lies on the end of the crease that is formed when the thumb and the index finger are joined together. It stimulates elimination of toxins through bowels. Pregnant women should not use this point.

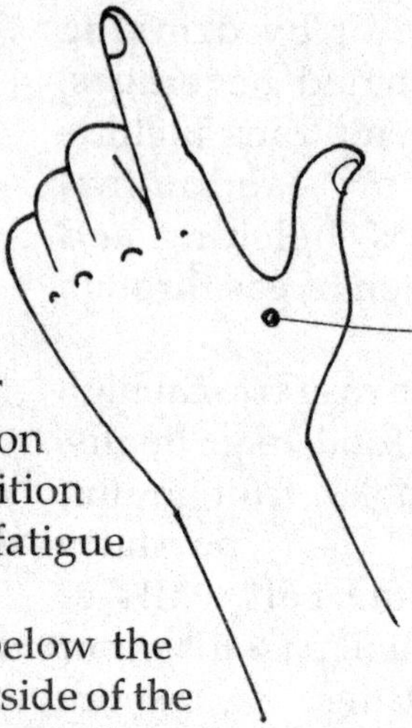

CV 6 known by the name 'Sea of Energy', is located three finger widths below the naval. Pressure on this point can be given in lying position (empty bladder). Relieves general fatigue and fortifies the immune system.

St 36 lies four finger widths below the kneecap, one finger width on the outside of the shin bone. This point strengthens the whole body, and tones the muscles.

St 27 is located three finger widths below the naval and same distance on the side of the middle axis on the front of the body. It relieves flatulence.

CV 8 is located on the belly button, helps relieve pain in the naval area and intestinal infections (both acute and chronic).

Sp 13 is located four thumb widths to the side of the middle axis, slightly above the pubic bone. Relieves tension and bloating in the stomach/intestines and flatulence.

For treating this condition using reflexology, focus on the reflex areas of small and large intestines, rectum and anus, stomach, pancreas, duodenum, liver, gallbladder, solar plexus, adrenal glands, diaphragm, and the spine reflexes, particularly the thoracic area. For precise location of these reflex areas, please refer to the figure at the end of the book.

Q. 61: What is a 'frozen shoulder'? Can acupressure help?

A. 61: Frozen shoulder is a condition in which the shoulder becomes stiff and painful. The condition may worsen to the extent that the patient may not be able to perform his/her normal day-to-day activities. Even putting on clothes or combing hair becomes a problem, i.e. normal arm movements become difficult, hence it is given the name 'frozen shoulder'. The patient is not able to lift his/her arm above elbow height. The pain may radiate

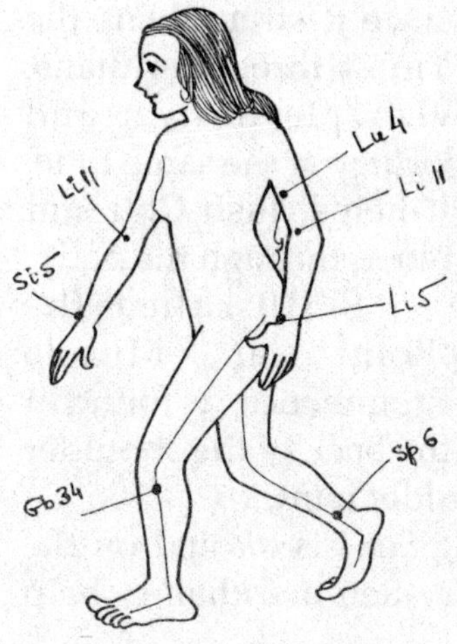

to the neck, down the arm and across the back and the chest. This condition can be caused by no apparent reason and even from a minor injury to the shoulder or at times in case cervical spondylitis is neglected beyond a particular stage. Lack of movement and exercise may also lead to this disease.

Giving pressure to the following pressure points helps overcome the pain as well as improve mobility:

Lu 2 'Cloud Door' can be found in the hollow below the outer end of the collarbone as shown in the figure. Very effective for its healing effect on the shoulder.

Lu 4, 'Broken Clouds', lies above the bony prominence on the thumb side of the wrist. This point strengthens the Ch'i of the lungs.

Li 4, known as 'Adjoining Valley', is known for its ability to relieve pain and circulate Ch'i. It lies on the end of the crease that is formed when the thumb and index finger are joined together. It stimulates elimination of toxins through bowels. It relieves stagnation of Ch'i too. Pregnant women should not use this point.

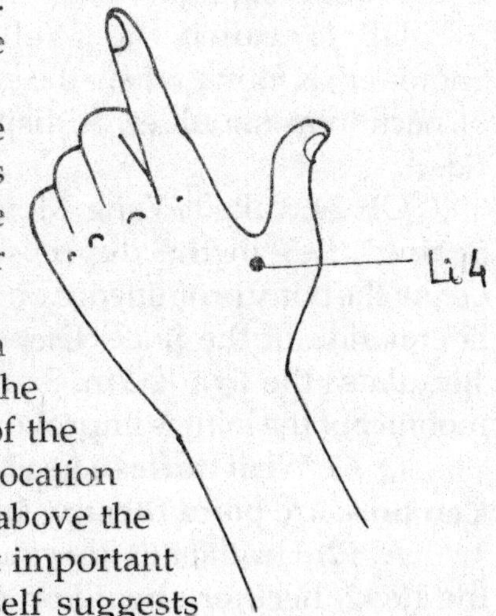

Li 5 is given the name 'Corner of Shoulder', and is located just below the joint of the shoulder. This point is specific for pain in the shoulder joint.

Sp 6, also 'Called Three Yin Meeting Point', is located above the ankle bone towards the inside of the leg on the back side. The exact location being about four finger widths above the ankle bone. It is one of the most important pressure points as its name itself suggests

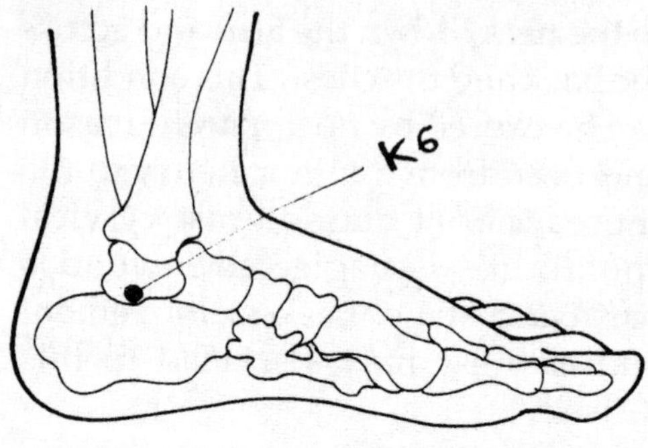

since it strengthens the Yin of three meridians, viz. spleen, liver and kidney at the same time. It helps flush Ch'i and blood through the body.

Si 10 called the 'Point at Muscle Prominence', is found at the back of the shoulder joint and is specific for pain in the shoulder joint.

K 6, known by the name 'Shining Sea', is located on the inner side of the ankle. It opens the Yin-Ren meridian to help counteract Yin deficiency.

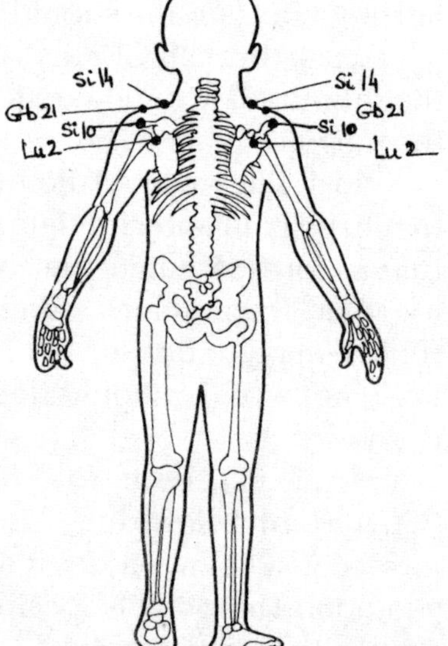

Sj 5, called 'Lateral Pass', is at a short distance above Sj 4 which is on the lateral side of the humerus bone. This also relieves the stagnation of Ch'i.

Sj 14, known as 'Shoulder Opening', lies in the hollow below the bone at the back of the shoulder and is specific for pain in the shoulder joint.

GB 21, called the 'Well of Shoulder', is found where the base of neck joins shoulder. It dispels wind.

GB 34, called 'Yang Mound Spring', lies in the depression below the bony prominence on the lateral side of the knee. Dispels wind, clears damp heat and stimulates the liver's Yin. Since liver Yin nourishes the joints, mobility of the joint is improved by giving pressure to this point.

Q. 62: What causes a headache, the most common ailment? Can pressure point therapy (acupressure) provide a solution?

A. 62: Headaches are caused by tension in the muscles of the head, neck or shoulders etc., due to the stress (physical, mental or emotional), poor posture, anger, anxiety and worry, which may constrict the blood vessels that supply oxygen to the nerve cells in the brain. The muscle tension can even block the flow of energy to the head. When there is inadequate supply either of oxygen or of life energy, the body presents this condition in the form of pain, i.e. headache. Often, people choose to repress this signal offered by the body to indicate inadequate supply of oxygen or life force by taking pills. Though these pills are said to be providing a remedy, yet as a matter of fact they do nothing to remove the cause of the pain and simply provide a temporary relief. Whereas a pain-killer may help overcome the sensation of pain for a while, it does nothing to remove the cause of the pain which may be due to constipation, anxiety or insufficient oxygen or an improper posture.

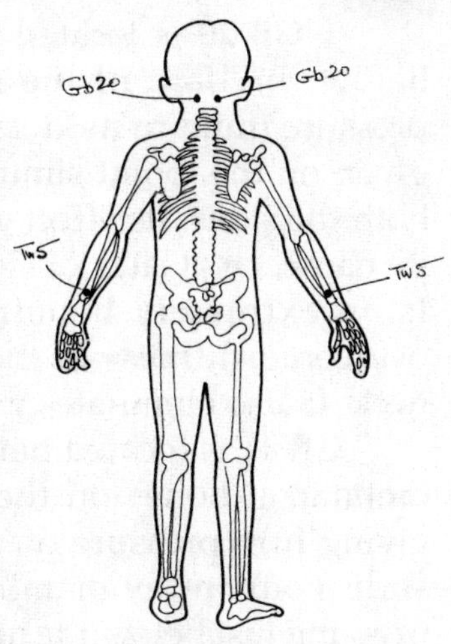

Pressure point therapy, i.e. acupressure helps us to remove the cause of the pain by relaxing the muscles, releasing block of flow in energy channels, relieving the tension and improving the supply of much required oxygen to the brain cells. The following schedule will be found to be helpful:

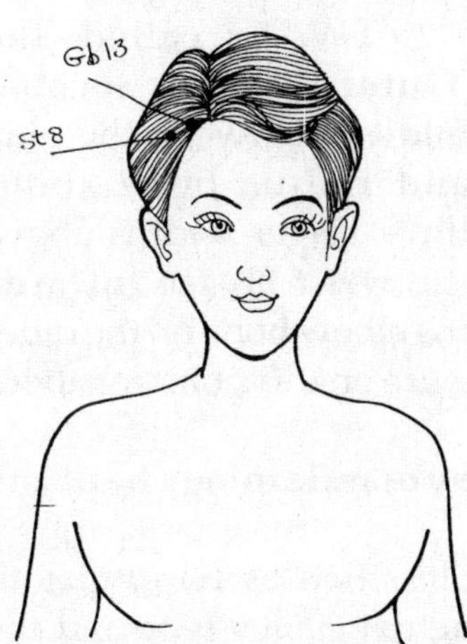

Li 4, known as 'Adjoining Valley', is known for its ability to relieve pain and circulate the Ch'i. It lies on the end of the crease that is formed when the thumb and index finger are joined together. It stimulates elimination of toxins through bowels. It relieves stagnation of Ch'i too. Pregnant women should not use this point

GB 20 is located in the hollow below the base of the skull. Steady pressure (mild to moderate) should be given on this point simultaneously on both the sides. Its effect goes well with its name, i.e. 'Gates of Consciousness'. Is an extremely beneficial point to overcome stiffness in the region of the neck. It also eliminates wind and cold.

GB 41 is located between the 4th and 5th metatarsal bones on the top of the foot. For giving firm pressure on this point you have to slide your index or middle fingers upwards, pressing just below the juncture. This point restores the flow of Ch'i, and relieves headache.

GB 13, 'Mind Root', is just inside the hairline above the forehead, in line with the outer edge of the eye. It calms the mind and removes headache. Apply firm pressure steadily for a minute or two.

St 8, known by the name 'Skull Support', is about an inch outside on the same level as point GB 13, and is an extremely effective point for relieving headache. This point has also to be pressed firmly for one to two minutes.

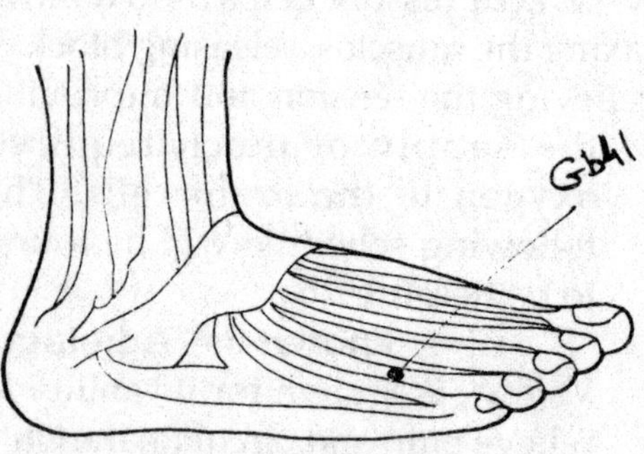

TW 5, called the 'Outer Gate', is located midway between the ulna and radius bone about three finger widths above the wrist crease towards the elbow bone on the outer side of the wrist (back side). Give pressure on this point for about a minute.

Q. 63 Can pressure point therapy or reflexology be of any help in case of hearing problem?

A. 63: Hearing problems are classified as two types in Chinese medicine. The first one is the deficiency type and the other is excess type. The deficiency type is caused by the improper functioning of the kidney's Ch'i. It takes the form of a gradual loss of hearing ability as we age. Weakening of kidney energy in the associated meridian is the causative factor behind this. To come out of this condition, all that is required is to tonify the kidney's Ch'i.

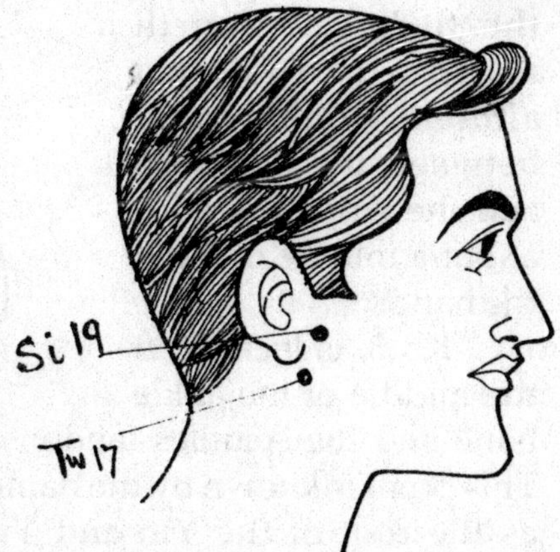

Excess type is considered to be due to an excess of stagnated Ch'i in the liver or gallbladder meridians. This condition at times results in an abrupt loss of hearing ability over a few days. For coming out of this situation we have to drain out the excess accumulation of energy from the liver/gallbladder meridians as the case may be, to correct the balance. Going by the pressure point therapy, the following schedule of pressure points shall be useful:

TW 5, 'Called the Outer Gate', is located midway between the ulna and radius bone about three finger widths above the wrist crease towards the elbow bone on the outer side of the wrist (back side). Give pressure on this point for about a minute. Stimulating this point in conjunction with Tw 17 has been found to be beneficial for any type of ear problems. This is considered to be a very effective and potent point in acupressure.

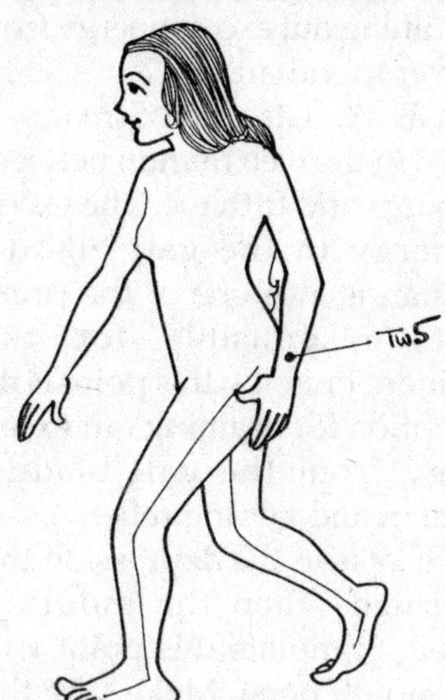

Tw 17 is located in the natural depression behind the earlobe. Apply mild pressure as this point may be tender.

Tw 3 is located on the back of the hand in the channel between

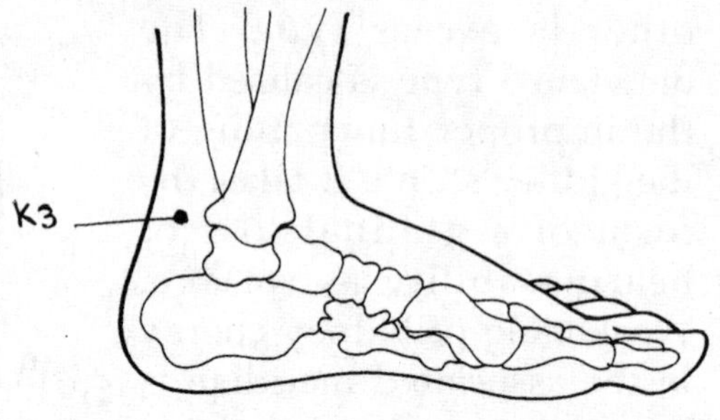

the little and fourth finger, in the depression almost half way between the knuckles and the wrist. Press for about a minute on both the hands.

Kd 3, is located in the middle of the ankle bone and the Achilles tendon on the back edge of the ankle. This point is known by the name 'Supreme Stream'. It is known as the root of the Yin and Yang of the entire body and is considered to be the prime source point in respect of the kidney meridian. This point has a powerful tonifying effect on the meridian and the entire body. Pressing this point shall be very useful in this condition.

B23 can be located in the middle of the waist, half way between the rib cage and the hip bone on the inner edge. This point in association with Kd 3 strengthens the kidney Ch'i.

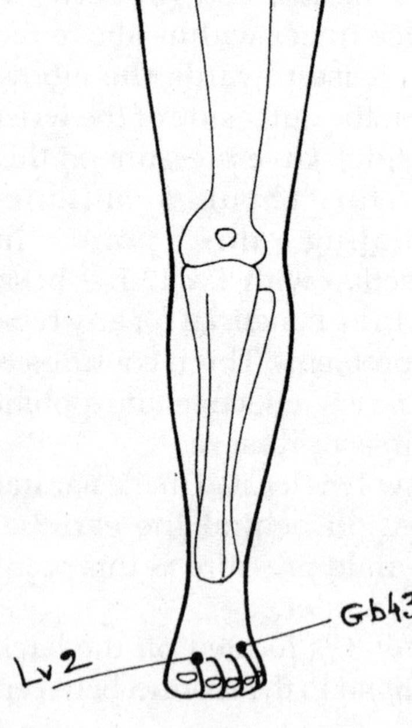

Lv 2 lies at the junction of the big and the second toe. This point is considered to be the best point for draining out excess energy from the liver meridian.

GB 43, 'Clamped Stream', is located in the web margin between the fourth and fifth toe. The excess of energy in the gall bladder meridian is also one of the prime causes responsible for this condition. Pressing this point is the best option for draining out excess energy from the gall bladder meridian and getting relief.

Si 19 is in the depression that is formed when the mouth is opened. Stimulate this point with your mouth open. Make sure that

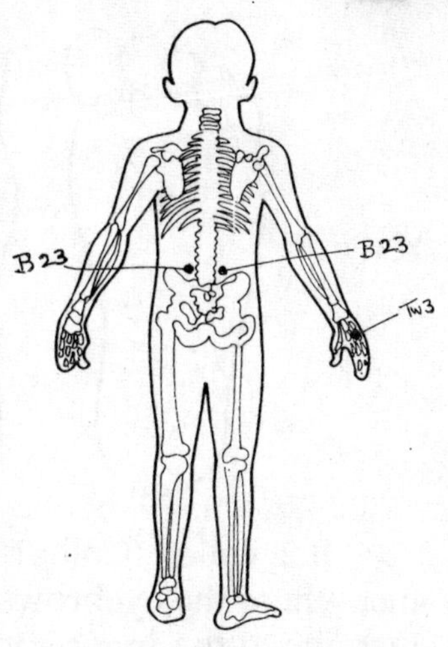

you are pressing in the centre of the depression thus formed. Apply pressure on this point using the three fingers of your hand joined together so that two more points about half an inch above and below this point are also pressed simultaneously. This is the crossing point of the gall bladder and triple warmer meridians and has a beneficial effect on the hearing power of the ears.

Q. 64: Why are hiccups caused? Can acupressure be of any help?

A. 64: Hiccups is a very annoying condition. They are rhythmic spasms in the diaphragm, lungs and at times the throat. No specific explanation is perhaps available to explain as to why and how hiccups are caused. They commence and after some time automatically stop. Sipping a little bit of lukewarm water and sitting in a relaxed position and breathing deeply could be the easiest way to get away with this condition most of the times. However, in case this problem persists or is repeated time and again, the following schedule of pressure point therapy shall be found to be useful. Again, we would like to

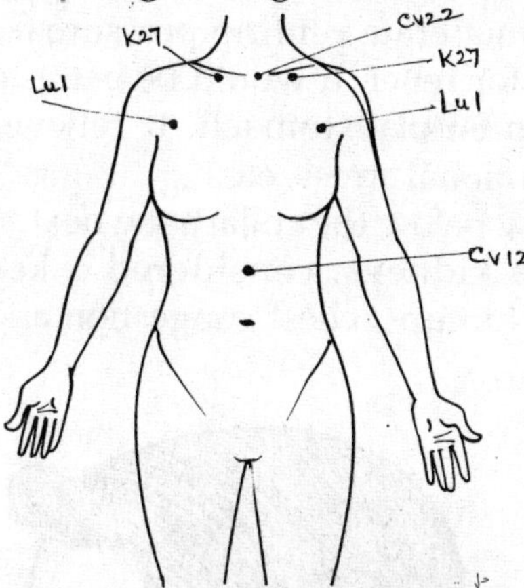

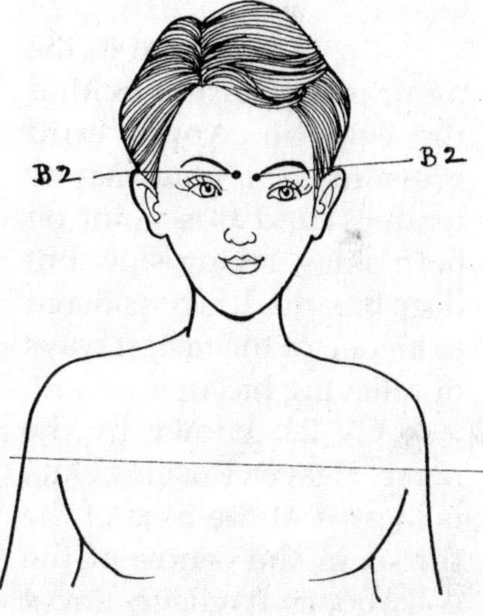

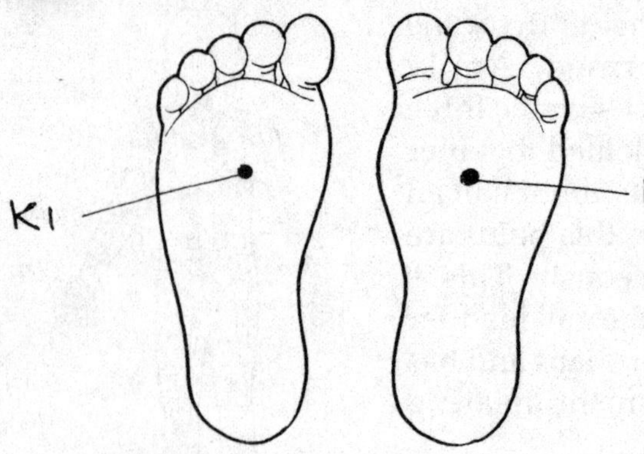

impress upon the importance of sitting or lying in as comfortable and relaxed a position as possible as well as deep breathing while pressure is being given on the prescribed pressure points:

B 2, called 'Collecting Bamboo', is located just above B 1 just where the eyebrows start near the bridge of the nose. It is just above the inner corner of your eye socket. Press for 2-3 minutes, giving moderate pressure.

Cv 12 is midway between the notch at the bottom of the breastbone and the naval. Give moderate yet firm pressure for about one minute on this point for relief. It would be better if pressure on this point is given empty stomach. It relieves hiccups, abdominal spasms, emotional stress, etc.

K 27 is located in the hollow below the collarbone next to the breastbone. It tonifies the kidneys, considered a key detoxification organ. It relieves hiccups, chest congestion and anxiety.

Tw 17 is located in the natural depression behind the earlobe. Apply mild pressure as this point may be tender. Hold this point on both sides, taking slow but deep breaths. It is considered to be one of the fastest ways of relieving hiccups.

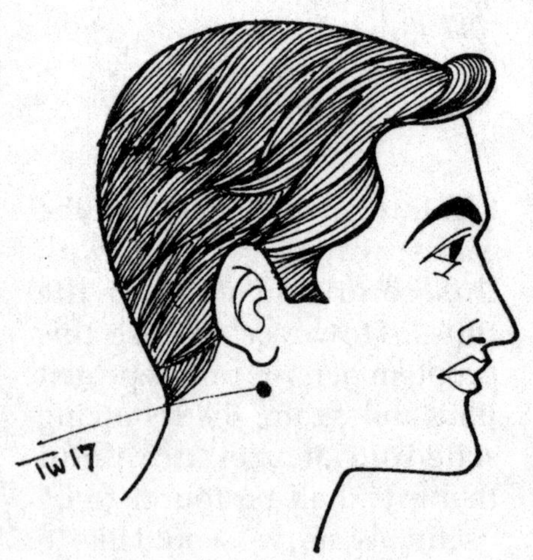

CV 22, known by the name 'Heaven Rushing Out', is located at the base of the throat in the centre of the collarbones. It relieves throat

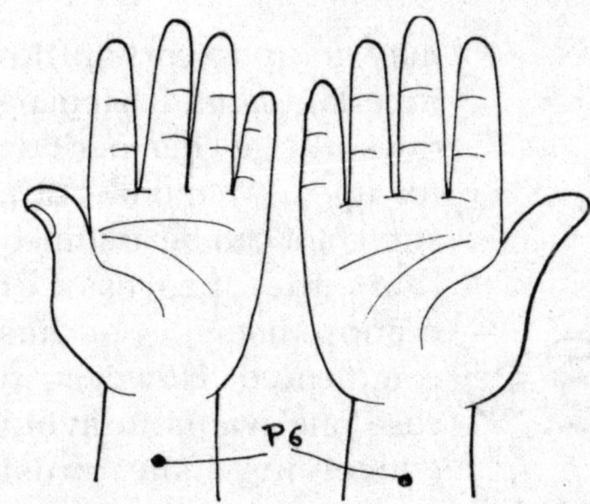

spasms, chest congestion and hiccups.

CV 17 called 'Sea of Tranquillity' lies on the centre of the breastbone about a palm width up from the base of the breastbone. It relieves, anxiety and hiccups besides panic attacks.

Lu 1, called 'Letting Go', is located on the outer side of the chest, about two and a half finger widths over the crease of the armpit, about an inch inside. It helps relieve hiccups and breathing difficulty.

Pc 6 is known by the name 'Inner Gate', and is located on the palm side of the wrist, about three finger widths above the wrist crease in the centre of the arm. It helps restore proper functioning of the diaphragm and consequently relief from hiccups.

Q. 65: What are hot flushes? Could acupressure help alleviate this condition?

A. 65: Hot flushes, cold feet and mood swings, etc., are some of the accompanying symptoms of menopause. This is the transition period in the life of a women, or it would not be incorrect to say that menopause, i.e. cessation of the monthly cycle signals the end of a women's fertile period and she attains freedom from painful periods, hassle of taking birth control measures and fear of pregnancy, etc., or to say, the beginning of a new phase of life. There is no hard and fast time frame, yet usually it commences any time after attaining the age of forty plus and

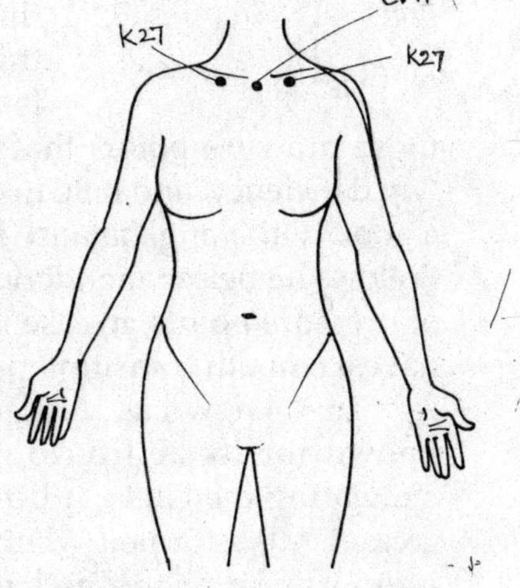

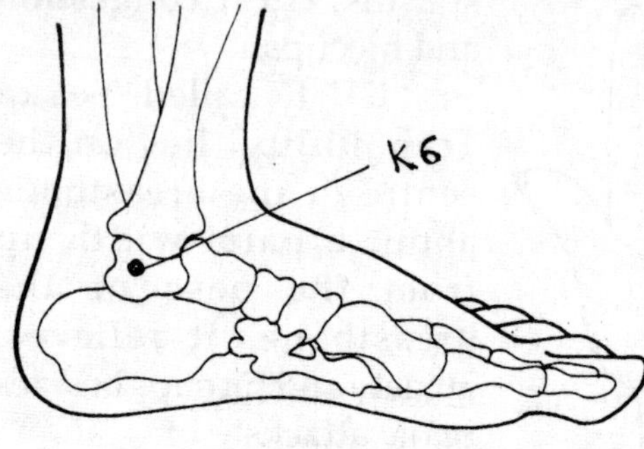

may go up to early fifties in certain cases. If a female does not get her periods for up to six months at a stretch, it can be assumed that the process of menopause has commenced. However, in case one wants to avoid conceiving, she must continue to take some form of birth control measures until one full year passes without menstruation.

The symptoms vary widely with various women. Whereas some have a comfortable passage of this transit period, others have symptoms like hot flushes, night sweats, vaginal dryness, mood swings, irritability and even depression at times. All this happens because of Yin deficiency. By attaining the age of menopause, majority of follicles have been exhausted which results in heavily reduced hormone levels. Lack of internal cooling ability caused by yin deficiency results in symptoms, like hot flushes, etc. The only way to alleviate this condition is to stimulate those pressure points that nourish the 'yin deficiency' and help in establishing a good 'yin/yang' balance in the body. Follow the below mentioned schedule of pressure points, in case you want to have a smooth transition period:

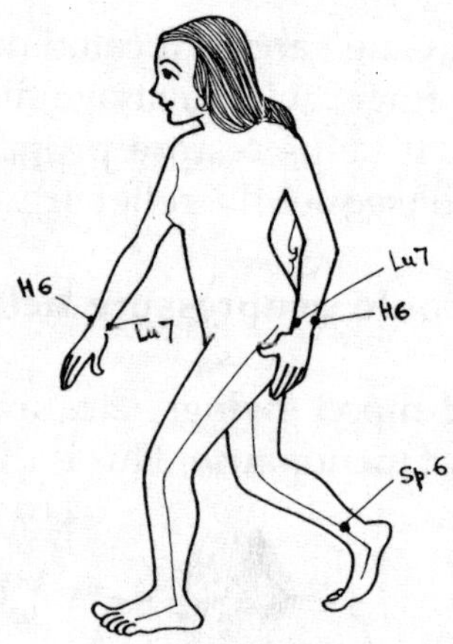

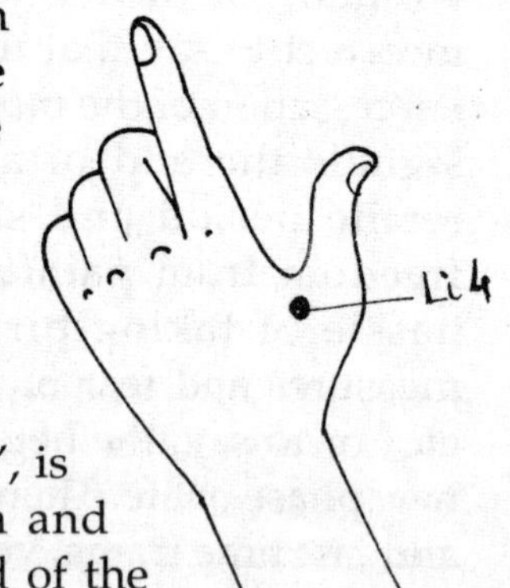

Li 4, known as 'Adjoining Valley', is known for its ability to relieve pain and circulating the Ch'i . It lies on the end of the crease that is formed when the thumb and the index finger are joined together. It relieves

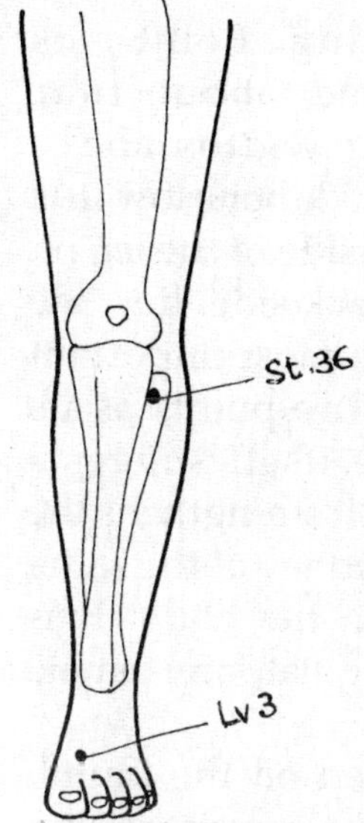

stagnation of the Ch'i and consequently hot flushes.

K 1, known as 'Bubbling Springs', is located on the sole of the foot in the centre between the two pads. It is a very useful point for getting relief from hot flashes.

K 27 is located in the hollow below the collarbone next to the breastbone. It tonifies the kidneys, considered a key detoxification organ. It relieves hot flushes, anxiety and depression.

GB 20 is located in the hollow below the base of the skull. Steady pressure (mild to moderate) should be given on this point simultaneously on both the sides. Its effect goes well with its name, i.e. 'Gates of Consciousness'. It is an extremely beneficial point to overcome hot flashes, irritability and stress.

CV 17, called 'Sea of Tranquillity' lies on the centre of the breastbone about a palm width up from the base of the breastbone. It relieves, anxiety calms nerves and alleviates hot flashes.

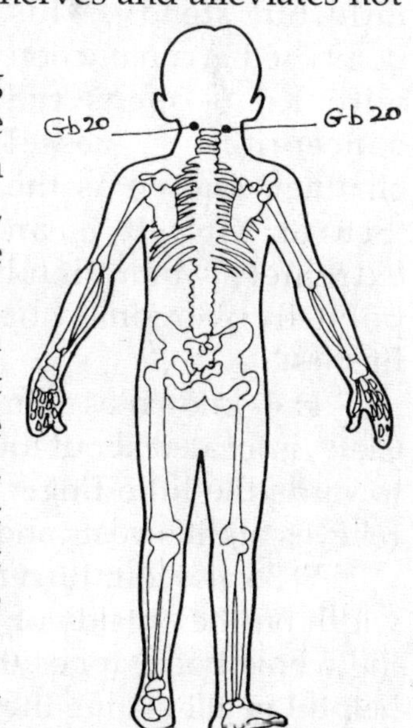

K 6, known by the name 'Shining Sea', is located on the inner side of the ankle. It opens the Yin-Ren meridian to help counteract Yin deficiency, thereby removing the basic cause behind the hot flushes.

Lv 3, lies between the big and second toe on the top of the foot. It regulates and tonifies the liver and the flow of Ch'i in the liver meridian, which is considered to be the most powerful organ for detoxification. It can be used for alleviating menopause symptoms of all kinds.

Sp 6, also called 'Three Yin

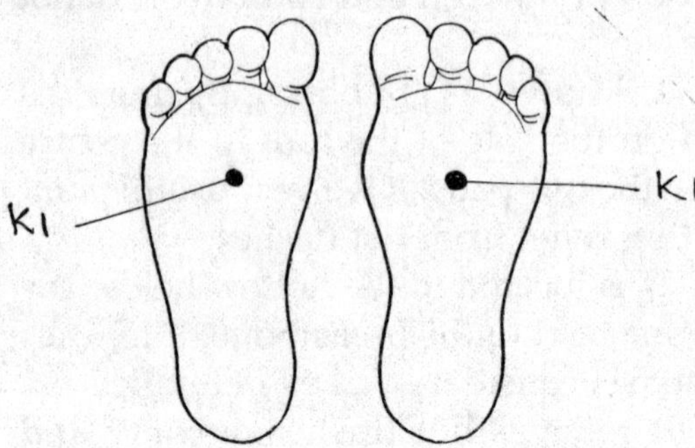

Meeting Point', is located about four finger widths above the ankle bone towards the inside of the leg on the back side. It is one of the most important pressure points as its name itself suggests since it strengthens the Yin of three meridians viz. spleen, liver and kidney at the same time. It helps flush Ch'i and blood through the body. It is considered one of the best pressure points to regulate any female problem.

Lu 7, called 'Broken Sequence', is located on the thumb side of the hand about two finger widths above the wrist crease, towards the elbow. As there is no flesh and pressure has to be given on the bone, it has to be mild but steady. This point used in conjunction with Kd 6 opens the conception vessel channel, known as the 'Sea of Yin'. It is an extremely beneficial point to overcome hot flushes.

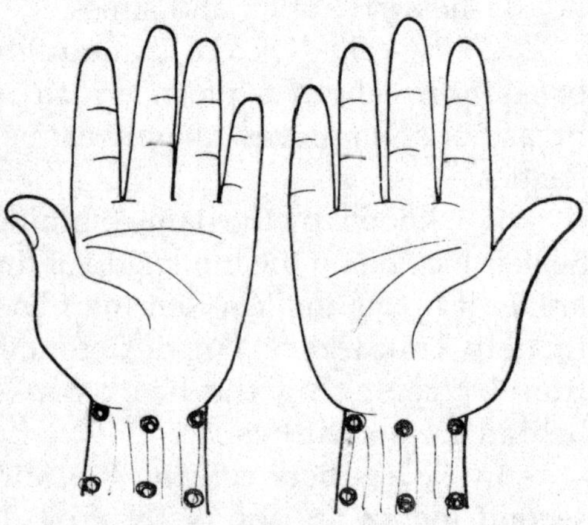

H 6, known as 'Yin Cleft', is located about four finger widths above the wrist crease towards the little finger side on the palm side of the arm. It relieves night sweats and irritability.

St 36, lies four finger widths below the kneecap, one finger width on the outside of the shin bone. This point strengthens the whole body, tones the muscles and has been found to be helpful in alleviating the condition of hot flushes.

Q.66 : What is hypertension, and how is it caused? Can acupressure be of any help in controlling this condition?

A.66: Heart is one of the vital organs in our body. It is considered to be the strongest organ made up of a muscle known as 'cardiac muscle' which keeps on constricting and relaxing a few days after conception and this process continues till death. When this muscle constricts, it pushes the blood through the chambers, into the vessels and then it relaxes to fill. This action is termed as a 'heart beat'. The speed of contraction and relaxation is regulated by the nervous system. This heart rate is fastest in case of infants; by the time one becomes an adult, it stabilises at around 72 beats per minute. It keeps varying in different situations, e.g. fever, anger, anxiety or exercising, etc. Where as a good number of conditions can affect our heart, one of the diseases that can adversely affect the heart is hypertention. The symptoms of this disease include a dull headache, nosebleeds (at times), dizziness, heaviness in the head, etc., but at times this disease does not produce any significant symptoms and that is why it is also called a 'silent killer'. The best course is to keep on checking your blood pressure once in a while and the moment the blood pressure (i.e. Systolic 115-130 and Diastolic 75-85) is found to be away from the indicated range, you must seek medical advise for the reason that the fluctuation in the B.P. range can affect not only your heart, it may also become the cause of other problems, e.g. kidney ailments, brain hemorrhage, eye problem or even paralysis.

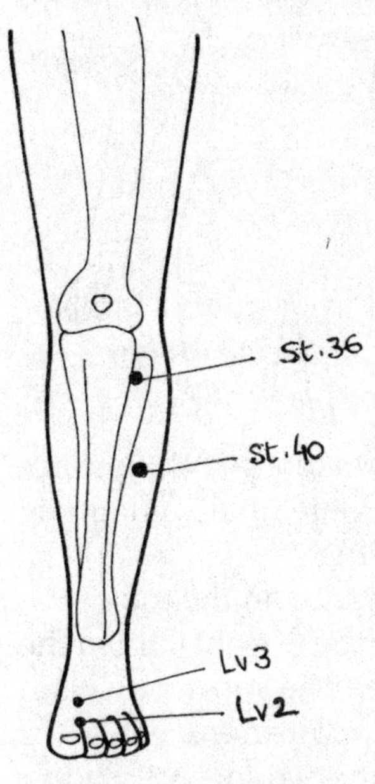

Faulty eating habits (i.e. consumption of a high fat and high cholesterol diet), mental stress, excessive physical strain, lack of exercising, alcohol consumption/smoking, inadequate sleep may be some of the causes behind this condition. Hypertension is also said to be caused either due to excess of Yang or an excess

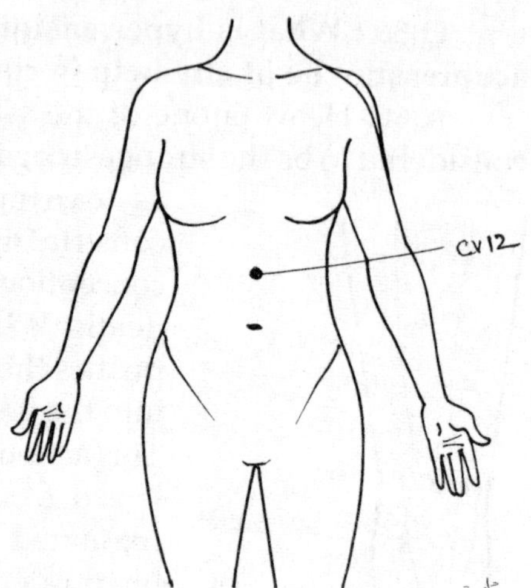

of phlegm and damp. Such a deficiency may occur in kidney or liver which control the circulation of Ch'i.

Hypertension can be kept under control with the help of the use of the pressure points that are being discussed here. Besides, it will be of help to the patient in case he follows a regulated life style and starts taking morning and evening walks, reduces consumption of salt in case he is used to taking more salt, resorts to a fat/cholesterol free diet with emphasis on green leafy vegetables, adequate consumption of water and proper exercising.

Lv3, lies between the big and second toes on the top of the foot. It regulates and tonifies the liver and the flow of Ch'i in the liver meridian, which is considered to be the most powerful organ for detoxification. One of the prominent cause of hypertension is blockage in the liver meridian and giving pressure on this point removes the blockage.

St 36, lies four finger widths below the kneecap, one finger width on the outside of the shin bone. This point strengthens the whole body, tones the muscles and has been found to be helpful in rejuvenating the Ch'i and blood. Used in combination with Li 11 this point yields good results.

GB 20 is located in the hollow below the base of the skull. Steady pressure (mild to moderate) should be given on this point simultaneously on both the sides. Its effect goes well with its name, i.e. 'Gates of Consciousness'. It is an extremely beneficial point to overcome stiffness in the

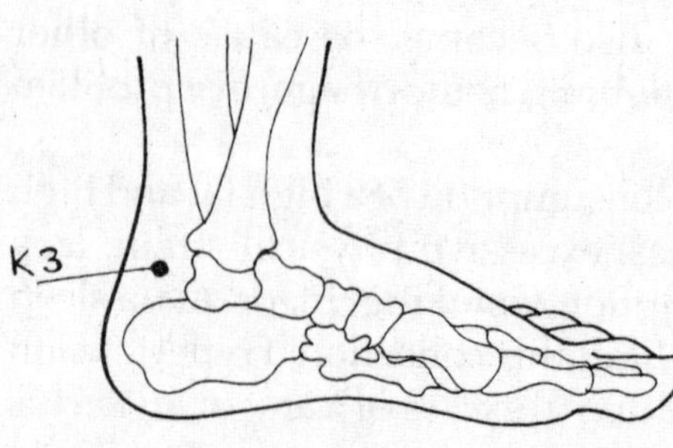

region of the neck. It also eliminates wind and cold.

K 1, known as 'Bubbling Springs' is located on the sole of the foot in the centre between the two pads, below the ball of the foot. Give firm pressure for a minute.

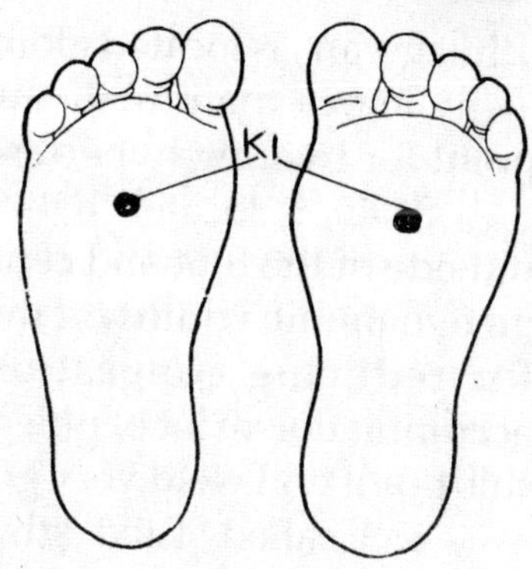

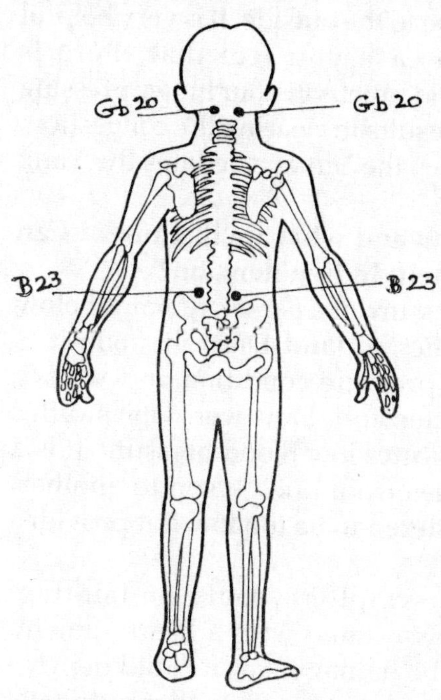

LI 11 is located at the outer end of the elbow crease. This point is very effective in relieving symptoms of cold, fever and in strengthening the immune system to help develop resistance from future colds. As this points gets very tender on touching, mild or massage like pressure only should be given on this point. Hold this point together with Ht 3 which lies on the elbow crease on the little finger side, exactly opposite Li 11.

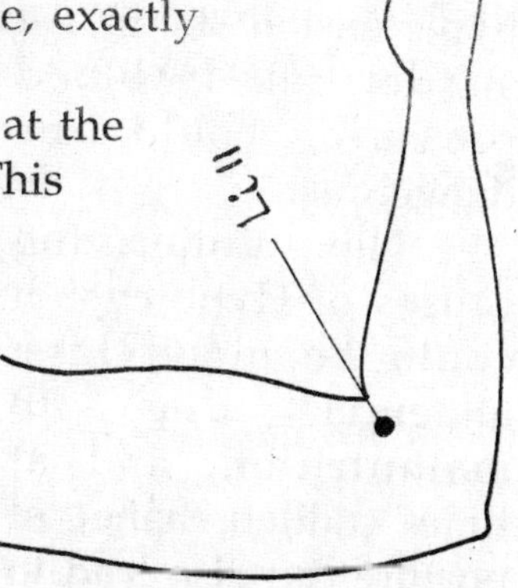

Lv 2, known as 'Xingjian', lies at the junction of the big and second toes. This point stimulates Yin and sedates Yang. It is used with Lv 3 for controlling hypertension.

B 23, as shown in the figure, stimulates the function of the Kidney.

Ren 12 (cv12) called

'Zhozgwan', is located along the mid line of the abdomen, a little away above the umbilicum, and is considered to be a specific point for treating hypertension.

St 40, is located half way between the ankle bone on the outside of the foot and centre of the kneecap. Find the tibia and go two thumb widths off the bone to the outside. It is very helpful for reducing congestion. In case you feel that there is accumulation of lot of phlegm and mucus in your lungs, pressing this point will yield very good results in clearing the congestion.

K 3, called 'Taixi' stimulates the Yin and sedates the Yang of liver and kidney.

Q. 67: What is hypotension and what are its causes? Can acupressure/reflexology also help in hypotension?

A. 67: In case the blood pressure of a person remains below the range of 90-60, i.e. Systolic '90' and Diastolic '60', it is considered to be a low blood pressure condition and we say that he is suffering from hypotension. However, views differ on the subject as to what constitutes low blood pressure. It is a relative phenomenon and varies from one person to another. Blood pressure has to be considered to be too low if it provides noticeable symptoms.

Some of the prominent symptoms could be fainting, dizziness, or some condition associated with a heart ailment. Very low blood pressure may be damaging as it could deprive the brain and other vital organs of oxygen and other nutrients. It could be fatal too, as such this condition, which is generally neglected by the people as compared to those suffering from hypertension, should get due care to avoid any complication. A sudden fall in blood pressure could be dangerous.

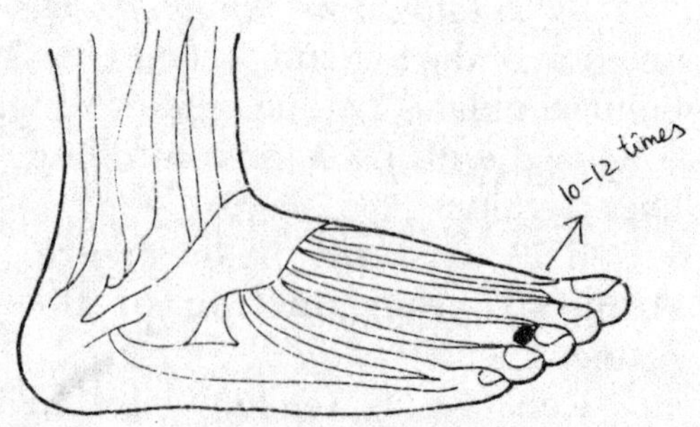

The underlying causes of Hypotension could be blood loss, anaemia due to malnutrition, and at times sudden change of posture can also lead to

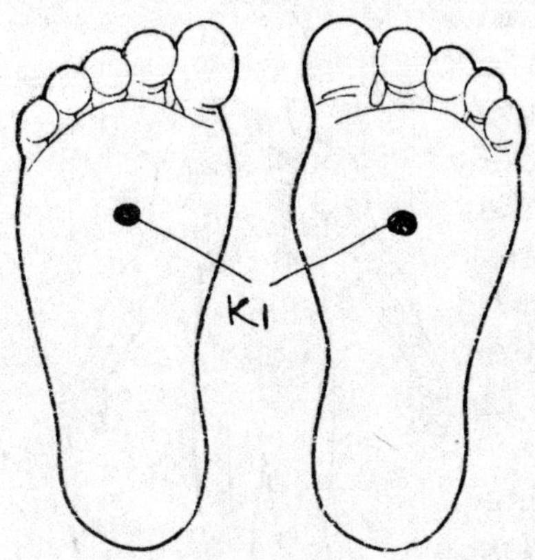

low B.P, which may result in dizziness or a temporary loss of consciousness.

Lv 3, lies between the big and second toes on the top of the foot. It regulates and tonifies the liver and the flow of Ch'i in the liver meridian, which is considered to be the most powerful organ for detoxification. One of the prominent causes of hypotension is blockage in the liver meridian and giving pressure on this point removes the blockage.

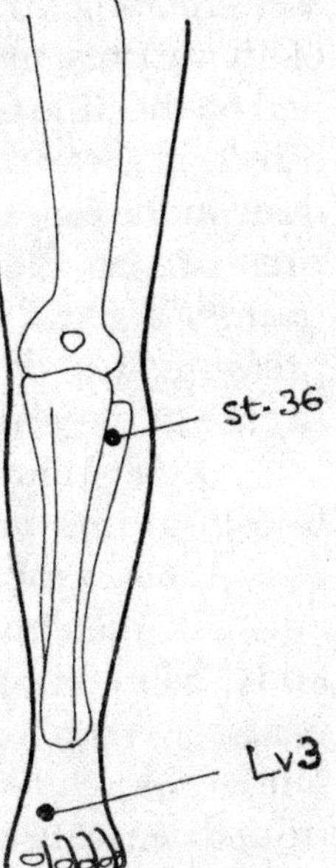

St 36, lies four finger widths below the kneecap, one finger width on the outside of the shin bone. This point strengthens the whole body, tones the muscles and has been found to be helpful in rejuvenating the Ch'i and blood. Used in combination with Li 11, this point yields good results.

GB 20 is located in the hollow below the base of the skull. Steady pressure (mild to moderate) should be given on this point simultaneously on both the sides. Its effect goes well with its name, i.e. 'Gates of Consciousness'. It is an extremely beneficial point to overcome stiffness in the region of the neck. It also eliminates wind and cold.

K 1, known as 'Bubbling Springs' is located on the sole of the foot in the centre between the two pads, below the ball of the foot. Give firm pressure for a minute.

LI 11 is located at the outer end of the elbow crease. This point is very effective in relieving symptoms of cold, fever and in strengthening the immune system to help develop resistance from future colds. As this points gets very tender on touching, mild or massage like pressure only should be given on this point. Hold this point together with Ht 3 which lies on the elbow crease on the little finger side, exactly opposite Li 11.

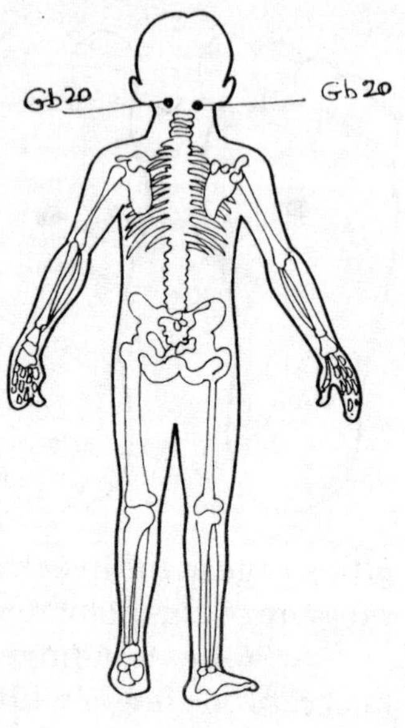

For treating this condition using reflexology, give pressure on the reflex areas relating to heart reflexes. Instead of giving pressure on the skin over the nail on the little fingers and toes in the direction away from the thumbs as is done in the case of hypertension, give pressure on the middle fingers and little toes towards the thumb/big toe rubbing this area 10-15 times with average pressure. Rest of the areas to be stimulated shall be the same as in case of hypertension.

Q. 68: What is immune system? Can acupressure help boost our immune system?

A. 68: Our immune system is a complex network that involves every aspect of our body. Skin being the first defence against viruses, lymph glands produce and store numerous white blood cells that protect us from disease. Even our thoughts, positive or negative, can affect increasing or decreasing our immune system. It locates, identifies and destroys bacteria and viruses as soon as they enter our body. Energy imbalance weakens our immune system. If we eat proper diet, do enough exercise and get enough rest and do not over stress ourselves, our immune system, i.e. capability to resist disease remains strong. It has been found that excess

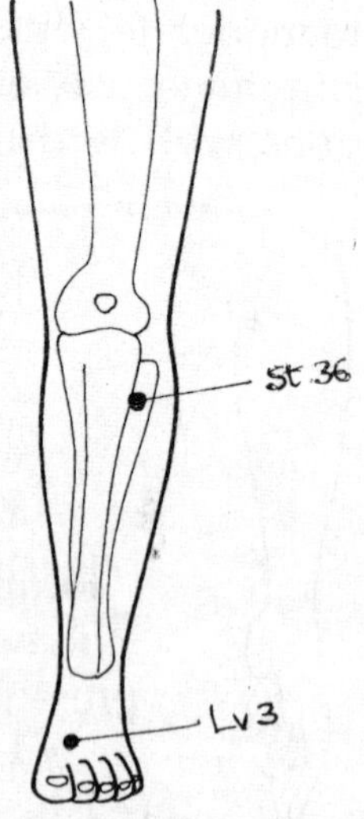

of a particular activity weakens the immune system, viz.

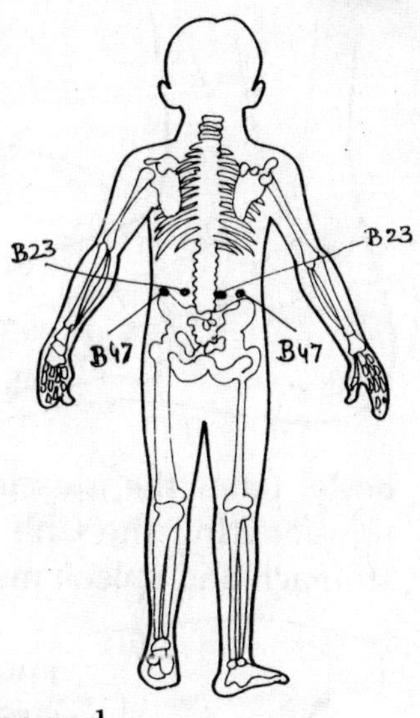

(i) Excess standing damages the bladder and kidney meridians, and may cause fatigue and backaches
(ii) Excess sitting adversely affects the stomach and spleen meridians
(iii) Excess lying has a direct impact on large intestines and the lung meridians
(iv) Putting excess strain on our eye or emotional stress has an adverse effect on small Intestines and heart meridians and
(v) Excess of physical exertion effects gallbladder and liver meridians.

The following pressure point schedule if followed up meticulously shall be of great help in keeping healthy by keeping this mechanism functioning at its best:

To restore the bladder and kidney meridians, stimulate B 23 and B 47 points. B 23 can be located in the middle of the waist, half way between the rib cage and the hip bone on the inner edge. B 47 lies in the middle of the waist four finger widths outside of the spine. These points not only provide relief in lower back pain but also reduce muscle tension, fatigue, depression, fear and trauma. Follow it up by holding K 27, 'Elegant Mansion', which is directly below your collarbone. Finally hold the 'Bigger Stream', K 3, called 'Taixi'. This stimulates the Yin and sedates the Yang of liver and kidney.

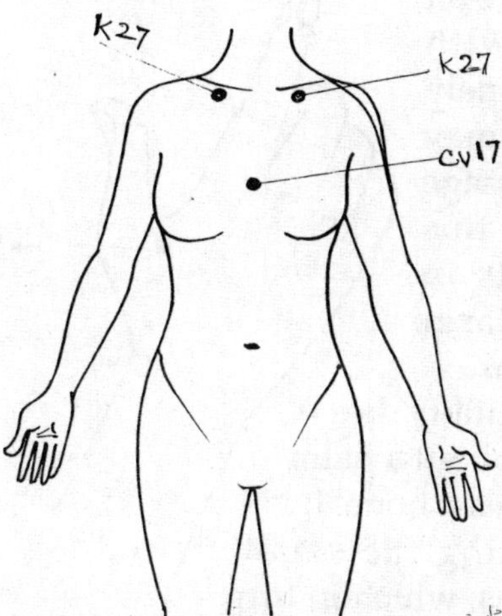

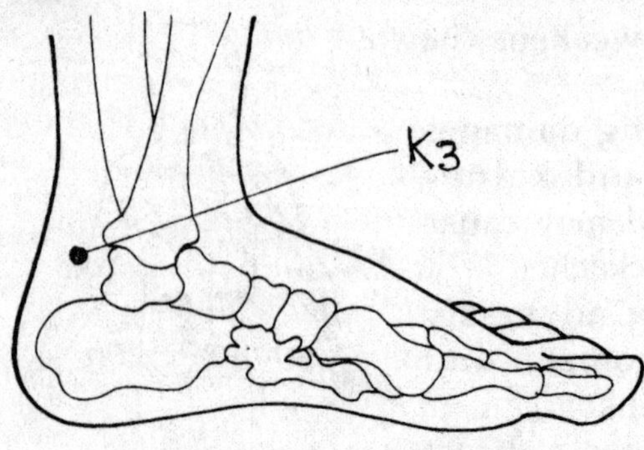

Hold all these points for one minute each as you breathe deep and exhale slowly.

St 36, lies four finger widths below the kneecap, one finger width on the outside of the shin bone. This point strengthens the whole body, tones the muscles and has been found to be helpful in rejuvenating the Ch'i and blood. Stimulate it to benefit the stomach and spleen meridians.

Li 4, known as 'Adjoining Valley', is known for its ability to relieve pain and circulate the Ch'i. It lies on the end of the crease that is formed when the thumb and index finger are joined together. It stimulates elimination of toxins through bowels. It relieves stagnation of the Ch'i too. Pregnant women should not use this point.

LI 11 called 'Crooked Pond' lies on the top outer edge of the elbow crease. It is considered to be one of the most effective points to control allergy and is also highly sensitive, therefore pressure on this point should be given with utmost care lest it becomes extremely tender. Even the touch of cloth may hurt once it gets tender. Even massage like pressure can be given on this point. Press these two points in conjunction to benefit the large intestines and the lung meridians.

CV 17, called 'Sea of Tranquillity' lies on the centre of the breast bone about a palm width up from the base of the breast bone. It is an excellent point for balancing the small intestine and the heart meridians, which in turn results in creating emotional balance in our body.

Lv 3, lies between the big and second toes on the top of the foot. It regulates and tonifies the liver and the flow of Ch'i in the liver meridian, which is considered to be the most powerful organ for detoxification. Pressing this point helps control damage caused to the gall bladder and liver meridians by excessive physical exertion, which could result in cramps and spasms.

Q. 69: Can acupressure help in improving memory and concentration?

A. 69: Yes, acupressure can help in a big way. As a matter of fact all of us need a sharp mind and memory so that we are able to concentrate better, in this age of cut throat competition.

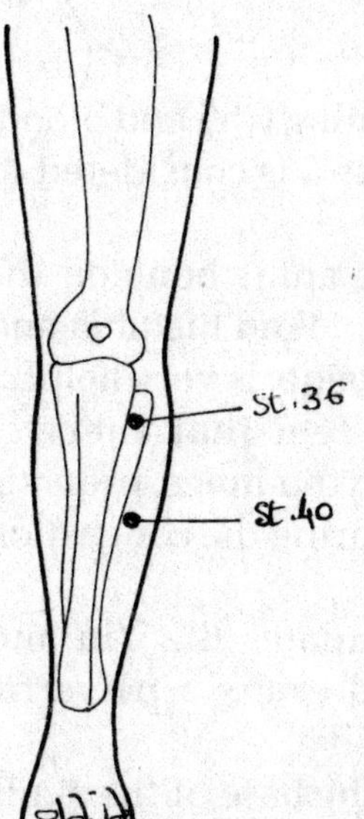

The cause behind the loss of memory or weak memory could be due to stress or some problem with the gastrointestinal system. Eating habits can also be a big factor in case our food is not balanced. Shoulder tension or tension in the neck also can be a causative factor. As a first step towards improving your memory, start eating food having complex carbohydrates, e.g. fresh vegetables, whole grains, sprouts, fresh wheat grass juice, etc., for benefiting memory. You must consult your physician in case your poor memory does not improve even after making amends with your diet and exercising, to rule out an underlying condition such as a heart disease or high blood pressure, etc.

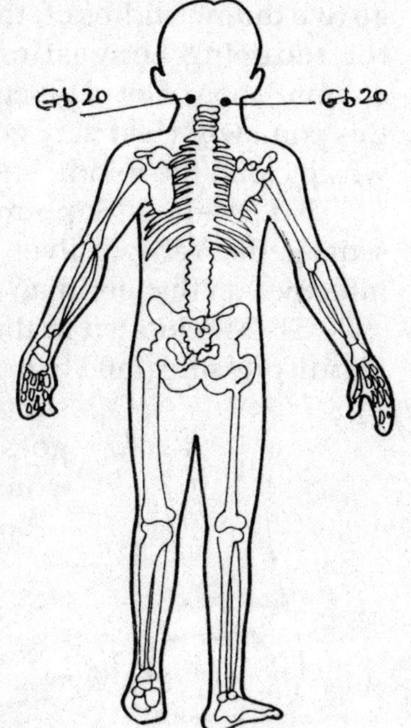

As per traditional Chinese

Medicine, brain function is directly related to the healthy flow of Ch'i in the kidney meridian. The following schedule of pressure point therapy (acupressure) shall be found to be greatly beneficial, as it will help tonifying the kidney's Ch'i and improving memory and concentration power of the brain:

St 36, lies four finger widths below the kneecap, one finger width on the outside of the shin bone. This point strengthens the whole body, tones the muscles and has been found to be helpful in rejuvenating Ch'i and blood. It also helps in clearing excess dampness and is considered to be the point that clears 'brain fog'.

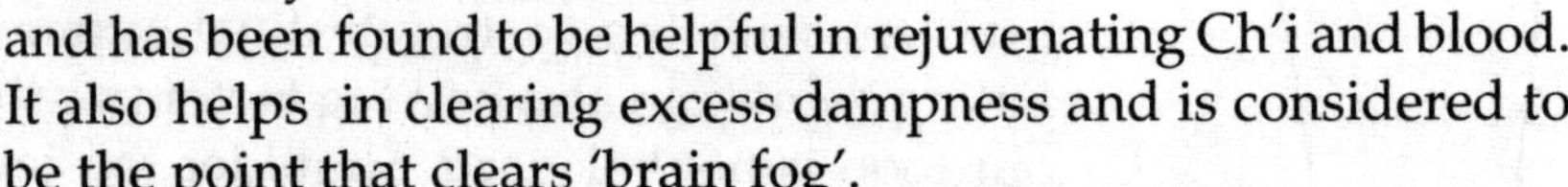

St 40 is located half way between the ankle bone on the outside of the foot and centre of the kneecap. Find the tibia and go two thumb widths off the bone to the outside. Is very helpful for reducing congestion. In case you feel that there is accumulation of lot of phlegm and mucus in your lungs, pressing this point will yield very good results in clearing the congestion which cloud the mind.

Kd 3 called 'Supreme Stream', stimulates the Yin and sedates the Yang of liver and kidney, and exerts a powerful influence on the meridian and the entire body.

GB 20 is located in the hollow below the base of the skull. Steady pressure (mild to moderate) should be given on this point simultaneously on both the sides. Its effect goes well with its name, i.e. 'Gates of Consciousness'. It is an extremely beneficial point to overcome stiffness in the region of the neck. It also eliminates wind and cold. A good point for mental concentration and improving memory.

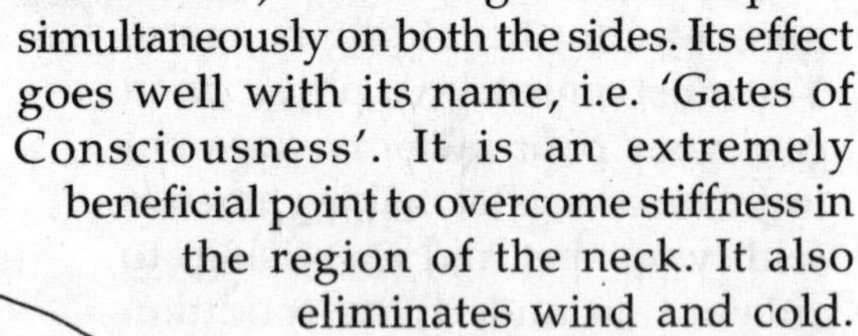

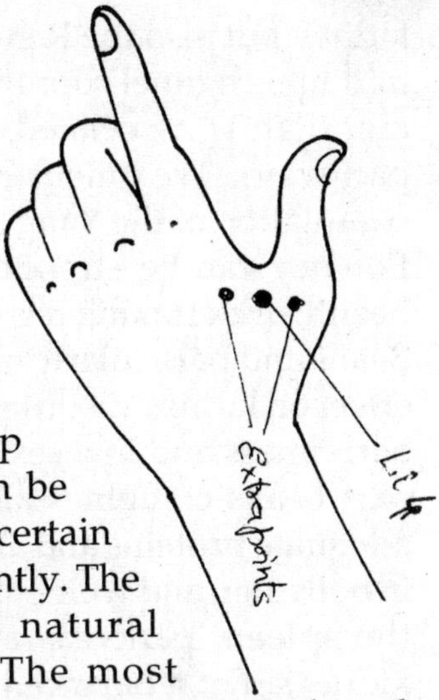

Ex 2, the 'Sun Point' is located in the depression of the temples, one and a half inches to the outside of the eyebrows. It helps improve memory and concentration.

In acupressure, pressure points are used to rebalance and rejuvenate the body. Of many revival potent points, GV 26 is the most useful. It is located in the middle of the upper lip right below the nose. This point can be used in itself or in conjunction with certain other points to revive the patient instantly. The point also stimulates the body's natural mechanism for restoring health. The most important thing to be done in this context is to strengthen the nervous system.

Q. 70: Can acupressure help in overcoming the sex-related problems, particularly impotency?

A. 70: Despite vastly increased openness about sex and related issues, sexual dissatisfaction remains one of the basic causes of disharmony in relationships. For most of the people, sex is an expression of love and belongingness. Some of the sex-related problems may be organic and biological, e.g. low sex drive, cases of impotence, and rising cases of infertility which is perhaps the most distressing of all the sex-related problems. On the other hand, inner pressures, e.g. fear factor and performance anxiety in men and emotional stress and pressure in women can result in vaginal infections, cramps, lack of sex desire or other problems relating to the genitals. In case you suffer from either of the problems of this sort, first of all consult your family physician to find out if your problem is being caused due to some organic or physical factor.

Traditional Chinese Medicine considers potency and sexual activity as governed by the kidneys. A depleted energy level of the kidneys can adversely affect your health and in turn, also your sexual life. Fatigue and low back problems can also be contributing factors. The deficiency may involve not only the kidney but also the Ren meridian (i.e. 'Conception Vessel' – the mid line channel running down the front of the body. The Ren meridian is associated with the sexual organs because of its pathway). Treatment of impotency comprises basically the stimulation of the Yang of the kidney in order to restore balance. Potency can be strengthened by improving overall physical health, undertaking regular exercises and eating a balanced diet. Beans and particularly black beans are known for their beneficial effect on kidney disorders and help overcome irregular menses, barrenness and low sex drive. Eating three parts grain and one part beans combines all the essential amino acids to provide adequate proteins and also strengthens the reproductive system in both men and women. Avoid excess sugar, as it can imbalance the spleen, pancreas and liver function which will tax the kidneys. Eat a balanced diet of whole grains, fresh food, fresh fruits (an apple a day) to improve overall health and energy level. Both of them are necessary for sexual competence.

Pressure point technique helps in alleviating muscular tension in the pelvic region which can in turn overcome problems relating to impotence, lack of sex drive, weak erection, premature ejaculation, vaginal infections and menstrual cramps, etc. Recent research has brought to light that factors, e.g. tight clothing, keeping mobile phones in the front or back pockets (radiation effect), lack of exercise and poor posture besides emotional stress are the major factors leading to this serious problem. With the removal of tension in the pelvic region, pleasurable sensations and the experience of orgasm can be better. Follow the following schedule of acupressure and feel the change in your life:

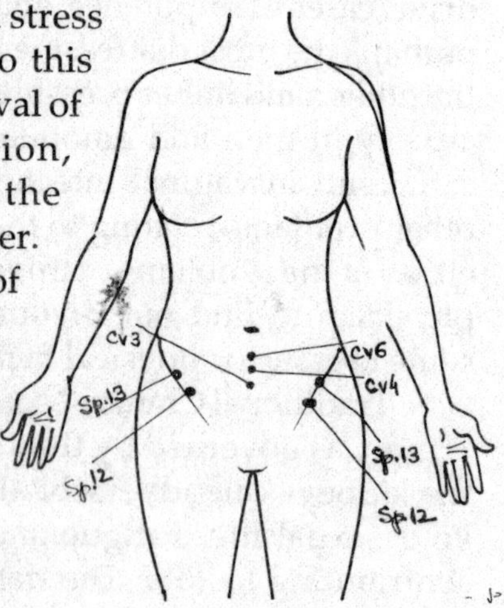

B 23 can be located in the middle of the waist, half way between the rib cage and the hip bone on the inner edge. It relieves depression and fear.

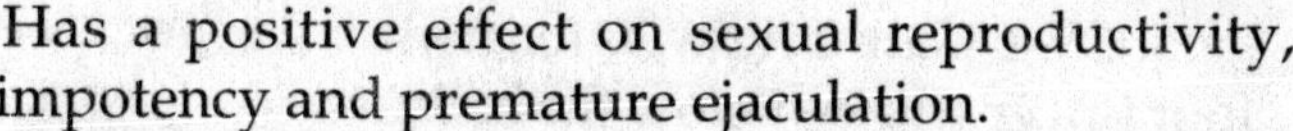

Has a positive effect on sexual reproductivity, impotency and premature ejaculation.

B 47, lies in the middle of the waist four finger widths outside of the spine. These points, not only provide relief in lower back pain but also reduce muscle tension, fatigue, depression and fear. It has a positive effect on sexual reproductivity, impotency and premature ejaculation.

K 1 known as 'Bubbling Springs', is located on the sole of the foot in the centre between the two pads. This is an important point for overcoming impotency and hot flushes.

St 36, lies four finger widths below the kneecap, one finger width on the outside of the shin bone. This point strengthens the whole body, tones the muscles and aids the reproductive system. Also overcomes impotency.

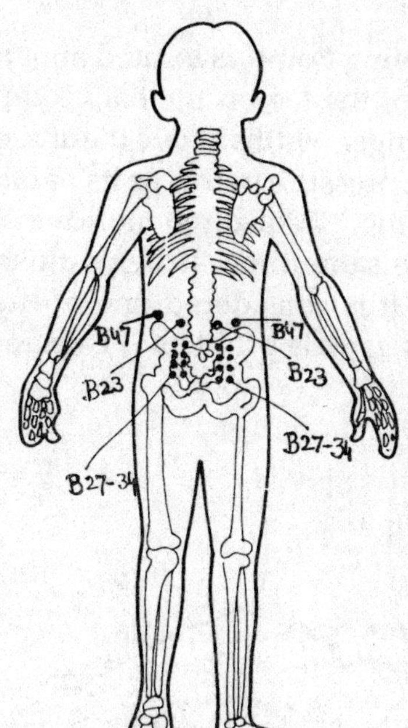

B 27 to B 34 are the pressure points located on the sacral part of the spine and can be managed even with the help of the fists of both the hands either sitting or lying on your belly. In the present context, these points help strengthen the reproductive system, relieve impotence, sterlity, irregular vaginal discharge and genital pain, etc.

Kd 3, lies midway between the inside of the ankle bone and Achilles tendon in the back of the ankle. It helps overcome sexual tensions, menstrual irregularity, etc.

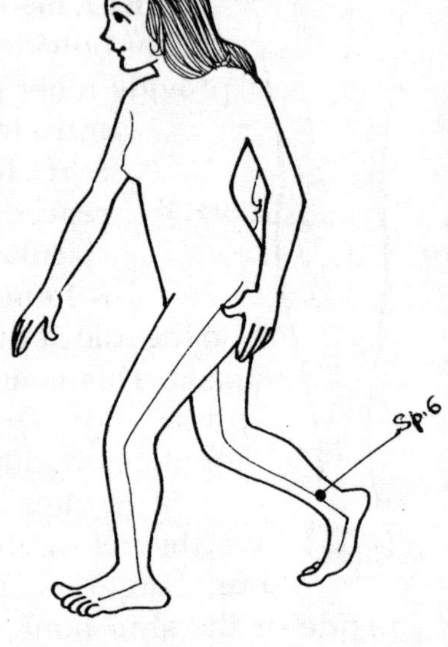

CV 4 'Gate Origin', is located four finger widths below the belly button or the navel. It helps relieve impotency and the irregular menstrual periods.

CV 6, 'Sea of Energy', lies three finger widths below the navel, it relieves reproductive problems, irregular periods and impotency. It strengthens the overall reproductive system.

Sp12 'Rushing Door' and Sp13 'Mansion Cottage' are in the pelvic region in the middle of the crease where the legs join the trunk of the body. These points are very effective for relieving impotency. These two points are specially effective for overcoming menstrual discomforts of any kind.

Sp 6, also called 'Three Yin Meeting Point', is located above the ankle bone towards the inside of the leg on the back side. The exact location being about four finger widths above the ankle bone. It is one of the most important pressure points as its name itself suggests since it strengthens the Yin of three meridians, viz. spleen, liver and kidney at the same time. It helps flush Ch'i and blood through the body. It is considered one of the best pressure points to regulate any female problem. Pregnant women should not press this point.

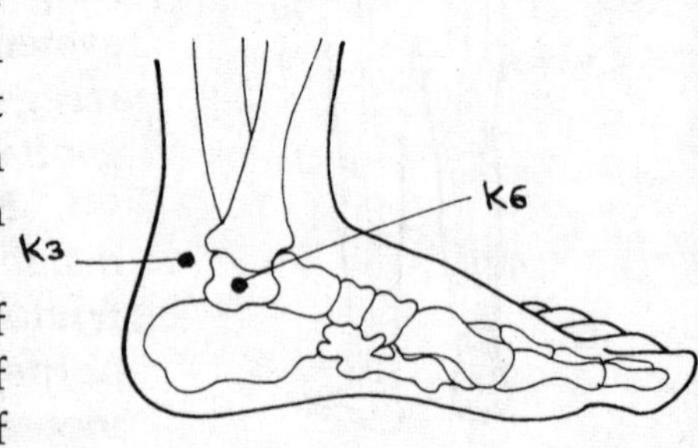

K 6 known by the name 'Shining Sea', is located on the inner side of the ankle. It opens the Yin-Ren meridian to help counteract Yin deficiency.

Du 4, called 'Gate of Life' lies along the midline of the back, at the level of kidney. It is an important point for reinforcing the Yang of the kidneys.

Du 20, called 'Many Meetings' lies at the crossing point of the urinary bladder, liver and Du meridian on the 'Crown of the Head'. It regulates and activates Yang Ch'i.

Ren 3 is a major point for treating disorders of urogenital system and is used for its direct effect on kidney. Also press Ren 4, on midline of the abdomen, above Ren 3. It strengthens the yang of kidneys.

Q. 71: What is meant by incontinence? How acupressure overcoming this problem?

A. 71: Inability to control urine is known as incontinence. It is a problem that is found more in the elderly people, and women in particular for the reason that their urethra is shorter. Some of the women suffer this problem after giving birth. This embarrassing condition, which is not a disease, keeps people confined to their homes for the fear factor, in case there is no immediate access to the toilet.

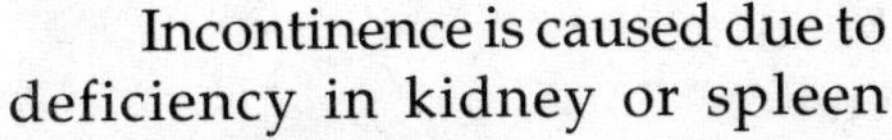

Incontinence is caused due to deficiency in kidney or spleen energy. This can lead to urinary or bowel incontinence. Spleen energy regulates the body's muscle tone. As such a decreased muscle tone leads to incontinence. Most of the times this condition is the outcome of the deficiencies in both of these organs. The positive aspect is that almost all or most of the people suffering from this condition can be benefitted by acupressure treatment.

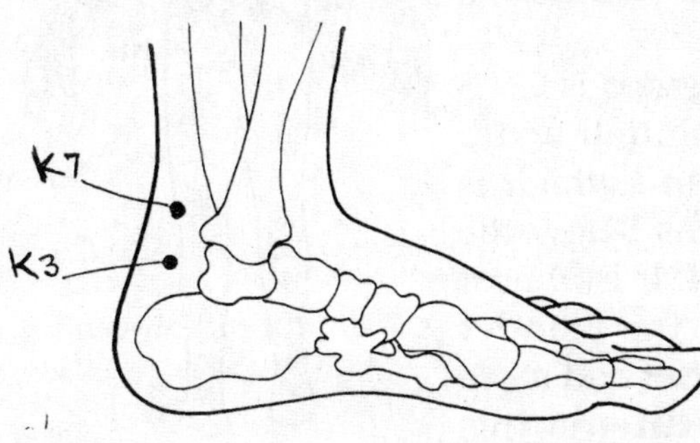

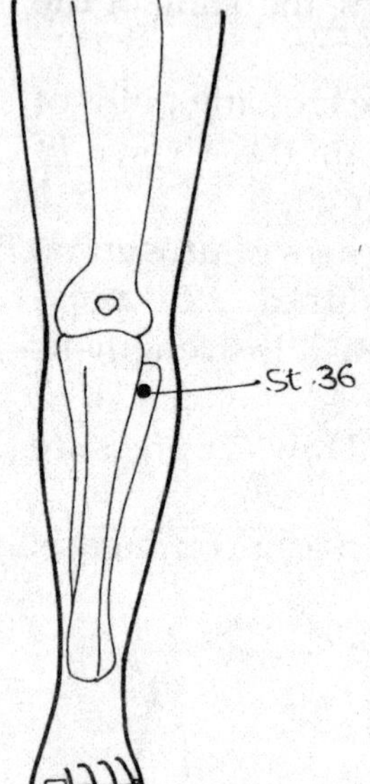

The following schedule will be found to be helpful:

Sp 6, also called 'Three Yin Meeting Point', is located above the ankle bone towards the inside of the leg on the back side. The exact location being about four finger widths above the ankle bone. It is one of the most important pressure points as its name itself suggests since it strengthens the Yin of three meridians, viz. spleen, liver and kidney at a time. It helps flush Ch'i and blood through the body. It is considered one of the best pressure points to regulate any female problem. Pregnant women should not press this point.

St 36, lies four finger widths below the kneecap, one finger width on the outside of the shin bone. This point strengthens the whole body, tones the muscles particularly in combination with Sp 6, and strongly revitalises the entire body.

Kd 3 lies midway between the inside of the ankle bone and the Achilles tendon in the back of the ankle. It helps overcome sexual tensions, menstrual irregularity, etc. From this point, three finger widths above towards the knees is the Kd 7 point. Press for about a minute with thumb pressure.

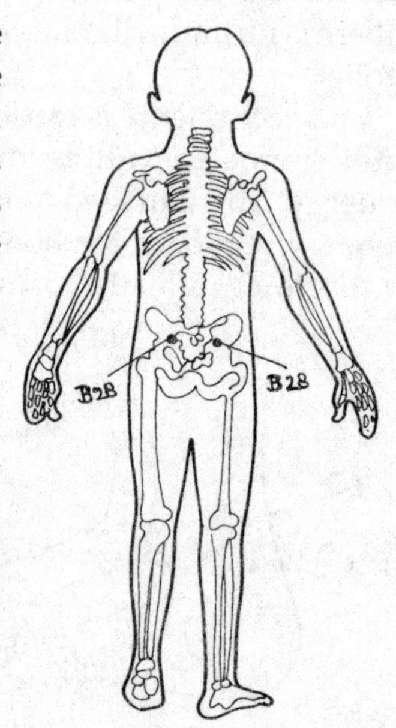

Next point to be pressed is CV 3 this point is about one thumb width below CV 4 'Gate Origin', which is located four finger widths below the belly button or the navel. It is almost specific in its effect on the bladder meridian. It would be better and more effective if steady pressure on this point is given for about a minute after emptying the bladder.

B 28 is an associated point of urinary bladder and is about one and a half inches on either side of the spine, in the mid-sacral area of the back. Spend several minutes stimulating CV 3 and B 28 which are almost specific to urinary bladder.

Q. 72: What is indigestion and heartburn, and what is the cause? How can acupressure/reflexology help?

A. 72: The main symptom of both indigestion and heartburn is a burning sensation in the oesophagus to the breastbone. Stress and tension can induce heartburn and overeating or eating too fast without chewing the food properly or consuming stale food or consuming food that does not go with our system may be the cause behind the aforesaid symptoms which can at times be associated with nausea and vomiting also. Consumption of food contaminated with bacteria may even cause food poisoning and cause cramps, vomiting, diarrhoea and at times dizziness.

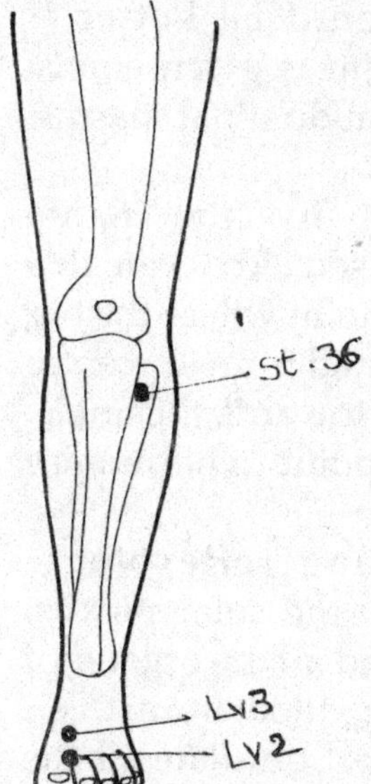

Most of the times indigestion or stomach upsets are caused due to overeating or the back flow of digestive acids from the stomach in the oesophagus that causes heartburn. Follow the following pressure point schedule to overcome this condition:

St 36, lies four finger widths below the kneecap, one finger width on the outside of the shin bone. This point strengthens the whole body and has a specific beneficial effect on digestion as well as on the Ch'i and blood.

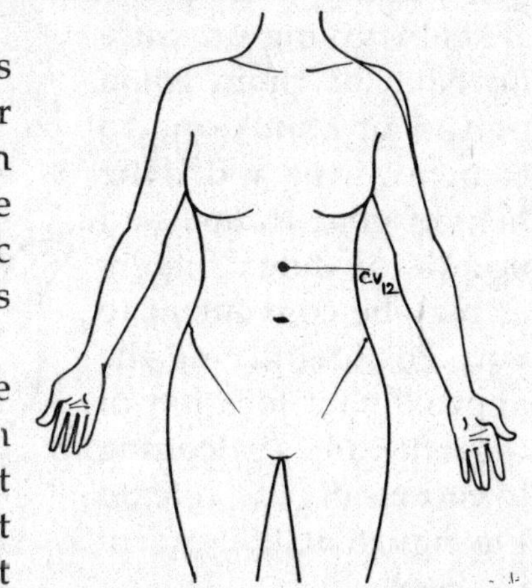

Pc 6, is known by the name 'Inner Gate', and it is located on the palm side of the wrist, about three finger widths above the wrist crease in the centre of the arm. It

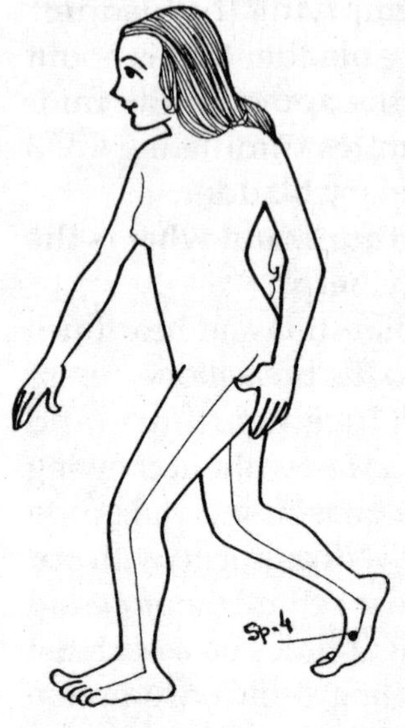

is known for its harmonising effect on the stomach. Use medium pressure for about a minute, building up slowly and releasing gradually at the end of the session. Repeat on the other hand too.

Cv 12, is midway between the notch at the bottom of the breastbone and the navel. Give moderate yet firm pressure on this point for relief for about one minute. It would be better if pressure on this point is given empty stomach. It relieves, abdominal spasms, emotional stress, etc.

Sp 4 known by the name 'Grandfather-Grandson'. To locate this point start from the joint where the big toe connects to the foot. Slide along the bone and from the centre of the joint move about three finger widths towards the ankle. Sp 4 is just below it. It is a very important point to harmonise the Ch'i of the stomach.

While treating this condition using reflexology, concentrate on the reflex areas relating to the solar plexus, diaphragm, the adrenal glands, the spine and all the organs of the digestive system, e.g. stomach, pancreas, duodenum, liver, gall bladder, large and small intestines, etc. Stimulate all the areas by giving pressure on each of them for a period of about one to two minutes with the help of your thumb and middle or index fingers as may be convenient to you. For identifying the approximate location of the reflex areas belonging to various organs, refer to the figure at the end of the book.

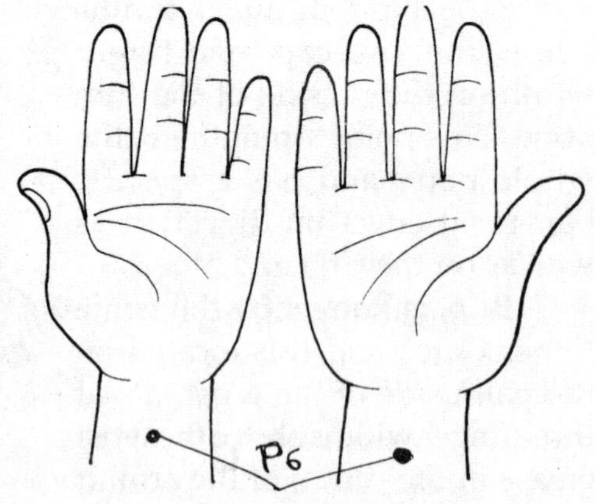

Q. 73: What is infertility, and what can the causes be? Can acupressure/reflexology be of any help?

A. 73: Inability to conceive is known as infertility. Infertility amongst both male and female is a common problem. Though this is a sufficient cause of tension and worry to the aspiring parents, yet it is also a fact that worry and tension further aggravate the condition. Other causes of infertility could be the blockage in the fallopian tubes or some disorder of the uterus or ovaries in the female partner or low sperm count in the male partner. In case, however, a women has problem in conceiving, both the partners should be examined and treated as per the requirement. It has also come to light over a period of time that in some cases very common problems, e.g. lower back pain, shoulder or neck tension/pain could also be the cause.

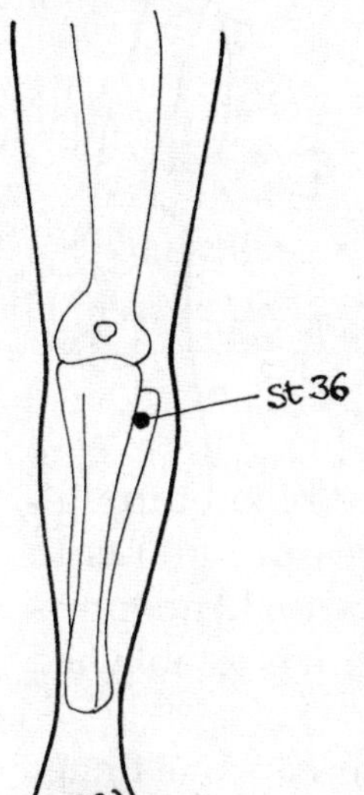

Acupressure and reflexology can both be extremely beneficial in treating this condition. Traditional Chinese Medicine also considers infertility to be the end result of several types of imbalances. There can be blockage in the pelvic area, leading to lack of proper menstrual cycle and even physical problems with the uterus and fallopian tubes (the tubes that connect the ovaries to the uterus), other factors can be deficiency of heat in the pelvis or a general lack of blood and energy. It would be better to treat the patient using both the techniques simultaneously. Applying pressure on the below mentioned pressure points in addition to stimulating the reflex points of all the organs relating to reproductive system as well as the points for overcoming stress shall be found to be highly productive.

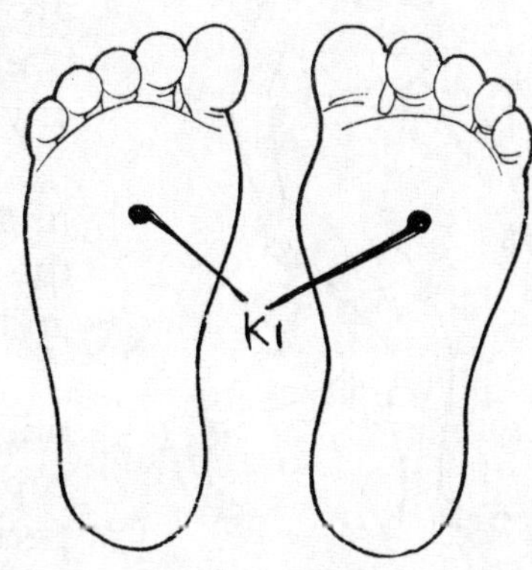

These are being described below:

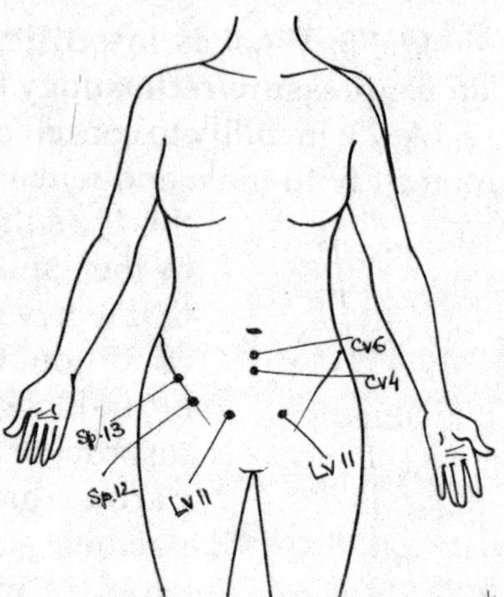

Sp 6, also called 'Three Yin Meeting Point', is located above the ankle bone towards the inside of the leg on the back side. The exact location being about four finger widths above the ankle bone. It is one of the most important pressure points as its name itself suggests since it strengthens the Yin of three meridians viz. spleen, liver and kidney at the same time. It helps flush Ch'i and blood through the body. It is considered one of the best pressure points to regulate any female problem. Pregnant women should not press this point. This point should not be pressed once it is established that the women has conceived.

St 36, lies four finger widths below the kneecap, one finger width on the outside of the shin bone. This point strengthens the whole body, tones the muscles particularly in combination with Sp 6, it strongly revitalises the entire body.

Sp12 'Rushing Door' and Sp13 'Mansion Cottage' are in the pelvic region in the middle of the crease where the legs join the trunk of the body. These points are very effective for relieving impotency and infertility problem. These two points are also specially effective for overcoming menstrual discomforts of any kind.

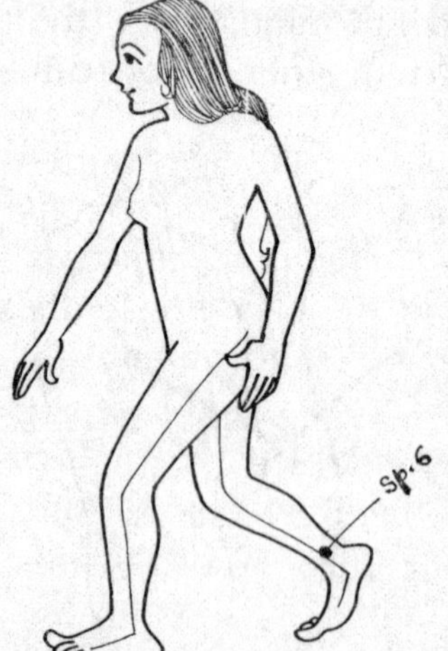

CV 4 'Gate Origin' is located four finger widths below the belly button or the navel. It helps relieve impotency and irregular menstrual periods.

CV 6, 'Sea of energy', lies three finger widths below the navel, it relieves reproductive problems, irregular periods and impotency and strengthens the overall reproductive system. This point is considered to be a 'Special Point' for toning the abdominal region and for enhancing fertility. This has to be pressed consistently for a period of 10 to 15 days or even more, every alternate day till the woman conceives, (not to be pressed during the periods).

B 23 can be located in the middle of the waist, half way between the rib cage and the hip bone on the inner edge. Relieves depression and fear. Has a positive effect on sexual reproductivity, impotency and premature ejaculation.

B 47 lies in the middle of the waist four finger widths outside of the spine. This point, not only provides relief in lower back pain but also reduces muscle tension, fatigue, depression and fear. It has a positive effect on sexual reproductivity, impotency and premature ejaculation.

K 1, known as 'Bubbling Springs' is located on the sole of the foot in the centre between the two pads. This is an important point for overcoming impotency and hot flushes.

Lv 11, known as 'Yin Corner', is located 2 thumbs widths below the upper edge of the pubic bone. It is also an important point to overcome infertility.

B47
B23
B47
B23

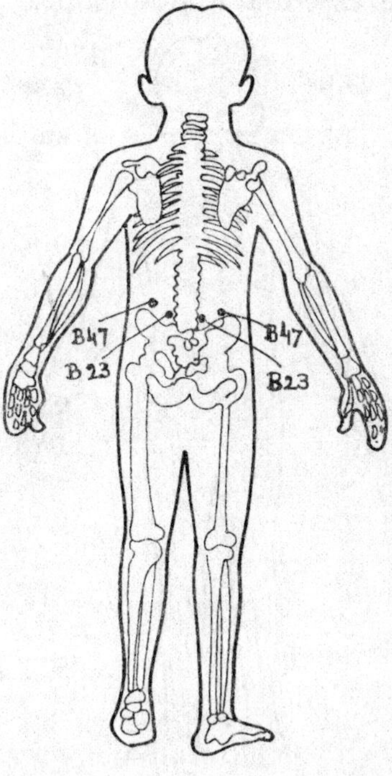

As has been discussed above, while giving a reflexology session to a patient who is trying to overcome infertility, stimulating the reflex points of all the organs relating to reproductive system as well as the points for overcoming stress shall be found to be highly productive. For doing so, stimulate all the reflex areas pertaining to the uterus, ovaries, fallopian tubes thoroughly, devoting time on each reflex area, giving rotating pressure with the help of thumb and middle finger or the index finger whatever is convenient. Also stimulate the reflex points of the ovaries and uterus on both sides of the wrists on both the hands as seen in the figures depicting the location of various reflex points of the body in the palms and the soles at the end of the book.

Q. 74: How can we overcome the disease known as insomnia using pressure point technique and reflexology?

A. 74: A person suffering from insomnia is generally unable to sleep peacefully for six to eight hours, which is essential for every human being depending upon age. This in turn leads to irritability and then to ill health in the absence of proper relaxation to our body that needs adequate rest after daylong hectic activity. At times, certain situations viz. pain, grief and anxiety may lead to disturbance in sleep.

As per traditional Chinese medicine, an uneven distribution of energy or in case the transition from Yang to Yin cycle is not smooth, or if the flow is interrupted, the result is insomnia. Sleep is essential to nourish the overall Yin of the body and to maintain a healthy balance of Yang and Yin. Lack of sleep makes us irritable and less efficient.

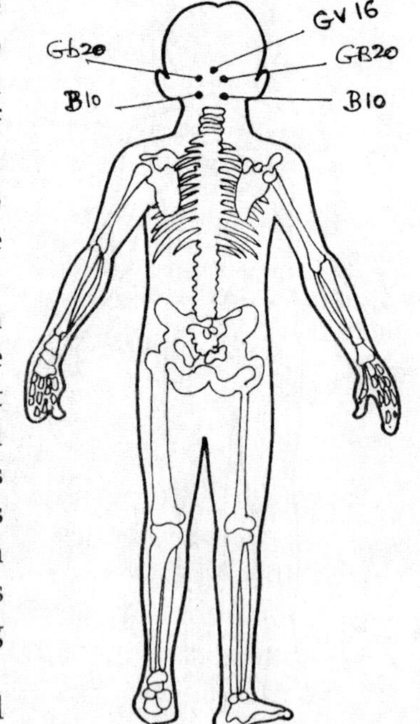

In such a situation, certain meridians become overloaded while others get blocked, but these can be corrected by a regime that includes acupressure, relaxation techniques to overcome stress and strain and a proper diet. In brief, acupressure is highly effective for relieving insomnia:

Lv 3, lies between the big and

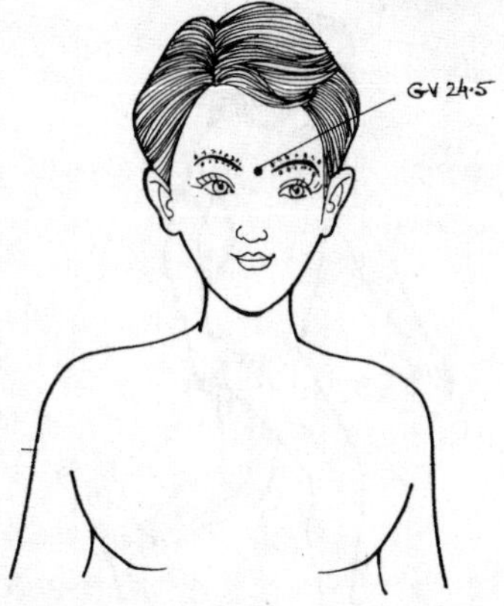

second toes on the top of the foot. It regulates and tonifies the liver and the flow of Ch'i in the liver meridian, which is considered to be the most powerful organ for detoxification. Pressing this point helps neutralise all types of stress and has a calming and relaxing effect on mind.

Sp 6, also called 'Three Yin Meeting Point', is located above the ankle bone towards the inside of the leg on the back side. The exact location being about four finger widths above the ankle bone. It is one of the most important pressure points as its name itself suggests since it strengthens the Yin of three meridians, viz. spleen, liver and kidney at a time. It helps flush Ch'i and blood through the body. The combination of the Yin nourishing and calming effect makes it important for getting rid of insomnia.

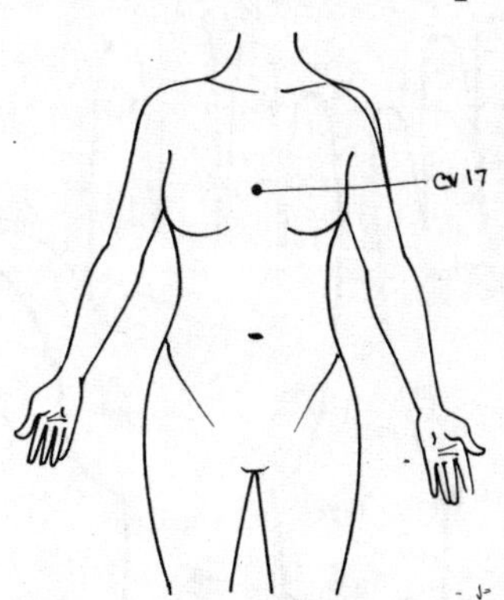

GB 20 is located in the hollow below the base of the skull. Steady pressure (mild to moderate) should be given on this point simultaneously on both the sides. Its effect goes well with its name, i.e. 'Gates of Consciousness'. It is an extremely beneficial point to overcome stiffness in the region of the neck. It also eliminates wind and cold. A good point for alleviating insomnia.

CV 17, called 'Sea of Tranquillity' lies on the centre of the breastbone about a palm width up from the base of the breastbone. It relieves anxiety, calms nerves and alleviates hot flushes.

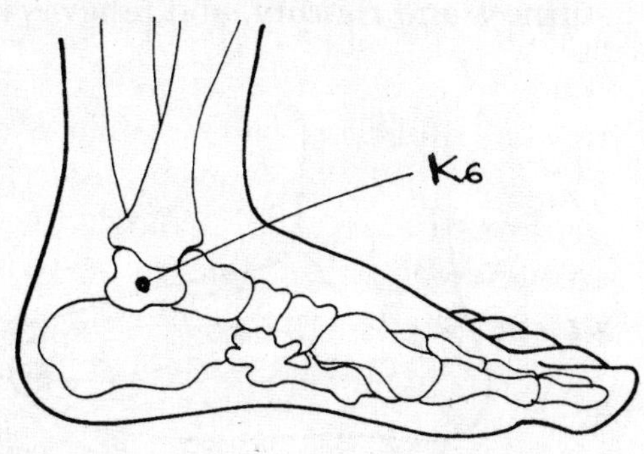

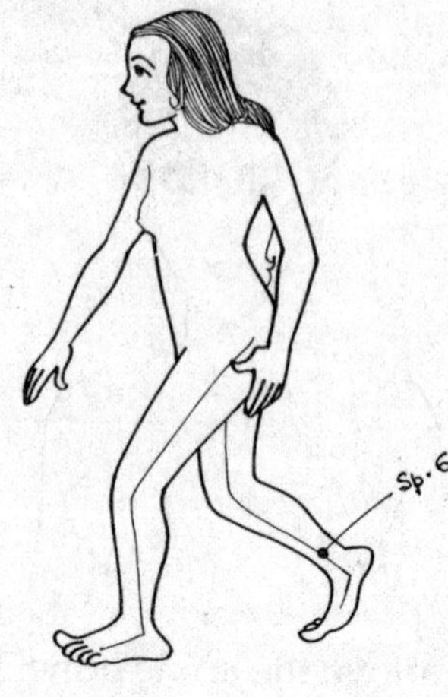

Helps overcome insomnia.

Pc 6, is known by the name 'Inner Gate', and is located on the palm side of the wrist, about three finger widths above the wrist crease in the centre of the arm. It helps relieve insomnia by its calming effect.

GV 24.5 is located between the eyebrows, in the indentation where the bridge of the nose meets the forehead. This tones up the endocrine system, particularly the pituitary gland. This also tones up the entire body, reduces stress and relieves head congestion, stuffy nose and headache, as also depression and emotional imbalances, thereby inducing relaxation for a good sleep.

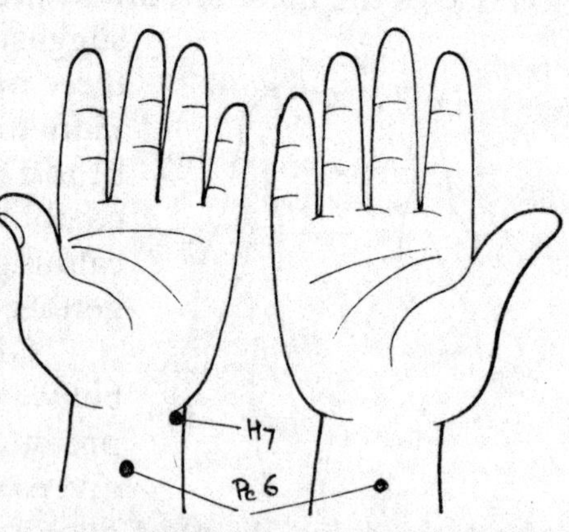

B 10 is located on the upper portion of the neck, about one thumb width outside the spine. Hold the back of your neck with one hand using all your fingers on one side and the thumb on the other to squeeze the neck muscle. It is considered as a key point for overcoming the stiffness and rigidity, and relieves insomnia.

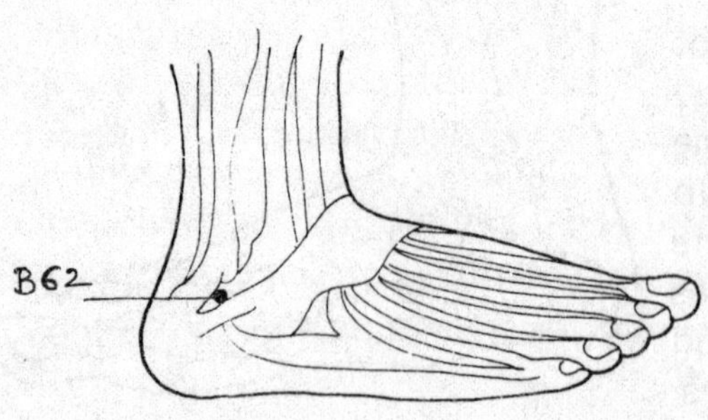

H 7, 'Spirit Gate' is located on the inside of the wrist crease towards the little finger side. It relieves anxiety which causes insomnia and is thus very useful.

GV 16, 'Wind Mansion' is located in

the centre of the back of the head in the hollow under the base of the skull. It relieves mental stress and insomnia.

K6 'Joyful Sleep' is found in an indentation below the inner side of the ankle. Relieves insomnia and anxiety.

B 62, 'Calm Sleep', is found on the outer side of the ankle in the indentation. It relieves back pain that makes it difficult to sleep.

As these repeated episodes of insomnia can make the patient feel exhausted, following reflex points if stimulated before retiring to bed will help induce relaxation and promote peaceful sleep. Stimulate the solar plexus area on both feet and palms by light thumb walking over the reflexes repeatedly. Follow it up by thumb walking over the head and brain reflex areas over the big toes of both the feet and the thumbs of both the hands, on the sides as well as on the stem of the toes and the thumbs.

Q. 75: What is irritable bowel syndrome (IBS)? Can acupressure/reflexology help?

A. 75: IBS is a term that describes a variety of conditions that affect the intestines and cause a lot of symptoms which may include alternating constipation and diarrhoea, excessive flatulence, nausea, loss of appetite, abdominal cramps and a general feeling of lethargy and weakness. There is no known cause of this condition, however, it is believed that stress and autonomic nervous system which responds to stress may be the causative factor. Certain foods may also irritate the bowel. According to Traditional Chinese Medicine, this condition may be caused because of some imbalance in the 'Earth Energy' in our body, which is one of the five vital elements of our body. In case your system is dominated by Earth Energy, you may love to eat or might have a tendency to overeat and this may aggravate digestive problems. As a consequence you may find it difficult to control your weight too. Once out of balance, you will have craving for sweets, chocolates, etc., which will further add to your woes.

A number of other conditions cause burning in the stomach area and chest, bloating, distension after eating, belching and difficulty in swallowing food. These include non-ulcerative dyspepsia, gastritis and peptic ulcer, etc. Although their physical symptoms appear to be similar, an acidy feeling in the stomach and throat that spurs the sufferer. Peptic ulcer often leads to an ulcer, which is an erosion of the wall of the stomach or the upper intestine. Gastritis is an irritation of the stomach membrane. Taking Aspirin could be the cause behind this irritation. Similarly, high degree of stress, smoking and other lifestyle related factors can be the cause of gastritis. An additional cause of digestive problems is invasion of microscopic pests, e.g. bacteria. Of course IBS can also present abdominal pain and digestive problems.

The ideal solution will be to get your dietary routine regulated and put in a better shape. That should be anybody's long term goal. As such add drinking enough water – say at least 8-10 glasses every day; avoid fatty foods; always eat well cooked food as raw food puts more strain on your spleen, an organ responsible for breaking down and extracting essential nutrients from food. Soups and stews are considered to be good spleen-nourishing foods. Reduce consumption of coffee, alcohol, pasta and cookies, etc., and look for ways to nourish yourself. Meanwhile, acupressure and reflexology can help you in alleviating your problems, as both these techniques have been found to be great stress busters, perhaps one of the main causes behind the condition. In other words acupressure and reflexology helps the body to do, what it is already trying to do i.e. heal itself.

Pc 6 is known by the name 'Inner Gate' and it is located on the palm side of the wrist, about three finger widths above the wrist crease in the centre of the arm. It helps relieve IBS (nausea in particular – in pregnant women to chemotherapy patients to sea going voyagers) by its calming effect.

Sp 6, also called 'Three Yin Meeting Point', is located above the ankle bone towards the inside of the leg on the back side. The exact location being about four finger widths above the ankle bone. It is one of the most important pressure points as its name itself suggests since it strengthens the Yin of three meridians, viz. spleen, liver and kidney at a time. It helps flush Ch'i and blood through the body. It is considered one of the best pressure points to regulate any female problem. Pregnant women should

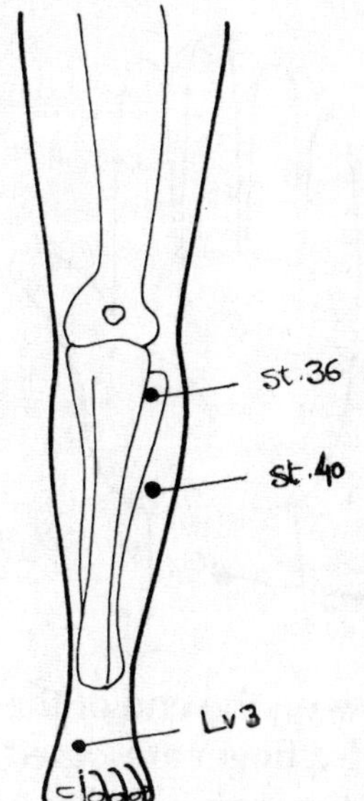

not press this point.

St 36, lies four finger widths below the kneecap, one finger width on the outside of the shin bone. This point strengthens the whole body, tones the muscles particularly in combination with Sp 6, it strongly revitalizes the entire body. It also quieten the rebellious Ch'i of the stomach, which causes nausea and vomiting

St 40 is located half way between the ankle bone on the outside of the foot and centre of the knee cap. Find the tibia and go two thumb widths off the bone to the outside. It is very helpful for reducing congestion. In case you feel that there is accumulation of lot of phlegm and mucus in your lungs, pressing this point will yield very good results in clearing the congestion which clouds the mind. This point is known for its capability of overcoming imbalance in Earth Energy.

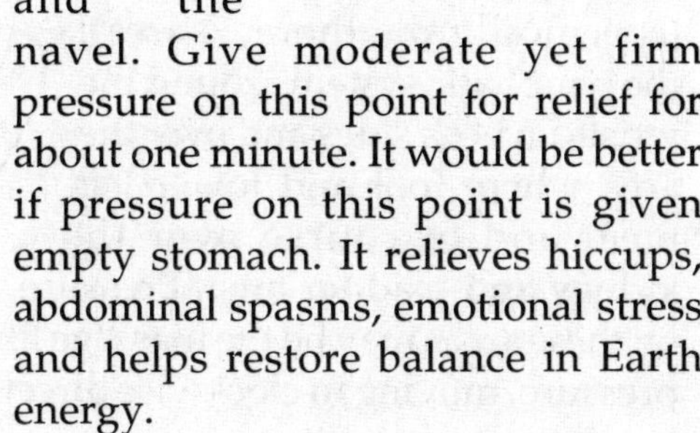

Cv 12 is midway between the notch at the bottom of the breastbone and the navel. Give moderate yet firm pressure on this point for relief for about one minute. It would be better if pressure on this point is given empty stomach. It relieves hiccups, abdominal spasms, emotional stress and helps restore balance in Earth energy.

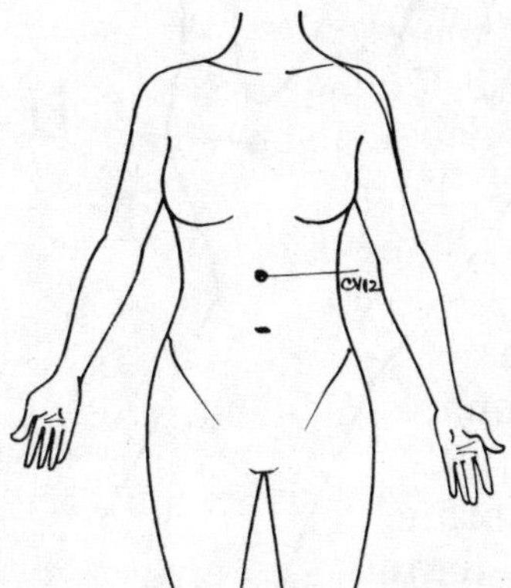

Lv3 lies between the big and second toes on the top of the foot. It regulates and tonifies the liver and

the flow of Ch'i in the liver meridian, which is considered to be the most powerful organ for detoxification. It improves the health of the gall bladder besides relieving nausea, vomitting, abdominal pain and distention.

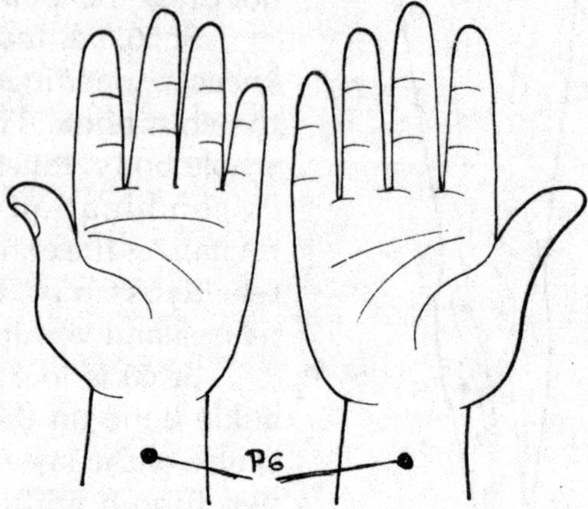

Li 4, known as 'Adjoining Valley', is known for its ability to relieve pain and help circulate the Ch'i. It lies on the end of the crease that is formed when the thumb and index finger are joined together. It stimulates elimination of toxins through bowels. A good point for improving overall intestinal function, including diarrhoea, constipation and abdominal pain. It relieves stagnation of the Ch'i too. Pregnant women should not use this point.

For treating this condition with the help of reflexology, focus on the following reflex points pertaining to all the areas of the digestive system, solar plexus, adrenal glands, the diaphragm, the spine (specifically the thoracic area), the lymphatic system around the wrists on both sides and over the area where foot and lower leg meet and of course over the kidney and bladder area. Pressure on these areas may be the massage like pressure, moving in clockwise direction, for about 2-3 minutes on each reflex area. The process should be repeated for some days and even twice a day in acute

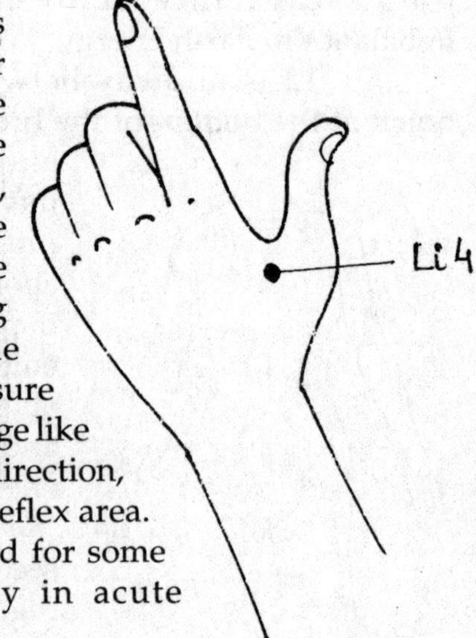

condition. For locating the areas to be worked on, look at the figures of palms and soles at the end of the book.

Q. 76: Can acupressure/reflexology help a knee pain condition?

A. 76: The knee joints absorb much of the body's weight when we stand or move. Persons engaged in sports activity or those who are overweight often suffer knee pain. Localised pain just below the kneecap may be a sign of patellar tendonitis. The knees are involved in some of the most common lower body injuries. Jumping may cause tearing of the tendon just below the kneecap or patella causing patellar tendonitis also known as jumper's knee. Knees may also suffer rupture of the cartilage in the knee joint between the femur and tibia. Excessive athletic activity may lead to tear of muscle fibres which may even result in accumulation of fluid in the muscle, causing pain, swelling and tenderness, etc. in the knee. Excessive jogging may also affect this joint adversely.

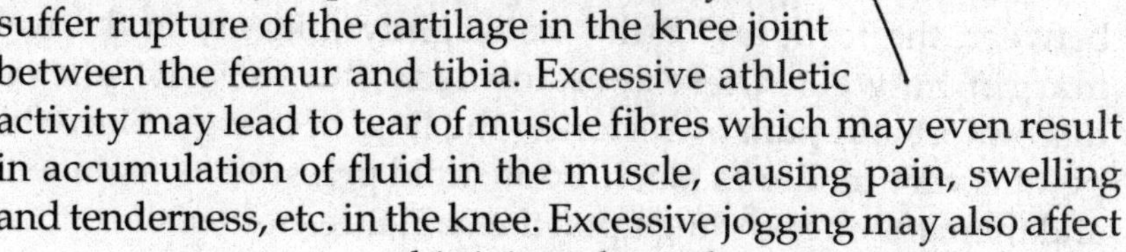

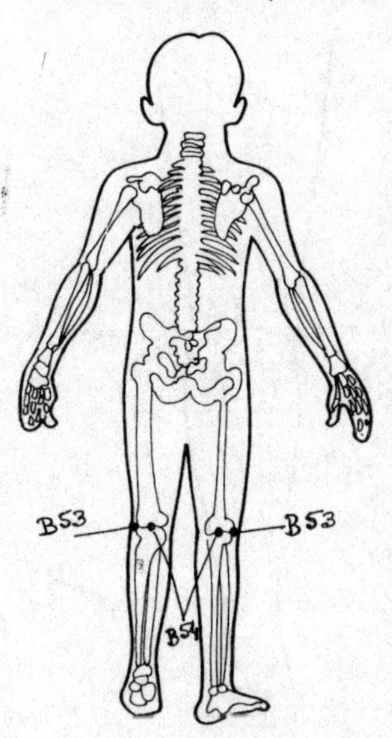

Both acupressure and reflexology can help overcome knee pain, reduce swelling and increase blood circulation in the knee area. Following schedule of pressure points will help:

Li 4, known as 'Adjoining Valley', is known for its ability to relieve pain and circulating the Ch'i . It lies on the end of the crease that is formed when the thumb and the index finger are joined together. It stimulates elimination of toxins through bowels. It relieves stagnation of the Ch'i too. Pregnant women should not use this point.

St 36, lies four finger widths below

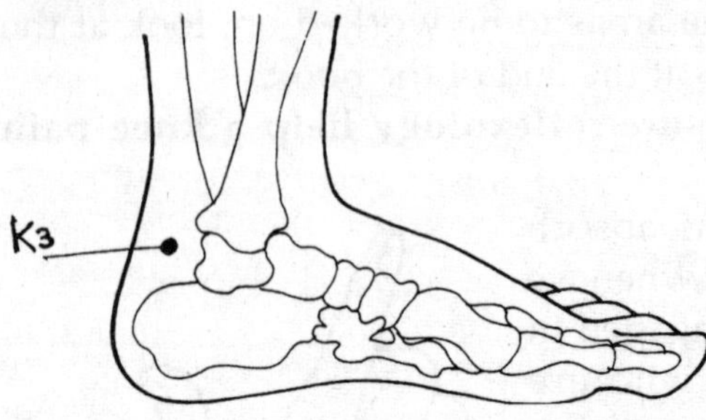

the kneecap, one finger width on the outside of the shin bone. This point strengthens the whole body, tones the muscles particularly in combination with Sp 6, it strongly revitalises the entire body. It also quiets the rebellious 'Ch'i' of the stomach. It also relieves knee pain.

Lv 2 known as 'Xingjian', lies at the junction of the big and second toes. This point stimulates Yin and sedates Yang. If possible try to give pressure on this point together on both the feet for better results.

Kd 3, lies midway between the inside of the ankle bone and the Achilles tendon in the back of the ankle.

GB 41'Falling Tears' is on the top of the foot, in the channel between the forth and fifth toes, slightly midway in the web margin between these toes towards the toes. It relieves discomfort and pain by restoring the flow of energy. Since this point is very tender to touch, apply mild pressure to begin with and thereafter depending upon the pain threshold of the patient gradually increase the pressure, hold and release gradually.

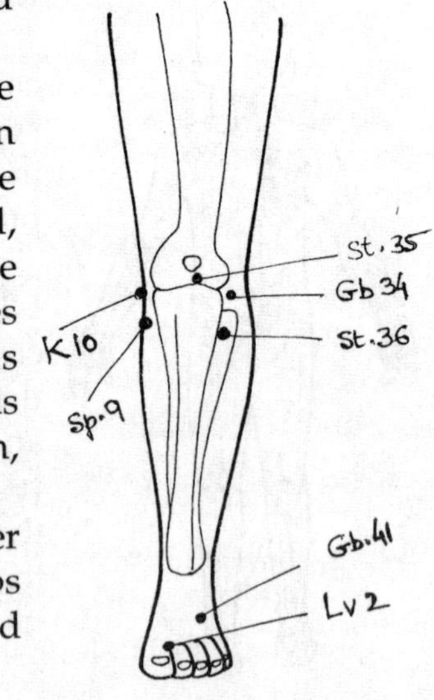

GB 34, called 'Sunny Side of the Mountain', lies in the depression below the bony prominence on the lateral side of the knee. Dispels wind, clears damp heat and stimulates the liver's Yin. Since liver Yin nourishes the joints, mobility of the joint is improved by giving pressure to this point. Relieves excessive knee pain, muscular strain etc.

St 35 'Calf's Nose', lies in the outer indentation below the kneecap. It helps reduce knee pain, stiffness and oedema.

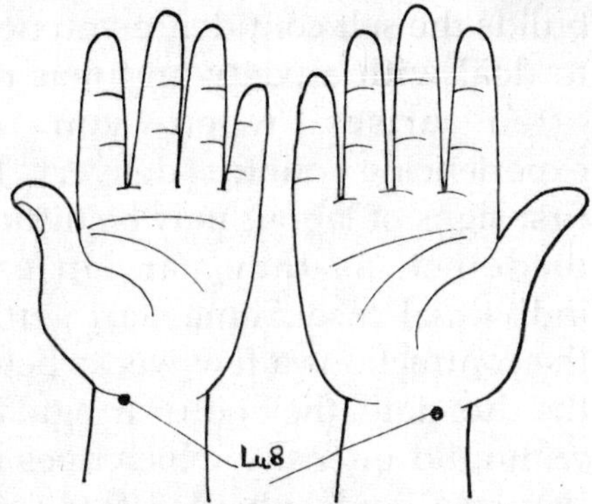

B 53 'Commanding Activity', is found on the outer side of the knee, at the end of the crease that is formed when the knee is bent. It helps overcome stiffness and pain in the knee.

B 54, lies in the middle of the back of the knee on the line formed (crease) when the knee is bent. This is a highly beneficial point for overcoming stiffness and pain in the knees as well as back. It is also very useful in alleviating sciatica pain.

K 10, known as 'Nourishing Valley', lies on the inner edge of the knee crease in the hollow between the two tendons. It helps relieve knee pain.

Sp 9, lies on the inside of the leg under the shin bone, just below the bulge. It helps in reducing oedema, water retention, swelling and other knee problems.

Lv 8 'Crooked Spring', is located on the inside of the knee, where the crease ends when the knee is bent. Relieves pain and swelling in the knees.

For treating this condition using reflexology, stimulate the reflex areas of the kidney, liver and spleen. Also stimulate the stomach and bladder reflex points. Giving pressure in the channel between the little and second toe on both the feet about a little less than half way on the dorsal portion of the foot and around the ankles on both anterior and posterior sides, on both the feet is highly beneficial. Also stimulating the area on the back of the knee and right below the patella bone about four finger widths below on the outer side, i.e. towards the little toe is considered to be highly beneficial. Stimulate these areas regularly, even twice a day in case you are doing it yourself for a couple of days to get maximum benefit.

Q. 77: What is meant by the term labour and delivery? Can acupressure help stimulating contractions and alleviate labour stress and pain?

A. 77: Participating in caring for yourself during labour builds the self confidence you need, to deal with anxiety and fear that often arises when you are experiencing your first delivery. The first signs of labour may be difficult to detect, as they vary in each individual case. Some start getting the contractions a few weeks before the due date, they occur irregularly with mild intensity which does not increase, and subside after some time. Active labour is indicated when the 'water breaks', this release of fluid that protects the baby can be just a trickle or a gush of fluid from the vagina. Other symptoms could be a light discharge of blood stained mucus or uterine contractions at a regular intervals.

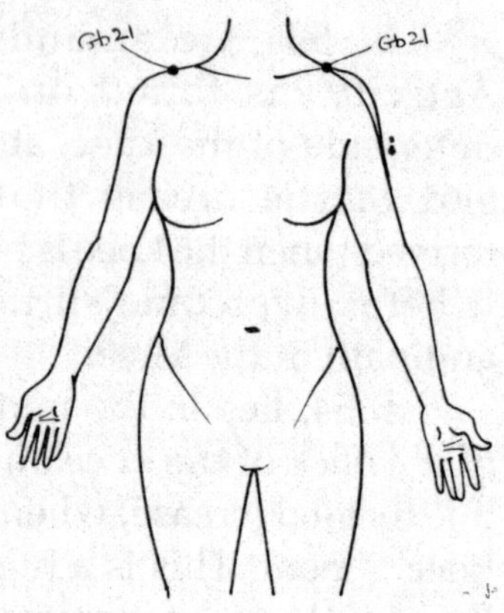

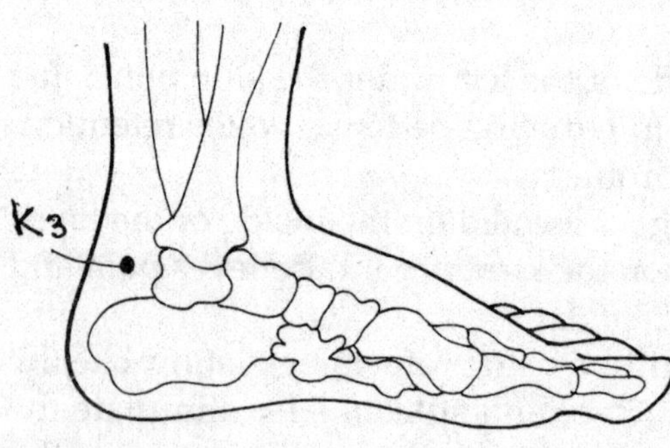

During normal delivery, the vaginal opening can be enlarged surgically, if necessary, by a procedure called episiotomy. In a Caesarean section, the baby is surgically removed from the womb. This procedure is generally used in an emergency when the life of the child or the mother might be at risk. Your doctor shall normally keep you informed about the status of your case and provide you with the information about all possible options.

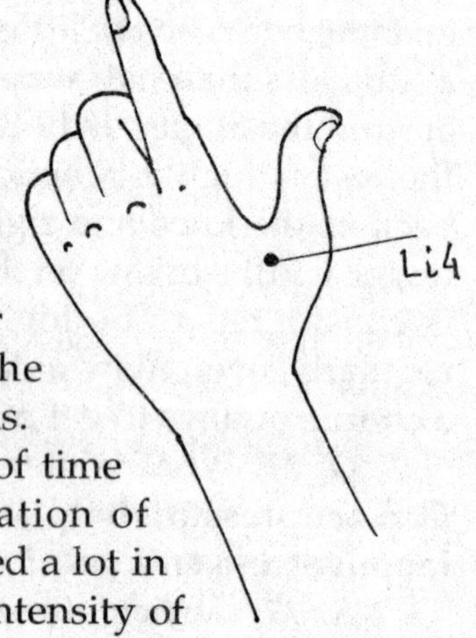

It has been seen over a period of time and in so many cases that stimulation of pressure points in certain cases helped a lot in increasing the regularity as well as intensity of

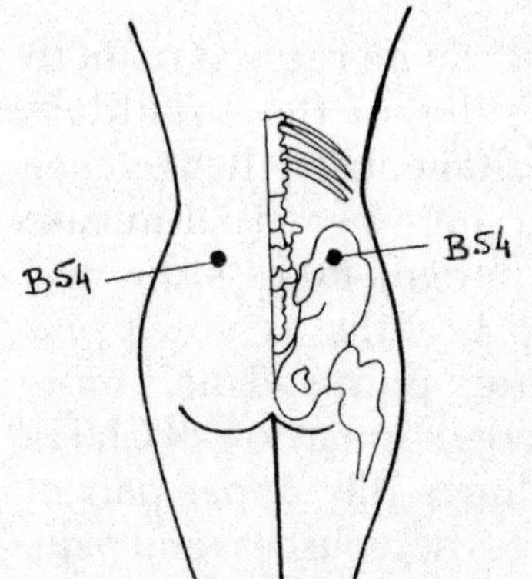

the contractions during labour, improved the confidence level of the mother-to-be by greatly reducing stress and giving relief from pain and exhaustion. The following is the effect of various pressure points shortly after they are introduced as part of the treatment to help labour:

B 67 located on the little toe of the feet just above the nail over the skin, press with firm pressure for about a minute, release gradually and press again. Repeat 3-4 times. This point is so effective that within no time the mother shall feel the baby drop into position. A highly effective point for difficult labour, capable of correcting the malposition of the foetus.

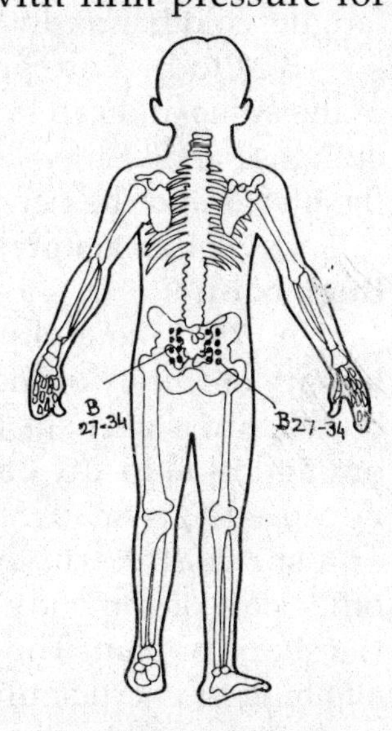

Kd 3 lies midway between the inside of the ankle bone and the Achilles tendon in the back of the ankle. It relieves labour pain, fatigue and back pain.

Li 4, known as 'Adjoining Valley', is known for its ability to relieve pain and help circulate the Ch'i . It lies on the end of the crease that is formed when the thumb and the index finger are joined together. It stimulates elimination of toxins through bowels. It relieves stagnation of the Ch'i too. This point brings in contractions and also helps alleviate labour pain.

Li 11

GB 21, known as 'Shoulder Well' is midway between the neck and the outer edge of the shoulder. This point is often found to be very tender. This

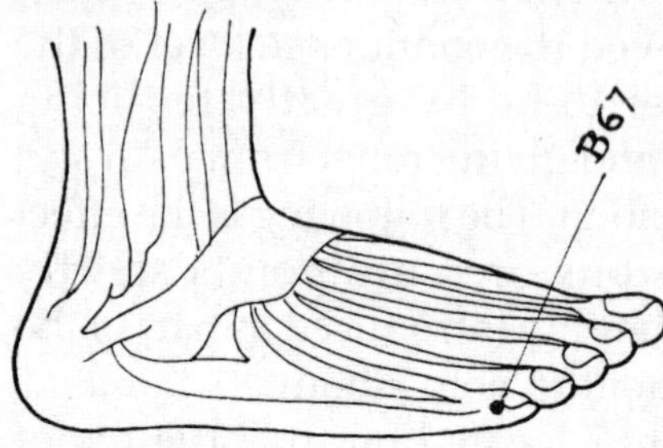

point can be pressed on both the sides of the shoulders simultaneously. It becomes even more beneficial in case the patient takes slow and deep breaths as you press various points. This points restores normal flow of Ch'i in the lungs (the upper part of the body). It assists childbirth and relieves nervousness and pain, fatigue, cold hands and feet.

B 27 to B 34 are pressure points located on the sacral part of the spine and can be managed even with the help of fists of both the hands either sitting or lying on your belly. It helps relax the uterus and the pelvic area to relieve pain during labour.

Q. 78: Can acupressure help overcome lower leg, hip and thigh pain?

A. 78: Like a child cries to draw attention when he is hungry or thirsty or there is some discomfort in any part of his body, pain is perhaps the expression of the body for drawing our attention to any part of it which needs attention. Pain can be caused by a small injury, by the pull or tear of some ligament or a sprain. Interrupted supply of blood to the brain or any other part of the body may also be expressed by our body in the shape of pain. The pain may be dull, throbbing, shooting, stabbing or excruciating type.

As we grow, it becomes a companion or a part of our life and at times people get so used to it that they learn to live with it. Leg, hip and thigh pain is also perhaps the most common form of pain we experience in our day-to-day life. It can be overcome without much effort or medication, in case it is being caused by any major injury to either of our bones or a big muscle tissue rupture where some medical intervention may become necessary. Acupressure can be of much help in overcoming routine sort of pains in legs, hip and thigh, as also alleviating pain caused due to some major injury as a result of some accident or fall, etc. The following pressure point regime shall be of help:

Li 4, known as 'Adjoining Valley', is known for its ability

to relieve pain and helps circulate Ch'i. It lies on the end of the crease that is formed when the thumb and the index finger are joined together. It stimulates elimination of toxins through bowels. It relieves stagnation of Ch'i too. Pregnant women should not use this point.

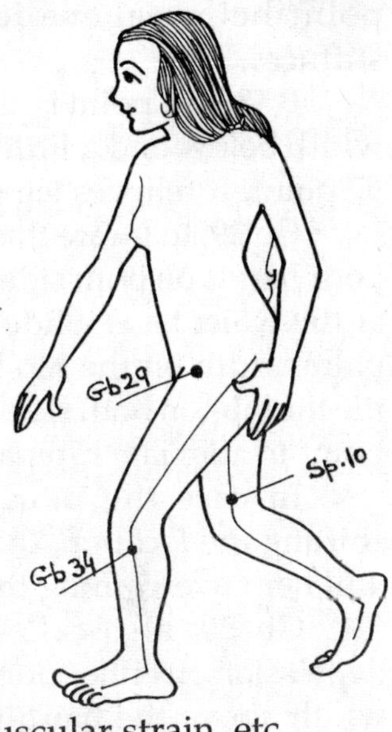

GB 34, called 'Sunny Side of the Mountain', lies in the depression below the bony prominence on the lateral side of the knee. Dispels wind, clears damp heat and stimulates the liver's Yin. Since liver Yin nourishes the joints, mobility of the joint is improved by giving pressure to this point. Relieves excessive knee pain, muscular strain, etc.

Gb 30, called the 'Jumping Circle', is the most important point for relieving hip pain. Stimulates circulation in the entire leg and lower back. This point can be found on the buttocks about one third of distance between the hip and tail bone. Needs to be pressed with sufficient pressure, if necessary with your elbow. Pressure should be given on both sides.

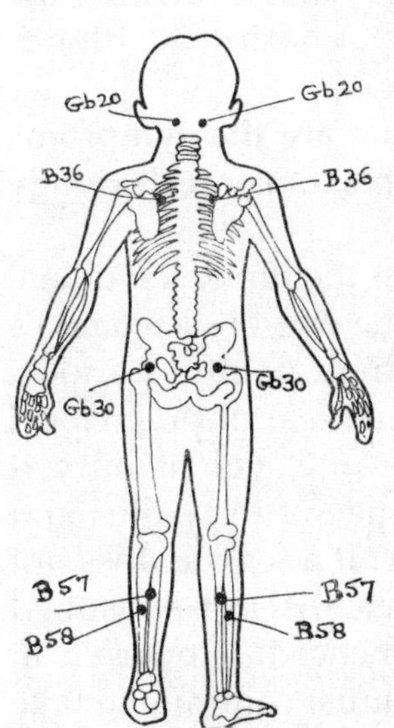

B 36, 'Receiving Support', is located on the back of the thigh just in the centre, below the buttock muscle. Pressure can be given on both sides at the same time with the help of thumbs. For taking self pressure lie down on your back with fists placed below this point and keep lying on the floor or hard bed for about 3 minutes.

B 57, 'Support the Mountain', is in the centre of the 'V' formed between the lower border of the calf muscle, almost half way between the ankle bone and the midpoint behind your knee. This pressure point helps relieve leg pain and stiffness.

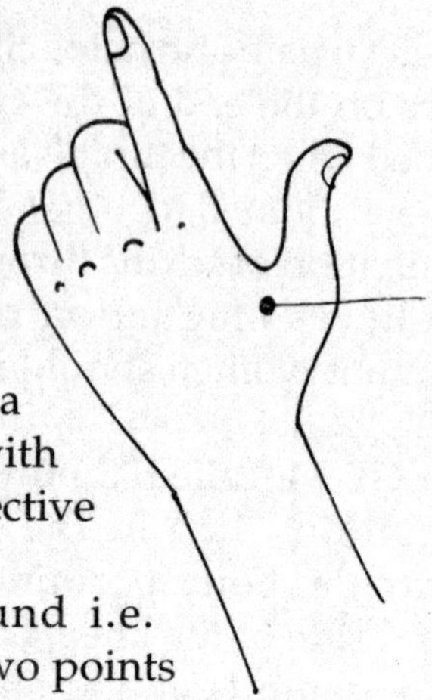

B 58, this point is about a thumb width below and a little outside of B 57 point. It relieves leg pain.

Gb 29, to locate this point, place your hands on both sides of your belt at the waist level. Slide down about a palm width on the hip bone. Press with the thumbs on both sides. Is a very effective point to alleviate hip pain.

In case the pain moves around i.e. shifting the location, the following two points will help overcoming the problem.

Gb 20, also called the 'Wind Pool', is located in the depression on either side of the vertebra of your neck, one thumb width above the hairline of the neck, at the base of the skull. Pressure can easily be given with the help of the thumbs of both the hands simultaneously. This point is very useful in relieving neck stiffness, headache, pain in shoulders/heaviness etc., and also regulating the internal movement of energy.

Sp 10, 'Sea of Blood' is found about two thumb widths above the knee on the bulge of the thigh muscle towards the anterior side. This points prevents stagnation of blood, particularly in the lower abdominal area.

Q. 79: What is menopause and what are the symptoms accompanying this condition? Can acupressure or reflexology help?

A. 79: This is the transition period in the life of a woman. Cessation of the monthly cycle signals the end of a women's fertile period and she attains freedom from painful periods, hassle of taking birth control measures and fear of pregnancy, etc. There is no hard and fast time frame, yet usually it commences any time after attaining the age of forty plus and may go up to early fifties in certain cases. If a female does not get her periods for up to six months at a stretch, it can be assumed that the process of menopause has commenced. However, in case one wants to avoid conceiving, she must continue to take some form of birth control measures until one full year passes without menstruation. The symptoms vary widely with various women. Whereas some have a comfortable passage of this transit period, others have symptoms like hot flushes, night sweats, vaginal dryness, mood swings, irritability and even depression at times. This is normally a gradual process with the changes associated with this condition taking place over a number of years.

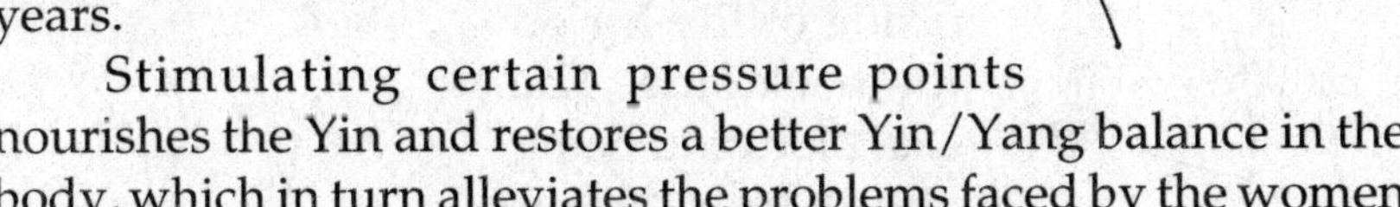

Stimulating certain pressure points nourishes the Yin and restores a better Yin/Yang balance in the body, which in turn alleviates the problems faced by the women

Pressure point therapy i.e. acupressure helps us to remove the cause of the pain by relaxing the muscles; release block of flow in energy channels, relieving the tension and improving the supply of much required oxygen to the brain cells. The following schedule will be found to be helpful:

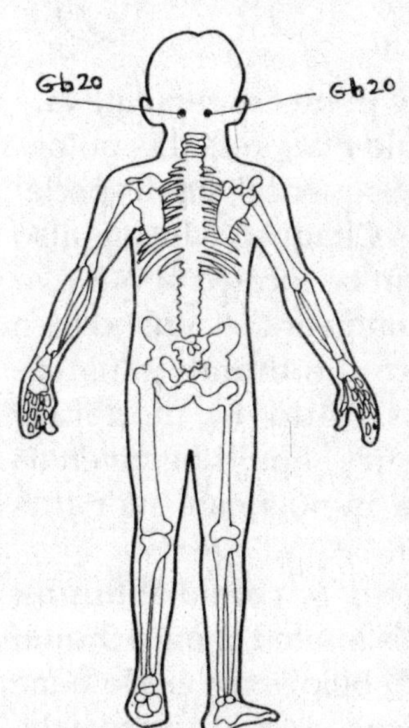

Li 4, known as 'Adjoining Valley', is known for its ability to relieve pain and help circulate the Ch'i. It lies on the end of the crease that is formed when the thumb and index finger are joined together. It stimulates elimination of toxins through bowels. It relieves stagnation of Ch'i too. Pregnant women should not use this point.

GB 20 is located in the hollow below the base of the skull. Steady pressure (mild to moderate) should be given on this point simultaneously on both the sides. Its effect goes well with its name, i.e. 'Gates of Consciousness'. Is an extremely beneficial point to overcome stiffness in the region of the

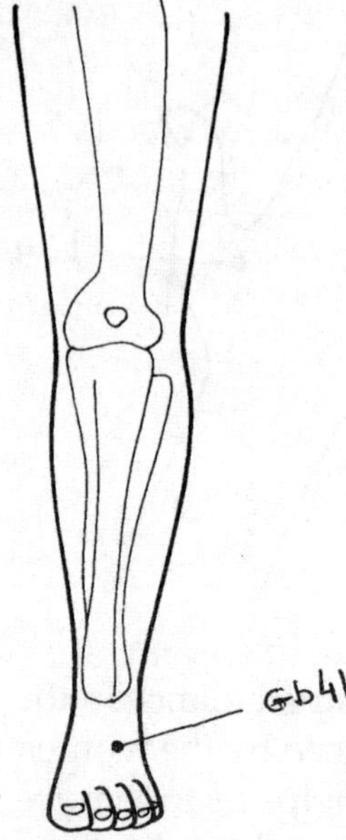

neck. It also eliminates wind and cold.

GB 41 is located between the fourth and fifth metatarsal bones on the top of the foot. For giving firm pressure on this point you have to slide your index or middle finger upwards, pressing just below the juncture. This point restores the flow of Ch'i, and relieves headache of menopause.

Sp 6, also called 'Three Yin Meeting Point', is located above the ankle bone towards the inside of the leg on the back side. The exact location being about four finger widths above the ankle bone. It is one of the most important pressure points as its name itself suggests since it strengthens the Yin of three meridians viz. spleen, liver and kidney at the same time. It helps flush Ch'i and blood through the body. It is considered one of the best pressure points to regulate any female problem. Pregnant women should not press this point.

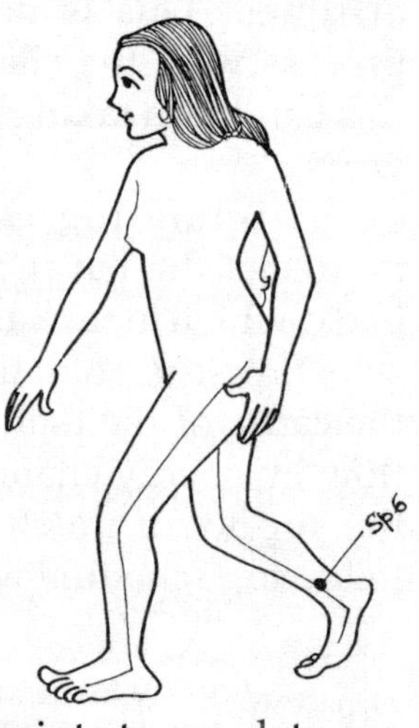

Lu 7, known by the name 'Broken Sequence', has a special function. It opens the Conception Vessel Channel, which is also known as the 'Sea of Yin'. This point can be located about two finger widths above a natural depression near the wrist crease where the thumb joins the wrist. Mild to moderate pressure should be given as there is no flesh over this point.

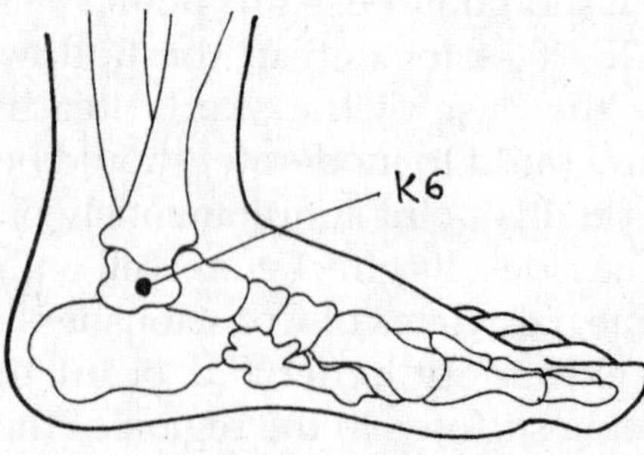

Kd 6, called 'Shining Sea', is located about a thumb width below the ankle bone (big toe side), towards the

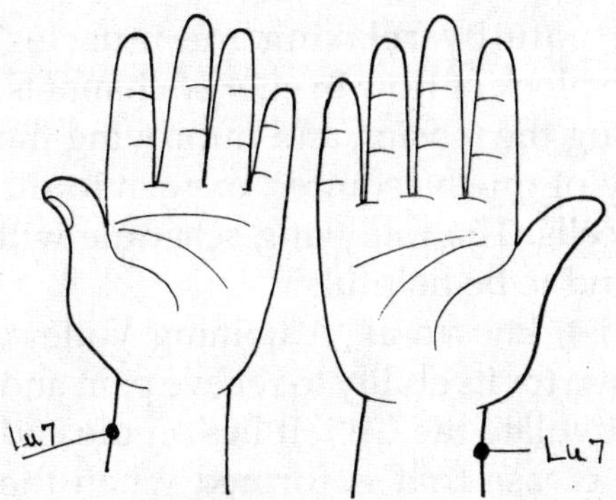

sole of the foot. Apply firm pressure. Because stagnation of kidney Yin is involved in menopause symptoms, pressing this point helps strengthen it. This is also helpful in opening 'Sea of Yin', if pressed after Lu 7.

While treating this condition using reflexology, stimulate reflex areas pertaining to the pituitary, uterus, adrenals, lymphatic system, kidney and bladder, ovaries, fallopian tubes, solar plexus, liver, spine, heart, brain, thyroid and parathyroid. Give pressure in clockwise movement on all the points except thyroid. Refer to the figures of palms and soles at the end of the book for location of reflex areas.

Q. 80: Can acupressure or reflexology be of any help in mitigating migraine? What are the symptoms accompanying this condition?

A. 80: A migraine is an extremely painful condition, which is at times only on one side of the head and is often accompanied with nausea, vomitting and visual disorders. Amongst its causes could be heredity , particular sort of food that does not go well with the system of the patient, and overexposure to sun or bright light can also trigger the condition. Besides stress and strain and erratic food habits (both content and timing) could be some other contributing factors. This condition, at times, requires professional medical intervention. However, acupressure and reflexology can be safely used in conjunction with medical intervention.

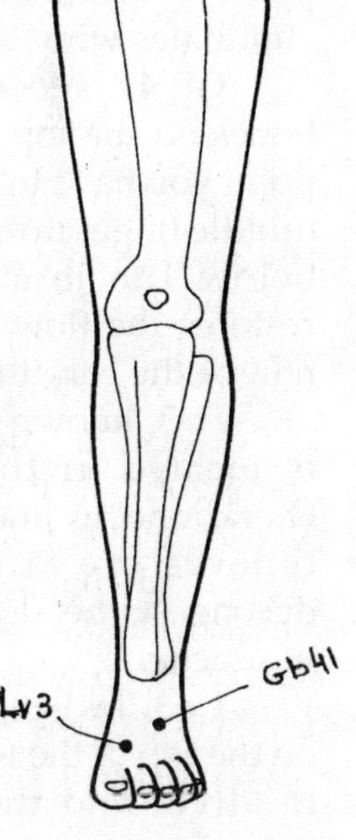

Pressure point therapy, i.e. acupressure helps us to remove the cause

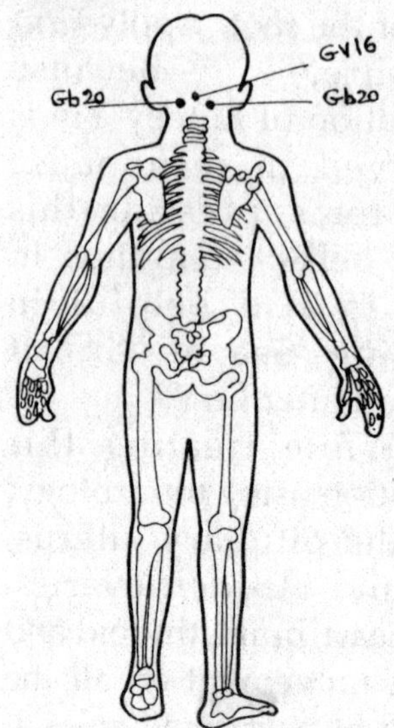

of the pain by relaxing the muscles, release block of flow in energy channels, relieving the tension and improving the supply of much required oxygen to the brain cells. The following schedule will be found to be helpful:

Li 4, known as 'Adjoining Valley', is known for its ability to relieve pain and help circulate the Ch'i. It lies on the end of the crease that is formed when the thumb and index finger are joined together. It stimulates elimination of toxins through bowels. It relieves stagnation of the Ch,i too. Pregnant women should not use this point.

GB 20 is located in the hollow below the base of the skull. Steady pressure (mild to moderate) should be given on this point simultaneously on both the sides. Its effect goes well with its name, i.e. 'Gates of Consciousness'. It is an extremely beneficial point to overcome stiffness in the region of the neck. It also eliminates wind and cold.

GB 41 is located between the fourth and fifth metatarsal bones on the top of the foot. For giving firm pressure on this point you have to slide your index or middle finger upwards, pressing just below the juncture. This point restores the flow of Ch'i, and helps relieve the condition.

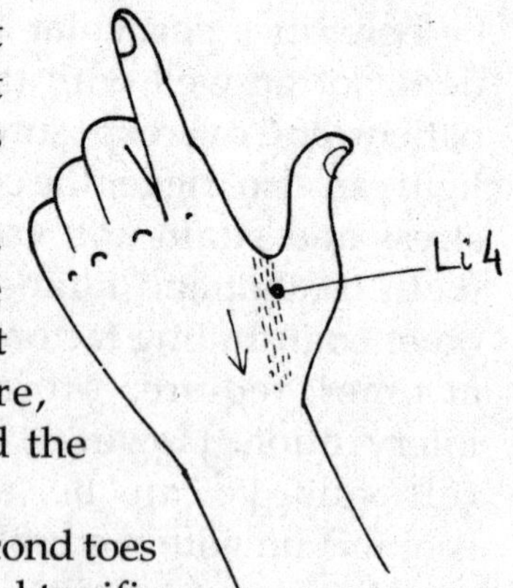

St 3, known as 'Facial Beauty', is located at the bottom of the cheekbone, in line with the pupil. It relieves eye fatigue and pressure, decongests head and eye strain and the headache.

Lv 3, lies between the big and second toes on the top of the foot. It regulates and tonifies the liver and the flow of Ch'i in the liver

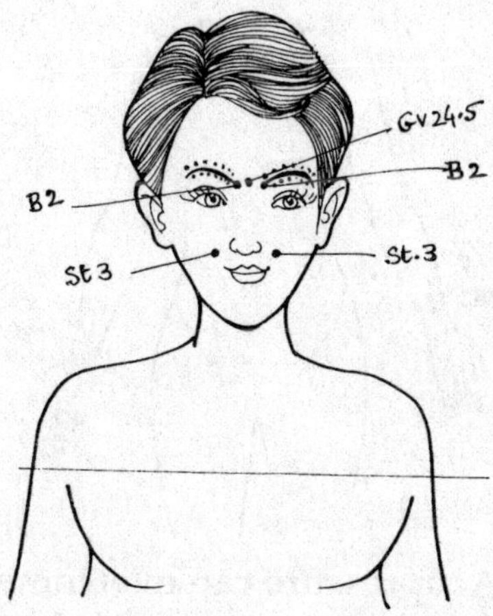

meridian, which is considered to be the most powerful organ for detoxification. It improves the health of the gall bladder besides relieving nausea, vomiting, abdominal pain and distention.

GV 16, 'Wind Mansion' is located in the centre of the back of the head in the hollow under the base of the skull. It relieves mental stress and insomnia.

B 2, 'Drilling Bamboo', lies in the indentation over the bridge of the nose between the eyebrows. It relieves, eye fatigue/pain and headache.

GV 24.5, 'Third Eye Point', between the eyebrows where the eyebrows and the bridge of the nose meet. This point balances the pituitary gland, headache and eye strain.

For healing this condition using reflexology, the reflex areas of the following organs/components of the body need to be stimulated giving thumb pressure for a period of 2-3 minutes on each reflex point. The areas to be worked upon are the head and brain, neck, adrenals, pituitary, lymphatic system, entire area of the digestive system, the spine (falling in the area of the big toe in particular), solar plexus, diaphragm, eyes, kidney and bladder. Also give pressure all over the eye brows starting from the bridge of the nose where eye brows start and going to the end till the temple bone pinching the eyebrows between the thumb and index finger. Giving clockwise movement if possible over the flesh area between the thumb and index finger. This area will hurt wherever you come across knot like formations. As these knots dissolve, the intensity of pain shall decrease and so shall the frequency of pain.

Q. 81: Can acupressure help in conditions like morning sickness and motion sickness?

A. 81: Many medical disorders, e.g. stomach ulcers, gastritis, diabetes, meningitis and even chemo-therapy given during the treatment of various cancers can induce nausea.

Morning sickness in pregnancy and motion sickness while travelling can also cause this condition. The person suffering from these conditions feels low and feels like vomitting. This condition is aggravated when tension accumulates in the stomach and obstructs proper abdominal circulation.

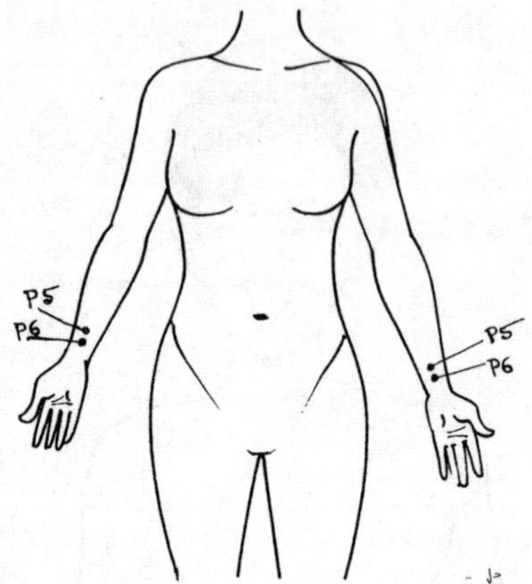

This leads to stress on the digestive system and related organs, that makes you feel sick. Acupressure can overcome this problem successfully within no time. Research has confirmed this line of action, both in respect of morning sickness in pregnancy, chemotherapy induced nausea, as well as problems arising out of motion sickness. As on date many doctors of conventional medicine have started adopting this non-conventional technique in overcoming this condition and many other conditions using pressure point therapy.

The following schedule of pressure points shall be found to be of immense help:

Pc 6, is known by the name 'Inner Gate', and it is located on the palm side of the wrist, about three finger widths above the wrist crease in the centre of the arm. It helps relieve IBS (nausea in particular-in pregnant women, in Chemotherapy patients, and even in sea going voyagers) by its calming effect.

St 36, lies four finger widths below the kneecap, one finger width on the outside of the shin bone. This point strengthens the whole body, tones the muscles particularly in combination with Sp 6, it strongly revitalises the entire body. It also quieten the rebellious Ch'i of the stomach, which causes nausea and

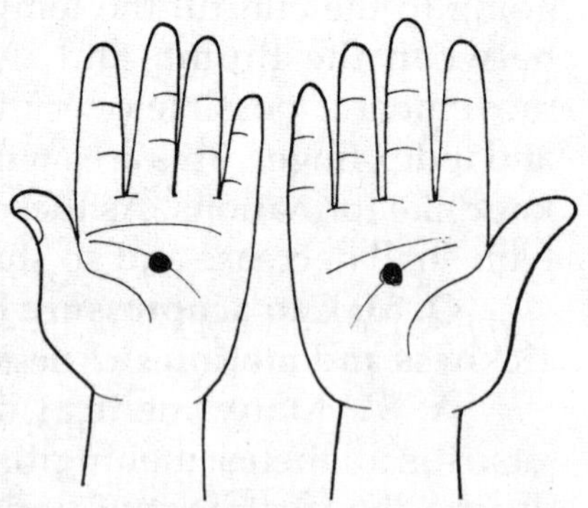

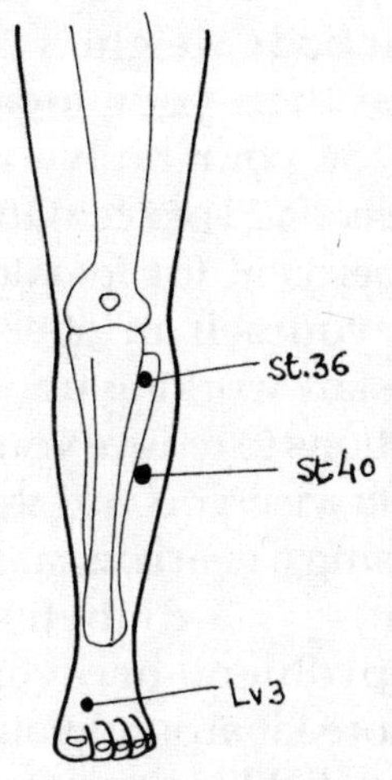

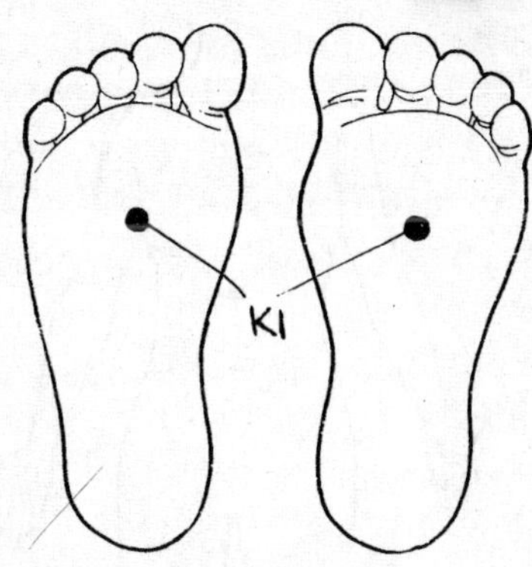

vomitting.

St 40 is located half way between the ankle bone on the outside of the foot and centre of the kneecap. Find the tibia and go two thumb widths off the bone to the outside. It is very helpful for reducing congestion. In case you feel that there is accumulation of too much phlegm and mucus in your lungs, pressing this point will yield very good results in clearing the congestion which cloud the mind.

P 5 is located four finger widths above the centre of the inner wrist crease, between the tendons. It relieves stomach upset besides nausea and vomitting.

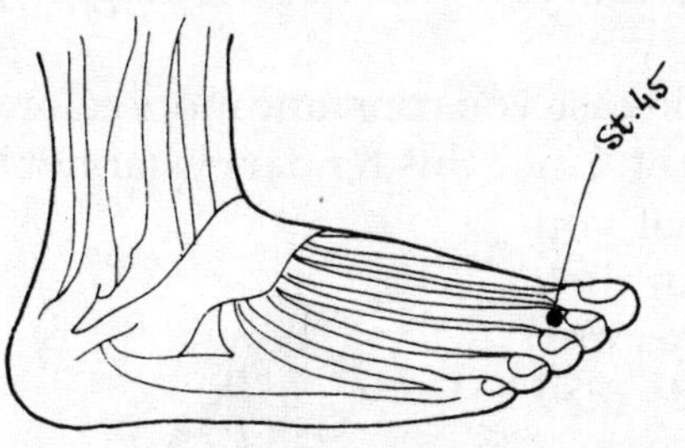

St 45, 'Severe Mouth' is located on the outside of the base of the nail of the second toe. It relieves nausea, indigestion, food poisoning and abdominal pain.

Lv 3, lies between the big and second toes on the top of the foot. It regulates and tonifies the liver and the flow of Ch'i in the liver meridian, which is considered to be the most powerful organ for detoxification. Pressing this point helps control damage caused to the gall bladder and liver meridians by excessive physical exertion, which could result in nausea, cramps and spasms.

Q. 82: What is obesity and what are the underlying causes? Can this condition be taken care of by acupressure or reflexology?

A. 82: Your ideal weight depends upon your height, age, sex (male or female) and the type of activity you are involved

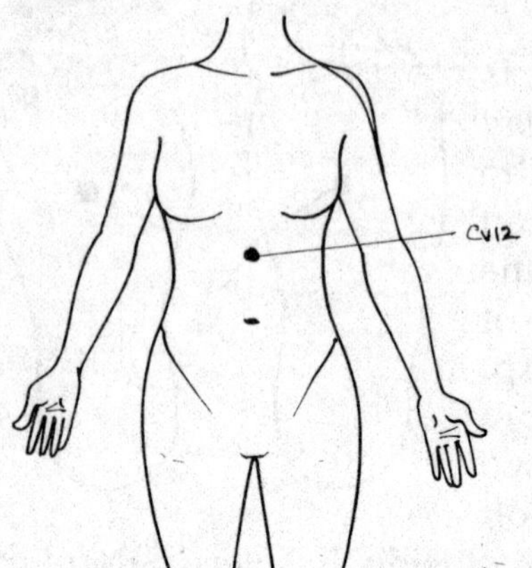

in. In case your body weight is 20 per cent more than your ideal body weight or your body fat percentage exceeds 25 per cent for male and 30 per cent for female, you can rate yourself in obese category and start working upon all possible options to reduce your weight as otherwise you run the risk of developing a heart disease, hypertension, diabetes, respiratory problem or even cancer. Particularly, if your body tends to store fat around your waist, unlike fat around the thighs. A more reliable measuring system is the BMI, the body mass index, which determines obesity based on the body fat content rather than the weight. You may be the same height and weight as someone considered to be obese, but in case you have thick bones and a lot of muscle and comparatively less body fat, you will not be diagnosed obese.

The simple theory is that in case you consume more calories than you burn, you gain weight. Since this tendency cannot be changed, you must realise that you have to be cautious about your diet, exercise in particular, besides any medical interference your body may require depending upon your condition.

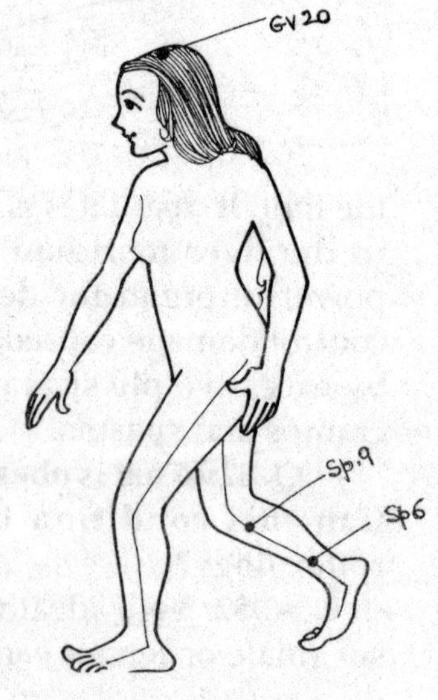

The causes behind this condition are primarily diet, insufficient exercise, heredity, besides thyroid problems. At times even diabetes leads to weight gain or loss. Certain drugs also attribute to obesity as a side effect. In addition to these factors, a recent study has shown that muscles as well as fat cells play a vital role in obesity. Your

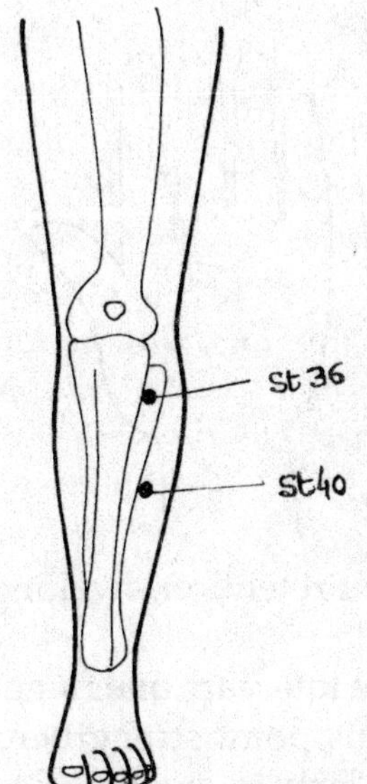

muscles become more efficient and burn lesser calories when you try to lose weight. In yet another study the findings were that 95 per cent of the people on a weight loss diet regained weight they had lost if it did not include exercise as a part of their programme. Though fat and fibre content in your diet play a major role, nothing is as important as exercise.

Therefore, you should think in terms of permanent change which you can continue and follow up rather than taking up crash control programmes and regaining weight the day you shun that programme. Draw out a programme in consultation with your doctor who will prescribe a good schedule of your calorie intake comprising of low fat, low sugar and high fibre diet for a long term and you shall have to maintain that level. To this add an exercise programme to your weekly routine. It is felt that a 30 minute walk at lunch, if morning walk is not possible shall be enough and effective.

Alternative therapies, e.g. acupressure and reflexology work well if practised as a complement to existing exercise and diet programme. Follow the following schedule of pressure point therapy in addition:

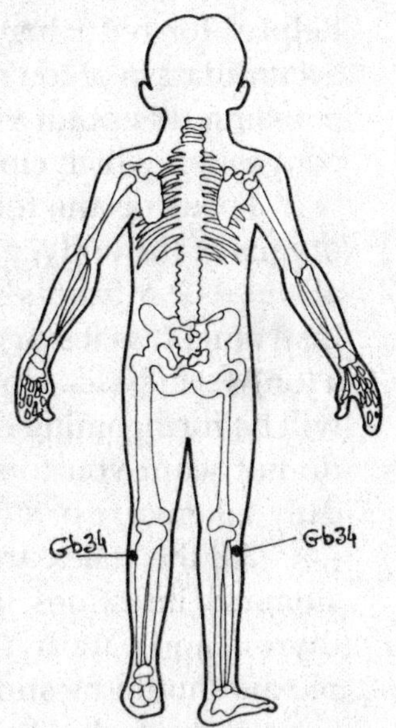

Sp 6, also called 'Three Yin Meeting Point', is located above the ankle bone towards the inside of the leg on the back side. The exact location being about four finger widths above the ankle bone. It is one of the most important pressure points as its name itself suggests since it strengthens the Yin of three meridians, viz. spleen, liver and kidney at the same time. It helps flush Ch'i and blood through the body. It is considered one of the best pressure points to regulate any female problem. Pregnant women should not press this point.

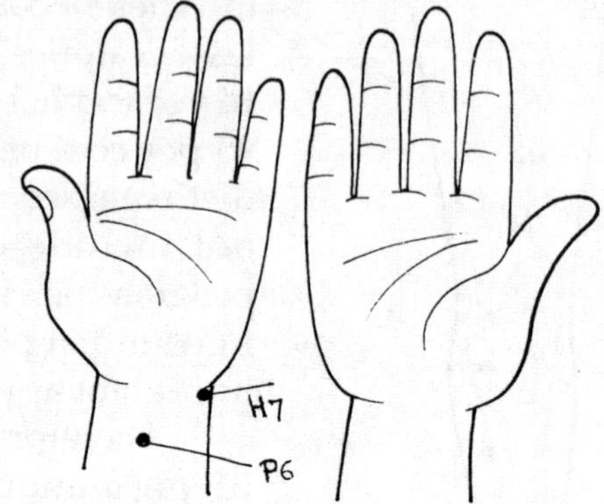

Sp 9, lies on the inside of the leg, under the shin bone, just below the bulge. It helps in reducing odema, water retention, swelling and other knee problems.

St 36, lies four finger widths below the kneecap, one finger width on the outside of the shin bone. This point strengthens the whole body, tones the muscles particularly in combination with Sp 6, it strongly revitalizes the entire body. It also quietens the rebellious Ch'i of the stomach

St 40 is located half way between the ankle bone on the outside of the foot and centre of the kneecap. Find the tibia and go two thumb widths off the bone to the outside. It it is very helpful for reducing congestion. In case you feel that there is accumulation of too much of phlegm and mucus in your lungs, pressing this point will yield very good results in clearing the congestion which cloud the mind.

Focus on the following reflex areas pertaining to various organs of the body, giving pressure on each area for a period of about 1-2 minutes with the help of your thumb or some instrument, as it suits you, for help in shedding some weight on a long term basis. However, as already stated above, the results will be forthcoming only if diet is controled (balanced diet); we do not want you to starve, and the exercise elements are also duly taken care of :

All the reflex areas related with the digestive system, e.g. stomach, intestines, liver, pituitary, adrenals, kidneys, bladder, thyroid and parathyroid, pancreas, lymphatic system and solar plexus should be stimulated. Refer to the figures of palms and soles at the end of the book for location of reflex areas.

Brisk rolling on the foot roller for 3 minutes (both morning and evening) shall help you reduce weight up to 2-3 kgs per month. See Q.9 for detailed description.

Q. 83: What is osteoporosis? Can acupressure be of any help in this condition?

A. 83: Osteoporosis means, 'porous bone'. It is a condition that causes the bone(s) to weaken gradually and in the process they become prone to fractures. Although bones of the entire body get affected yet the most affected are those of hip, spine and wrists. In elderly people hip bone fractures are very common. It generally gives way at the neck of the femur. Prolonged immobility often leads to bed sores which further complicates the issue.

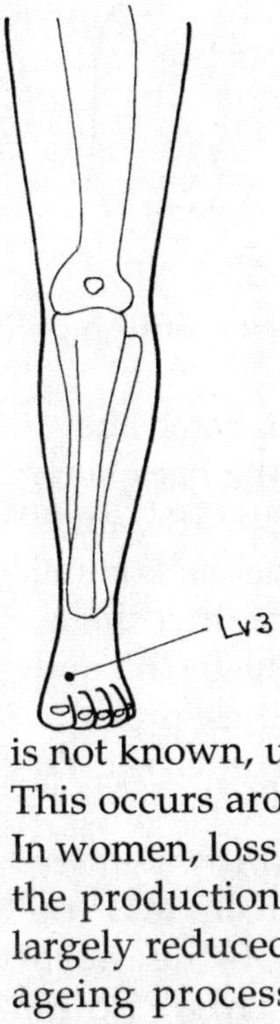

Lv3

Studies have revealed that women are more prone towards this disease because of the factors that their bones are lighter and as their body undergoes hormonal changes, particularly after menopause, loss of bone mass perhaps accelerates. In men the incidence of this ailment is comparatively much lesser.

Whereas the exact cause of this disease is not known, usually bones begin to lose calcium, the essence. This occurs around the age of 35-40 years in most of the cases. In women, loss of bone density, takes place after menopause, as the production of estrogen that keeps calcium in the bones is largely reduced. Though some loss in bone density is a part of ageing process, in certain women this disease is owing to heredity factor too. Women who get their ovaries removed for some reason before the age of forty years are at a greater risk of developing this condition. According to the findings of a research study, women whose hair turn more than 50 per cent grey before attaining the age of 40 years are almost four times more prone to this disease as compared to others.

Diseases like kidney problems or hyperthyroidism that effect the body's ability to absorb calcium also cause osteoporosis. Since osteoporosis is a condition which is difficult to reverse, the best alternative is prevention which is quite possible with the help of alternative therapies, e.g. acupressure and reflexology. Pressure in this condition has, however, to be given with utmost caution since the bones become very weak and excessive pressure may cause a fracture, particularly when giving pressure in the region of wrist or spine, etc.

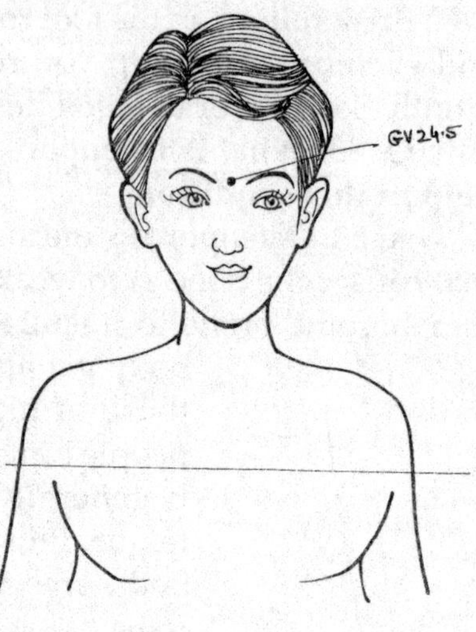

Press the following acupressure points for prevention of this condition much before it takes place:

Sp 6, also called 'Three Yin Meeting Point', is located above the ankle bone towards the inside of the leg on the back side. The exact location being about four finger widths above the ankle bone. It is one of the most important pressure points as its name by itself suggests since it strengthens the Yin of three meridians, viz. spleen, liver and kidney at a time. It helps flush Ch'i and blood through the body. It is considered one of the best pressure points to regulate any female problem. Pregnant women should not press this point.

GV 24.5 'Third Eye Point', between the eyebrows where the eyebrows and the bridge of the nose meet. This point balances the pituitary gland, which in turn stimulates and corrects the functioning of the thyroid gland also.

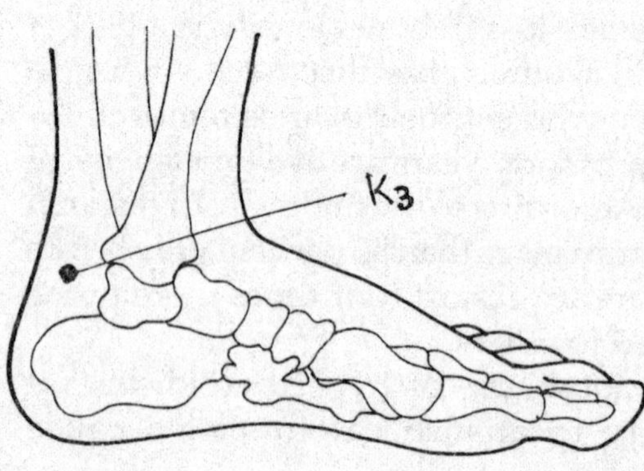

Lv 3, lies between the big and second toes on the top of the foot.

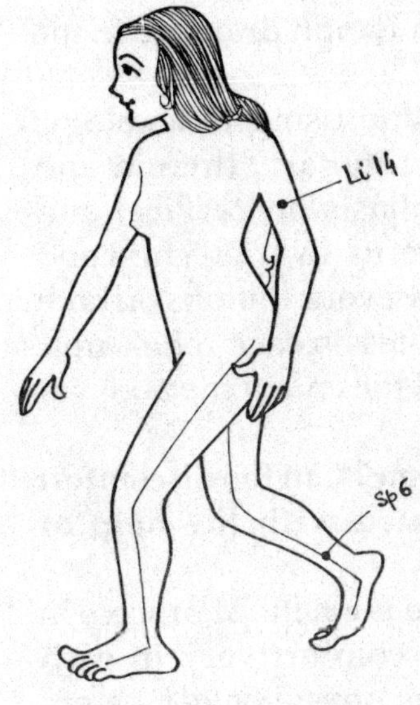

It regulates and tonifies the liver and the flow of Ch'i in the liver meridian, which is considered to be the most powerful organ for detoxification. It improves the health of the gall bladder.

Li 4, known as 'Adjoining Valley', is known for its ability to relieve pain and circulating the Ch'i. It lies on the end of the crease that is formed when the thumb and the index finger are joined together. It stimulates elimination of toxins through bowels. It relieves stagnation of the Ch'i too. Pregnant women should not use this point.

Kd 3, lies midway between the inside of the ankle bone and the Achilles tendon in the back of the ankle. It helps overcome sexual tensions, menstrual irregularity besides stimulating the kidneys.

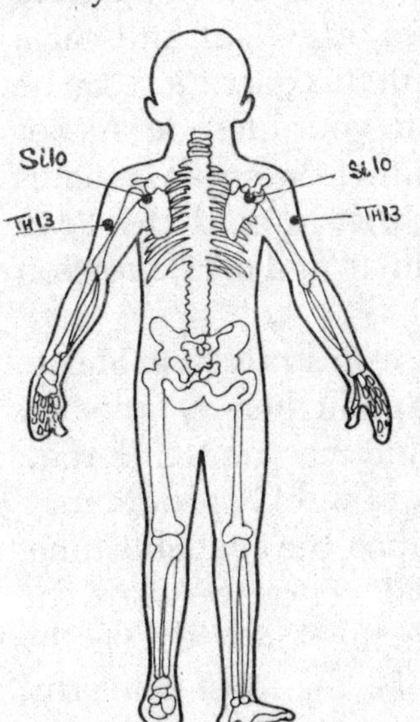

TH 13, lies on the back of the upper arm, directly below the shoulder. It takes care of problems related to the thyroid gland, infections of the lymph passages in the neck, throat or armpit area. Helpful in prevention of the condition in question.

SI 10 is found in line with SI 9, below the upper edge of the shoulder blade. It helps in lymph drainage problems in the neck and throat area.

LI 14 is about 7 thumb widths above the LI 11 on the outside of the upper arm. It is useful in problems with lymph drainage in the neck, throat or armpit, etc.

For the prevention of this condition using reflexology, concentrate on the reflex areas of the pituitary, thyroid and parathyroid, spine (with special emphasis on cervical and thoracic area), adrenals, solar plexus, uterus, ovaries, chest and lungs etc., giving pressure with the help of your thumbs on both soles and palms for a period of 1-2 minutes on each reflex area. Refer to the figures of palms and soles at the end of the book for location of reflex areas

Q. 84: What is premenstrual syndrome? Can the discomfort and associated conditions be alleviated with the help of acupressure or reflexology?

A. 84: As we know, menstrual cycle is a natural process in women and the associated pain or discomfort vary in each individual, both psychological as well as physiological, before the beginning of the cycle. The symptoms of premenstrual syndrome (PMS) include irritability, depression, lack of concentration, tenderness in the breast(s), mood swings, and weight gain or fluid retention. Though most of the women accept this as a part of their life, those who have poor diet or live a sedentary lifestyle (lack of exercise) suffer more as compared to those who are regular with their walks/exercises and eat a balanced diet. Discomfort associated with this condition can be greatly overcome by some adjustments in your lifestyle. As per the TCM, the entire liver meridian including the organ initiates the menstrual cycle. As such the culprit behind the PMS symptoms is imbalance in the Liver meridian and the stagnation of Liver Ch'i.

With a view to balance the imbalance, in addition to above, in case you follow the following pressure point therapy schedule and/or reflexology schedule, you will find that life is different. You can adopt this schedule as part of your weekly programme at least 3 to 4 times a week, depending upon the available time.

Lv 3, lies between the big and second toes on the top of the foot. It regulates and tonifies the liver and the flow of Ch'i in the liver meridian, which is considered to be the most powerful organ for detoxification. Pressing this point shall overcome the

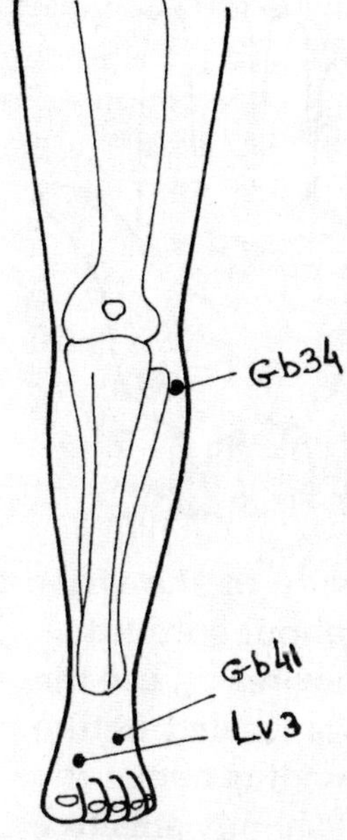

root cause and provide much relief.

Sp 6, also called 'Three Yin Meeting Point', is located above the ankle bone towards the inside of the leg on the back side. The exact location being about four finger widths above the ankle bone. It is one of the most important pressure points as its name itself suggests since it strengthens the Yin of three meridians viz. Spleen, Liver and Kidney at the same time. It helps flush Ch'i and blood through the body. It is considered one of the

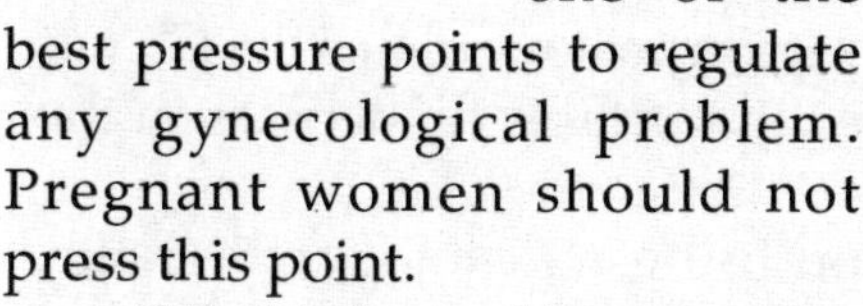

best pressure points to regulate any gynecological problem. Pregnant women should not press this point.

GB 41 is located between the

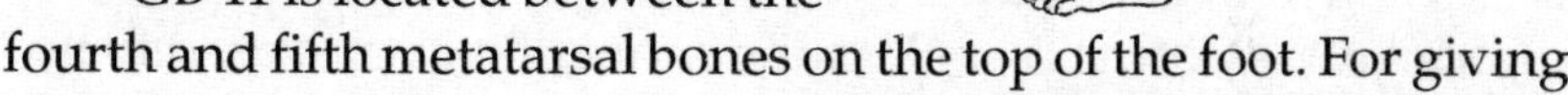

fourth and fifth metatarsal bones on the top of the foot. For giving firm pressure on this point you have to slide your index or middle finger upwards, pressing just below the juncture. This point restores the flow of Ch'i, and helps relieve the condition.

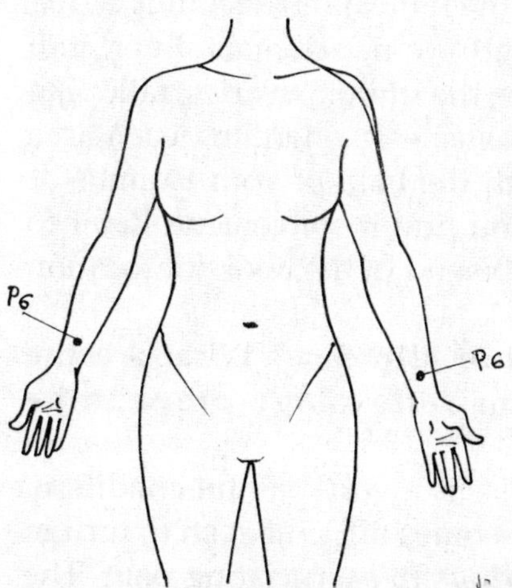

GB 34, called 'Sunny Side of the Mountain', lies in the depression below the bony prominence on the lateral side of the knee. Dispels wind, clears damp heat and stimulates the Liver's Yin. Since Liver yin nourishes the joints, mobility of the joint is improved by giving pressure to this point. It relives excessive knee pain, muscular strain, etc.

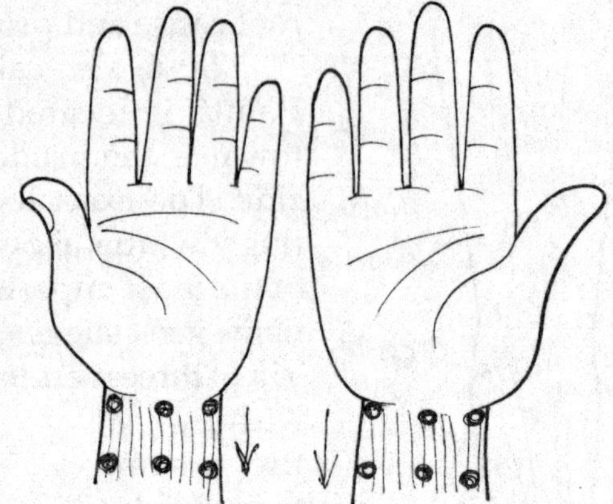

TW 5, called the 'Outer Gate' is located midway between the ulna and radius bone about three finger widths above the wrist crease towards the elbow bone on the outside of the wrist (back side). Give pressure on this point for about a minute.

In case there is excessive tenderness in the breasts, use the pressure point Pc 6, 'Inner Gate'. This point is located on the palm side of your wrist, about three finger widths above the wrist crease and in the centre of the arm. Pc 6 is highly effective for any sort of pain in the chest region as it regulates the Ch'i of blood as well as in the chest area that causes tenderness in the breasts.

For attending this condition using reflexology, the reflex areas of the organs falling in the digestive, nervous and reproductive systems as well as the endocrine glands need to be focused upon. For doing so, press the reflex points relating to the pituitary, pancreas, thyroid, parathyroid, adrenals, liver, gall bladder, large and small intestines, the uterus, ovaries, fallopian tubes, spine, kidney, the solar plexus, etc., attending each area for about one to two minutes with the help of your thumbs or index or middle finger the way you find it convenient. Refer to the figures of palms and soles at the end of the book for location of specific reflex areas.

Q. 85: What is a prolapse or slip disc? What are the symptoms? Can acupressure or reflexology prove to be beneficial in this condition?

A. 85: A prolapsed or slip disc is a very painful condition. The pain is so agonizing that it becomes difficult even to turn in the bed. Coughing or sneezing brings in excruciating pain. The patient is forced to confine to the bed. Ignoring this condition is not only difficult but impossible, but in case you do, it could lead to permanent damage and may even lead to paralysis.

The inter vertebral discs are actually flexible pads that are tightly fixed between the vertebrae that make the spinal column. Each is a flat, circular capsule made of a tough fibrous outer membrane. The discs are firmly embedded between the vertebrae and are held in place by ligaments. There is literally little room for them to slip or move. The point on which the vertebrae actually turn are called the facet joints, which stick out like arched wings on either side of the vertebrae and keep the vertebrae from bending or twisting far enough to damage the spinal cord. At times these discs are also called the shock absorbers for the spine. These discs also keep the vertebrae separate to prevent any damage through rubbing over each other. However, with ageing they begin to harden as the blood supply to these discs is considerably reduced. Under stress, at times the inner material either swells or herniates, pushing through the outer membrane of the disc. All or part of the material actually protrudes through the outer casing at a weak spot, causing pressing against the surrounding nerves. Further activity or injury may rupture or tear the membrane, the disc material may injure the spinal cord or the nerves that radiate from it. Such damage may be irreversible. While not all herniated discs press on nerves, it is possible for a person to have deformed discs without pain or discomfort.

This condition is usually caused by everyday activities e.g. lifting heavy weight the wrong way, stretching too hard, playing or even lifting phone receiver in a wrong lying position, jerking during an accident or as a result of jumping from some height. The problem may, however, at times appear without any apparent cause. Obesity also puts excessive strain on the spine and the ligaments that hold the discs in place.

Acupressure or reflexology treatment in conjunction with conventional medical treatment, which is generally based on rest and painkillers, has been found to be highly effective in this condition. Merely a few sessions provide relief in the pain to the extent that the patient is about 30 to 40 per cent relieved.

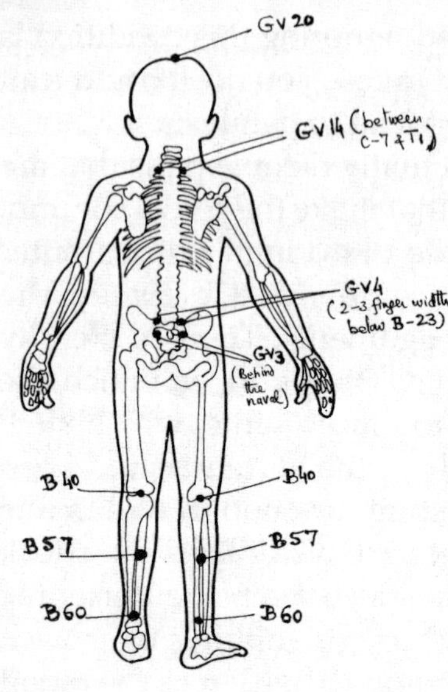

The following pressure points will be beneficial:

GV3, is located over the lower spine, just below the fourth lumbar vertebrae. Feel for the upper edge of the pelvic bone and locate this point at that area of the spine. Give pressure on this point for about a minute in clockwise direction with the help of your thumb. Thereafter you can give massage, like pressure with the pad of your palm for another minute of two. This point should not be stimulated in case the woman is pregnant.

GV4, This point is located between the second and third vertebrae directly behind the belly button. Press it with moderate to strong pressure with the help of your thumb on the midline of the spine about a thumb width on either side.

GV14, is located between the seventh cervical vertebrae and the first thoracic vertebrae and can be easily located by tilting your head downwards. The most prominent bone on the back (below your neck) when you bend your head is the seventh vertebrae. Press between C 7 and T 1 with moderate yet firm pressure for about a minute.

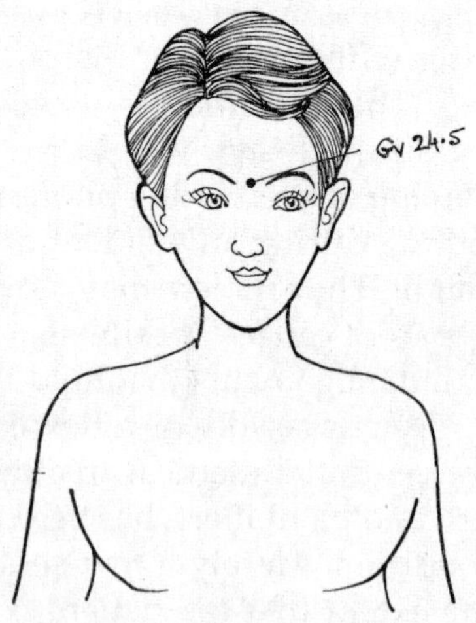

GV20, is located on the top of your head, midway along an imaginary line connecting the upper part of the ears. Give pressure using your thumb or index finger. Avoid pressure on this point if you are suffering from hypertension.

GV 24.5, 'Third Eye Point', is

between the eyebrows where the eyebrows and the bridge of the nose meet. This point balances the pituitary gland, which in turn stimulates and corrects the functioning of the thyroid gland also. Mild to moderate pressure may be given on this point for about 30 seconds.

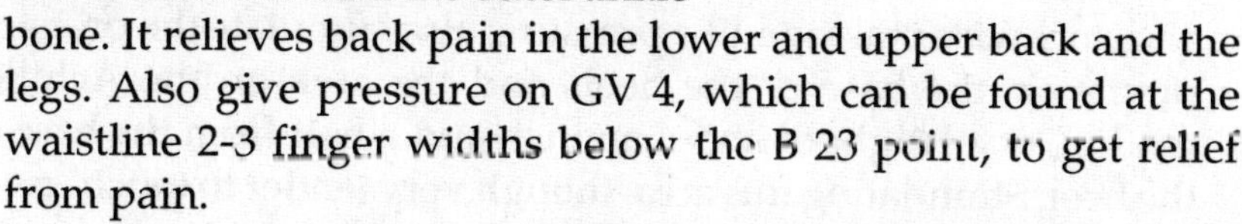

B 60, lies half way between the Achilles tendon and the outer ankle bone. It relieves back pain in the lower and upper back and the legs. Also give pressure on GV 4, which can be found at the waistline 2-3 finger widths below the B 23 point, to get relief from pain.

Since one may find it difficult to heal himself by giving pressure on the points which are on the back, pressure on the following points, on the back of the hand, may be given which have been found to be extremely beneficial.

Li 4, known as 'Adjoining Valley', is known for its ability to relieve pain and circulating the Ch'i. It lies on the end of the crease that is formed when the thumb and index finger are joined together. Pregnant women should not use this point. Just half inch above and below this point, there are two more points which are highly beneficial in relieving back pain. Apply sufficiently strong pressure on these points with the help of the thumb of the other hand. Repeat the process on the other hand. Two more extra points lie on the back of the hands. First between the second and third finger bones and the second between the fourth and fifth finger bones, half way between the knuckles and the wrist. In case you find that the pain comes back, repeat the process for some sessions, as it may take

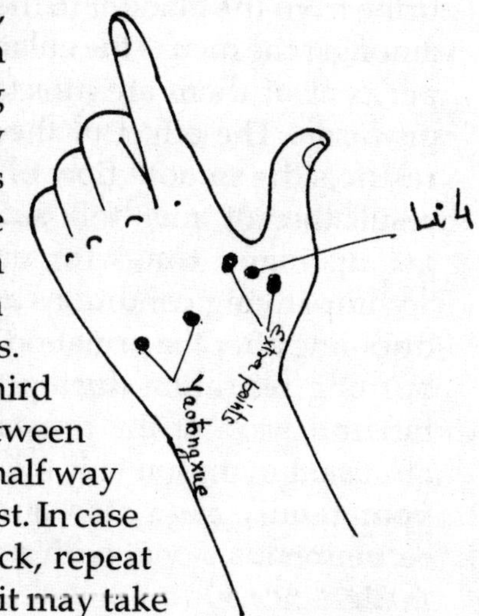

some time to be fully cured.

B 40, 'Middle of the Crook', is a very helpful point for relieving pain the lower back region, it is located in the back of you knee, right in the centre between the two tendons and on the crease that is formed when you bend your knee. This point is also called the 'Command Point' because of its powerful influence on all the lower back problems.

For attending this condition using reflexology, the reflex areas of the organs falling in the reflex area of the spine (the lumbar and sacral region in particular), behind the crease of the knees, on both sides of the ankle bones give clockwise and anticlockwise massage-like pressure; also stimulate the pressure points on the base of the heels and the area on the Achilles tendon, at a height of about an inch and a half from the base of the heel. Stimulating this area, though very tender to touch, gives immense relief. Refer to the figures of palms and soles at the end of the book for location of specific reflex areas.

Q. 86: Can acupressure or reflexology help resolve the prostate problem?

A. 86: Prostate is a gland located midway between the scrotum and anus, below men's bladder. It produces and secretes fluid that accompanies the sperm, protecting it on its way to the cervix. It surrounds the urethra, the tube that carries urine from the bladder to the penis. The most common problem amongst the men is the enlargement of this gland and at least 50 per cent of them are affected by it in the age group of 45-50 onwards. The effect of the enlarged prostate gland is that it restricts the smooth flow of urine through the urethra and as a result thereof, men folk suffering from this condition have to get up many times for urinating during the night. Other accompanying conditions are slow urination, difficult to start, dribbling after the urination or at times this is accompanied with burning sensation during urination. These conditions signal inflammation of the prostate. In case you have either of the aforesaid symptoms, it would be wise to get it checked from your family physician and get the tests, etc., what ever he recommends done, with a view to rule out the possibility of malignancy.

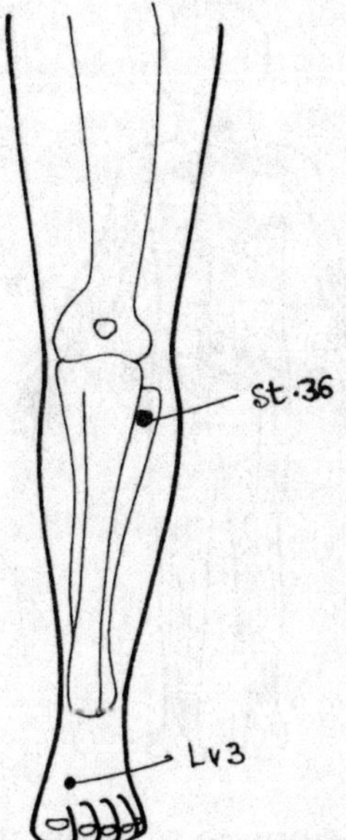

Attending this condition using acupressure or reflexology in conjunction or even with either method shall be found to be highly beneficial. Press the following pressure points:

Lv 3, lies between the big and second toes on the top of the foot. It regulates and tonifies the liver and the flow of Ch'i in the liver meridian, which is considered to be the most powerful organ for detoxification. Pressing this point shall overcome the root cause and provide much relief.

Sp 6 also called 'Three Yin Meeting Point', is located above the ankle bone towards the inside of the leg on the back side. The exact location being about four finger widths above the ankle bone. It is one of the most important pressure points as its name itself suggests since it strengthens the yin of three meridians viz. spleen, liver and kidney at the same time. It helps flush Ch'i and blood through the body

St 36, lies four finger widths below the kneecap, one finger width on the outside of the shin bone. This point strengthen the whole body, tones the muscles particularly in combination with Sp 6, it strongly revitalises the entire body. It also quiets the rebellious Ch'i of the stomach.

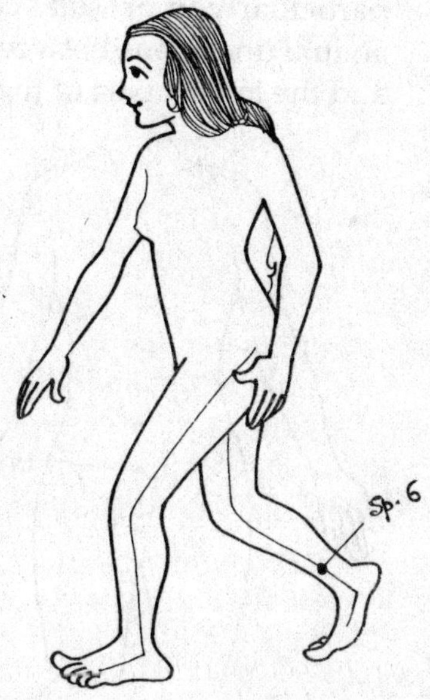

Next point to be pressed is CV 3 this point is about one thumb width below CV 4 'Gate Origin', which is located four finger widths below the belly button or the navel. It is almost specific in its effect on the bladder meridian. It would be better and more effective if steady

pressure on this point is given for about a minute after emptying the bladder.

B 28 is an associated point of urinary bladder and is about one and a half inches on either side of the spine, in the mid sacral area of the back. Spend several minutes stimulating CV 3 and B 28 which are almost specific to urinary bladder.

B 23 can be located in the middle of the waist, half way between the rib cage and the hip bone on the inner edge. It relieves depression and fear. Has a positive effect on sexual reproductivity organs and as such helps alleviate conditions, e.g. prostate, impotency and premature ejaculation, etc.

To handle this condition using reflexology, stimulate the reflex areas relating to the kidneys, adrenals, ureters, etc. There are two more areas to be stimulated which are highly beneficial particularly in prostate condition, to loctate these points make an imaginary line between the lowest bottom of the ankle bone and the lowest part of the heel and bisect this line into two. The point of intersection is the area to be stimulated. Repeat the process on the other side of the foot and stimulate the area which will be very tender to touch but is very effective. Give pressure on these points on both the feet by slowly moving the pad of your thumbs in this area as deep as possible for a period of about one minute or so. Thereafter stimulate the areas about 4-5 inches above the base of the

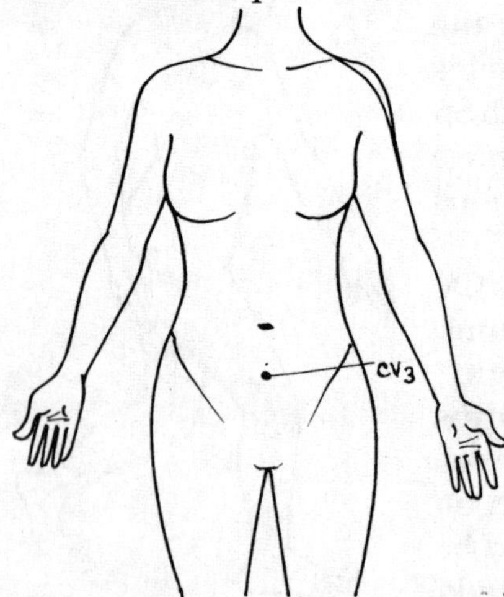

heel on the back side along the Achilles tendon. Give massage-like pressure on the entire area holding the Achilles tendon between your thumb and index finger. Stimulate this entire area for about 1-2 minutes on both the feet to get maximum benefit. Refer to the figures of palms and soles at the end of the book for location of specific reflex areas.

Q. 87: What causes sciatica? Can acupressure or reflexology help this condition?

A. 87: A majority of sciatica or lower back problems are accompanied by severe pain in the back or sides, most of the times radiating from hip joint region towards the ankle bone. Sometimes the situation is so aggravated that the patient finds it difficult to move the foot and is accompanied by excruciating pain in the entire leg. Most of the sciatica problems have stress, improper posture, injury or weak muscles as their underlying cause. Since back muscles and ligament strain are also amongst the probable causes, it would be better to keep our spine and back muscles strong as well as flexible, which can be easily done with a little bit of light exercising as a routine even thrice a week.

Sciatica is often caused by a ruptured or a slipped disc in the lower lumbar area. When the injured disc presses against the sciatic nerve, a burning pain radiates through the buttocks and down the thigh. The two sciatic nerves are the largest nerves in the body, running down each leg from the lower spine, where a network of nerves branches out from it on either side. For this reason, you may find that the reflex point on one foot is more tender and sensitive than the reflex point on the other side.

Acupressure has been found to be tremendously effective for relieving the stress and strain of the muscles which is the underlying cause of sciatica condition. The impact of pressure points can be increased by the use of heating pads or a hot water bottle (if there is no inflammation), in conjunction with acupressure for their lasting effect. Pressure on the following pressure points shall be found effective:

B 40, 'Middle of the Crook', is a very helpful point for relieving pain of the lower back region. It is located in the back of your knee, right in the centre between the two tendons and on the crease that is formed when your bend your knee. This point is also called the 'Command Point' because of its powerful influence on all the lower back problems.

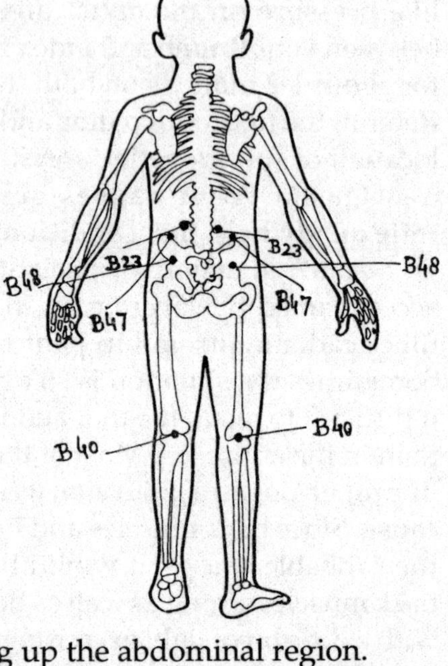

B 23 can be located in the middle of the waist, half way between the rib cage and the hip bone on the inner edge. It relieves depression and fear. Has a positive effect on sexual reproductivity organs and as such helps alleviate lower back pain, sciatica and fatigue caused owing to the severe pain.

CV 6, 'Sea of Energy', lies three finger widths below the navel. This point is considered to be a 'special point' for toning up the abdominal region.

B 47, lies in the middle of the waist four finger widths outside of the spine. These points, not only provide relief in the low back pain but also reduce muscle tension, fatigue, depression and fear as also alleviate sciatica pain in association with B 23 point.

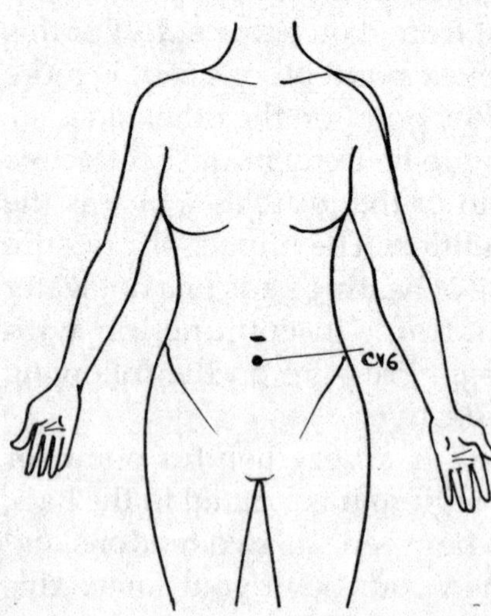

B 48 can be found about 1-2 finger widths outside the sacral region, midway between the top of the hip bone and the base of the buttocks. It relieves sciatica, hip pain, lower back pain and tension in the region.

Using reflexology to help overcome this condition, we shall have to work down the spine reflex area particularly in the lumbar and sacral regions to make sure that there

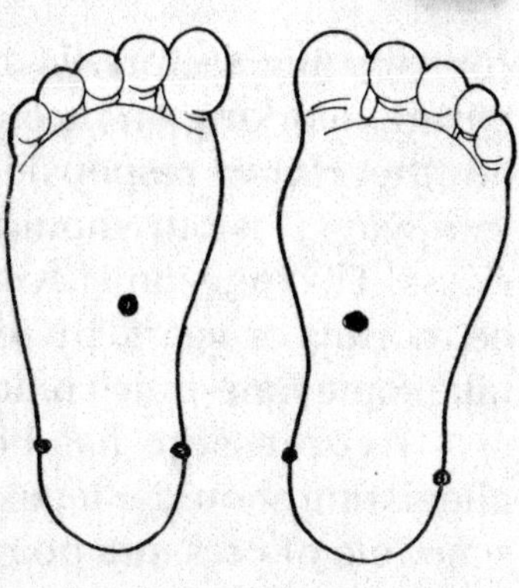

are no pinched nerves. Using both the thumbs, work simultaneously on both the sides, since the sciatic nerve comes down the spine. Concentrate working on the waistline down to the heels to send the healing forces to all the inflamed and strained parts of the lower lumbar region. Next job on hand is to find out the reflex where the sciatic nerve crosses the foot. This point is located on the base of the heel pad. This area of the foot corresponds to the sciatic nerve pressure point in the buttock. You will experience a sharp pain on pressing this area. However, it would be better to use an instrument to give pressure/stimulation to this part of the heel due to its thickness as thumb pressure may not be sufficient. Once you have located the sciatic reflex, work on it with a deep rolling motion, to your pain threshold. Ease up the pressure and roll gently to overcome the tenderness you might have developed. Thereafter work between the hip and buttock reflexes. Beginning with the foot on the outside with the thumb walking across the foot, working over the point where the sciatic nerve crosses the heel. This area will also be tender to touch therefore, work on them with caution and gentleness. Work on the lumbar and sacral reflex areas of the spine too; these you will find in the lower arch of the foot on both the feet. Look at the figures of soles at the end of the book for identifying the specific reflex areas.

Q. 88: Can acupressure/reflexology help alleviate shoulder tension/pain?

A. 88: Pain is a fact of life. It may be due to an injury, a result of hectic activity at home or during the course of the day due to driving or because of some weight you might have lifted during the day, a sprain or it may come from within the body owing to ill health or trouble within some organ, etc. It could as well indicate the overall emotional and physical state, due to which at times there is stiffness in the shoulder or neck area. Stressful lifestyle or emotional strain may also be the contributing factors. Working on computers for long hours, typing, working on machines/desks, watching television may be other factors responsible for pain or tension in the shoulders. In a way, it is our shoulder that take most of our tension and stress. This tension is accumulated over a period of time, may be months or years. By releasing shoulder tension, which may take some time, much relief can be felt in the arms and the hands.

Acupressure has been found to be highly effective in alleviating shoulder tension/pain. Follow the below mentioned schedule of pressure points to overcome this problem:

Li 4, also known by the name 'Adjoining Valley' is located at the crease of the mound that pops up when the thumb and index finger are joined together. Pressure on the left hand can be given by the right hand and on the right hand by the left hand thumb and index finger. This is considered to be one of the most effective acupressure and acupuncture points to relieve headache and pain in other parts of the body, to relax muscles and it also balances the flow of energy in the lower and upper part of the body. It also activates the bowel movement. Pregnant women should not press this point as it can cause miscarriage.

Li 11, known as 'Pool at the Crook' it is located at the outside end of the crease that is formed in case we bend our hand to touch our shoulder. Give pressure on both hands with the help of opposite hands. This point becomes very tender on pressing therefore utmost caution has to be exercised while pressing this point, which is very useful in clearing the excess heat and dampness from the body and also pain in the elbow, arm and shoulders. It is also an important point to combat allergy and to treat tennis-elbow.

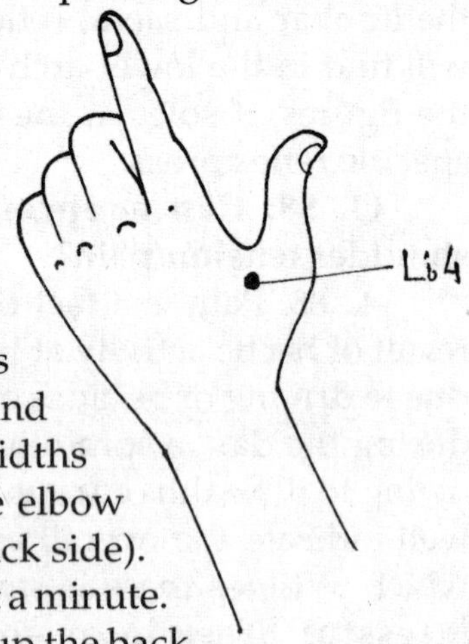

Li4

TW 5, called the 'Outer Gate' is located midway between the ulna and radius bone about three finger widths above the wrist crease towards the elbow bone on the outside of the wrist (back side). Give pressure on this point for about a minute. The 'Triple Warmer Channel' runs up the back of the arm to the shoulder and neck, then moves around to the side of the neck. This point is extensively used to treat any type of problem with the arm, shoulder and neck.

TW 10, 'Heavenly Well' is located one thumb width directly above the tip of the elbow, towards the shoulder. It helps relieve elbow pain, stiffness in the elbow and the shoulder. Press for about a minute with your thumb or middle finger firmly then release gradually. Deep breathing simultaneously shall further improve the effect of this point.

Gb 20, also called the 'Wind Pool' is located in the depression on either side of the vertebra of your neck, one thumb width above the hairline of the neck, at the base of the skull. Pressure can be easily given with the help of the thumbs of both the hands simultaneously. This point is very useful in relieving neck stiffness, headache, pain in shoulders/heaviness, etc., and also regulates the internal movement of energy.

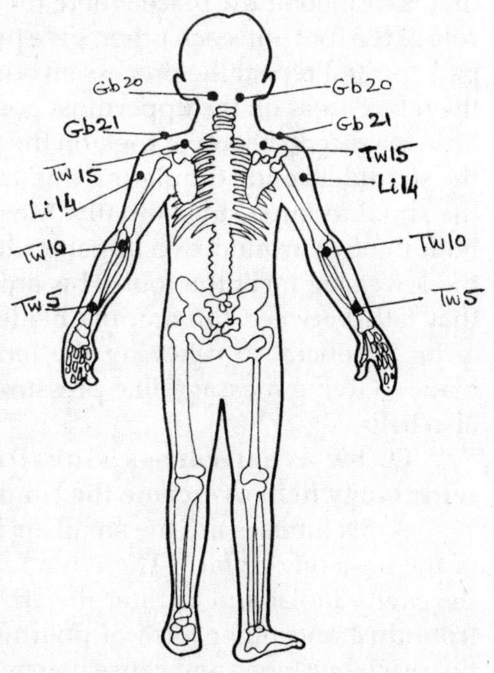

GB 21, known as 'Shoulder Well' is midway between the neck and the outer edge of the shoulder. This point is often found to be very tender. This point can be pressed on both sides of the shoulders simultaneously. It becomes even more beneficial in case the patient takes slow and deep breaths as you press various points. This points restores normal flow of Ch'i in the lungs (the upper part of the body). It relieves shoulder tension, nervousness and fatigue. Pregnant women should not press this point.

TW 15, 'Heavenly Rejuvenation', lies on the shoulders midway between the base of the neck and the outside of the shoulders, one half inch below the top of the shoulders. It relieves muscular tension, stiff neck and shoulder pain.

LI 14 , 'Outer Arm Bone', is found on the outer surface of the upper arm one third of the way down from the top of the shoulder to the elbow. Relieves aching in the arm, shoulder tension and stiff neck.

For overcoming this condition using reflexology, work on the reflex areas right under the big toes over the natural crease that is formed at the place where the big toe and the pad of the sole of the foot join each other, give pressure on and around the pad too and repeat the process on both the soles. Also stimulate the reflex areas on the uppermost portion of the soles where the little toe meets the lower foot, on the soles. This area pertains to the shoulders and stimulating this area helps reduce tension in the shoulder area substantially. Massage the upper portion of both the feet around two finger widths below the point where the lower leg meet the foot. This area also pertains to the area that falls between the scapula blades of the shoulders and is quite beneficial in relieving the tension/pain between these blades. Giving massage-like pressure around the big toes shall also help.

Q. 89: What causes sinusitis? Can acupressure or reflexology help overcome the condition?

A. 89: Sinuses are the small air filled spaces on either side of the nose on our face. There is a fine lining of mucus to keep the cavity moist and to filter the air we breathe, to keep it free from dust and other form of pollution so that these things do not reach our lungs and cause damage to them. Sinuses may get

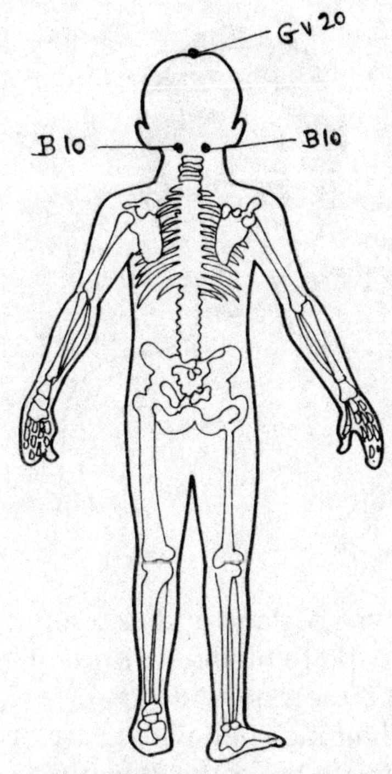

blocked or swollen due to factors e.g. bacterial infections, colds, pollens and we feel heaviness or pain in the head, blocked or dripping from the nose, etc. In certain conditions, the cavity becomes dry and the nose gets choked and crusty.

In case of chronic problems with your sinuses viz. loss of sensation of taste or smell, etc., consult your doctor as there may be some other cause, e.g. constipation, a poor diet which may require to be corrected based on medical advice. Acupressure and reflexology both can help improve this condition and in most of the cases it may not require medical intervention and surgery which is generally recommended in such cases can be avoided. Give a fair trial for say two to three weeks and you will generally succeed in securing a cure. The following schedule of pressure points may be followed:

Li 4 also known by the name 'Adjoining Valley', is located at the crease of the mound that pops up when the thumb and index finger are joined together. Pressure on the left hand can be given by the right hand and on the right hand by the left hand thumb and the index finger. This is considered to be one of the most effective acupressure and acupuncture points to relieve headache and pain in other parts of the body, to relax muscles and it also balances the flow of energy in the lower and upper part of the body. It also activates the bowel movement. Pregnant women should not press this point as it can cause miscarriage.

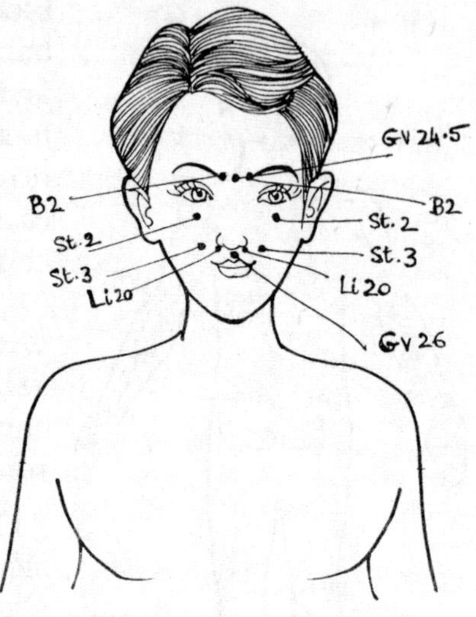

GV20, is located on the top of your head, midway along an imaginary line connecting the upper part of the ears. Give pressure using your thumb or index finger. Avoid pressure on this point if you are suffering from hypertension.

GV 24.5, 'Third Eye Point', between the eyebrows where the eyebrows and the bridge of the nose meet. This point balances the pituitary gland, which in turn stimulates and corrects the functioning of the thyroid gland and also sinus congestion, headache and eyestrain. Mild to moderate pressure may be given on this point for about 30 seconds.

B 10 is located about one and a half inch below the base of the skull, one half an inch on either side of the spine. It has been given the name 'Heavenly Pillars' and it relieves allergic reactions, e.g. swollen eyes, headache, exhaustion, etc. Pressure can be given by interlacing your fingers behind your head, grasping the neck and pressing firmly for about a minute.

B 2, known by the name 'Gathered Bamboo' is located at the inner end of your eye sockets, near the bridge of the nose, in the small indentation. It helps in relieving headache, sinus congestion and other allergy symptoms.

St 3 can be found at the bottom of the cheek bone in line with the pupil. It relieves stuffy nose, head congestion, discomfort in the eyes, e.g. burning and swelling.

GV 26 is located on the upper lip just in the middle below the centre of the nose. This point is very frequently used as a first aid revival point. This is also used to cure cramps, fainting and dizziness as also it relieves headache, sinus pain as well as head congestion.

LI 20, 'Welcoming Perfume', is on the side of the nostrils where they meet the upper lip. Relieves sinus pain, nasal congestion and swelling over the face.

For overcoming this condition using reflexology, give stimulation over all the finger tips including the thumbs on both feet and hands giving clockwise pressure for 20-30 seconds on each finger tip. Also stimulate the channels between the fingers. Stimulate the adrenals, stomach, liver, kidney and large as well as small intestine areas. Also stimulate the outer edges of both the big toes as well as the thumbs as stimulating these areas will help overcome nasal as well as head congestion, to overcome this condition.

Q. 90: Can acupressure help in overcoming skin problems too?

A. 90: Skin serves as the first line of defence of our body. It provides a sort of cover to our body and helps to throw out toxins through tiny sweat glands and thus purify our body. In the event, the kidneys are, for some reason, not able to detoxify through urine or an individual is constipated, the residual toxins may find way to the skin. Our skin has many type of problems and each problem may have a different cause. Oily or dry type skin are very common. Rashes appear over it frequently either owing to some allergic reaction to some medicine or some other factors, acne or dermatitis are also very prevalent.

The cause(s) could be ranging from poor diet, weak digestion, improper functioning of certain internal organs (e.g. kidneys, liver, etc.), hormonal disturbance, etc., can figure in the shape of some problem or the other over our skin. Like in other ailments, stress also plays a vital role on the nature of our skin.

To overcome these problems, a multi-pronged approach would be the best course. In minor problems, adequate exercise, yoga and meditation or any other approach to control stress, a balanced diet regime along with following schedule of pressure points should suffice. However, in case an aggravated condition exists, it would be advisable, to consult a skin specialist and carry on with acupressure in conjunction with the medical treatment to get faster and long lasting results:

Sp 6, also called 'Three Yin Meeting Point', is located above the ankle bone towards the inside of the leg on the back side.

The exact location being about four finger widths above the ankle bone. It is one of the most important pressure points as its name itself suggests since it strengthens the yin of three meridians viz. spleen, liver and kidney at the same time. It helps flush Ch'i and blood through the body. It is considered one of the best pressure points to regulate any gynecological problem. Pregnant women should not press this point.

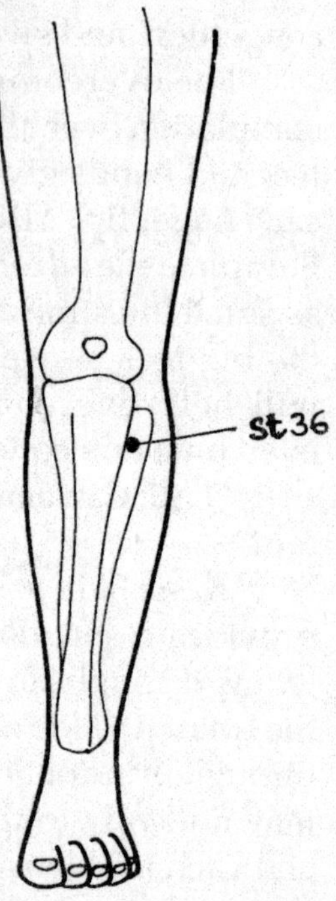

St 36, lies four finger widths below the kneecap, one finger width on the outside of the shin bone. This point strengthen the whole body, tones the muscles particularly in combination with Sp 6, it strongly revitalizes the entire body. It also quiets the rebellious Ch'i of the stomach, which causes nausea and vomiting

Li 11 known as 'Pool at the Crook' is located at the outside end of the crease that is formed in case we bend our hand to touch our shoulder. Give pressure on both hands with the help of opposite hands. This point becomes very tender on pressing therefore, utmost caution has to be exercised while pressing this point which is very useful in clearing the excess heat and dampness from the body and also pain in the elbow, arm and shoulders. It is also an important point to combat allergy and to treat tennis elbow.

TW 5, called the 'Outer Gate' is located midway between the ulna and radius bone about three finger widths above the wrist crease towards the elbow bone on the outside of the wrist (back side). Give pressure on this point for about a minute. The Triple Warmer Channel runs up the back of the

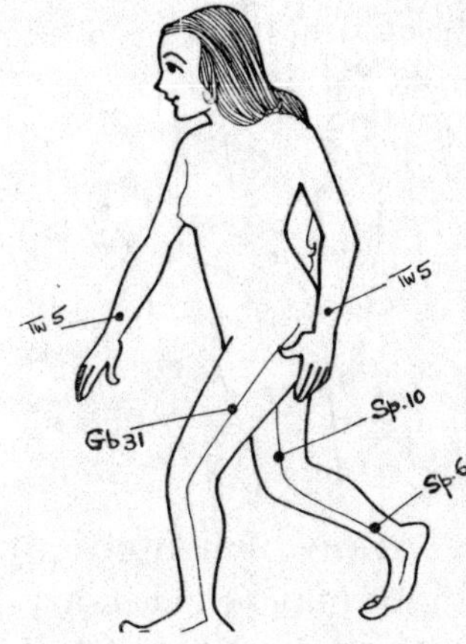

arm to the shoulder and neck, then moves around to the side of the neck. This point is extensively used to treat any type of stiffness/stress in the arm, shoulder and neck. It helps in expelling wind and heat.

Sp 10 is yet another important point that can be used with success for removing stagnation in the flow of blood, which in turn helps expel excess heat from the blood that causes skin disorders. It also promotes better blood circulation.

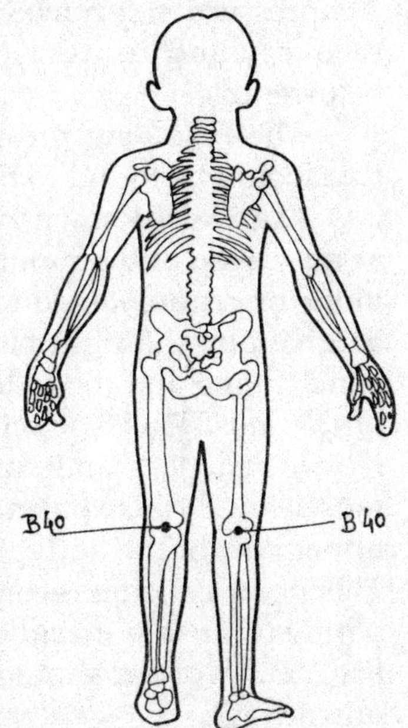

Gb 31, 'Wind market', can be found by standing, hands down touching your thighs on both the sides. This point is located on the place where your index finger touches the thigh. Firm pressure can be given on this point. It helps expel excess of wind and thus overcomes the itching problem.

B 40,'Middle of the Crook', is a very helpful point for relieving pain the lower back region, it is located in the back of your knee, right in the centre between the two tendons and on the crease that is formed when your bend your knee. This point is also called the 'Command Point' because of its powerful influence on all the lower back problems. This point also helps in expelling excessive heat from the blood thereby helping in curing skin diseases. It has been found specifically useful in the treatment of eczema.

Q. 91: What are the causes of a sore throat? Can acupressure help?

A. 91: Bacterial infections could perhaps be the prime cause of a sore throat, though there may be so many other causes like

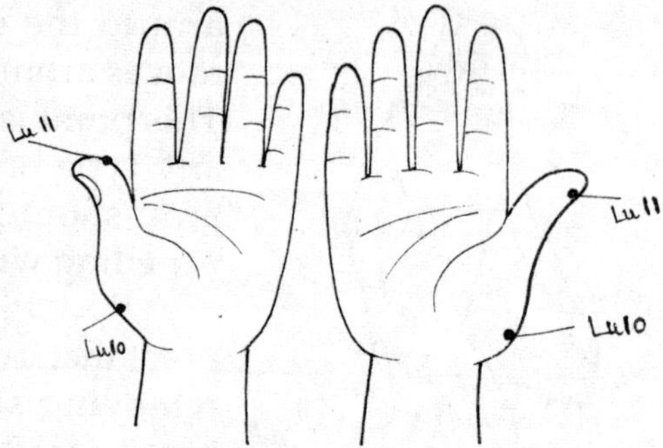

consuming very cold water or sudden exposure from hot to cold, over exertion of the vocal cords, pollens or allergens, etc. This condition can be easily cured with the pressure point therapy except if caused by bacterial infection, which may require intervention of a medical professional, as administration of an antibiotic may be necessary. Acupressure may however, be used in conjunction to get faster recovery and to develop immunity for preventing future recurrences.

The following pressure point schedule is recommended that would be found to be useful:

Li 4, is also known by the name 'Adjoining Valley' is located at the crease of the mound that pops up when the thumb and index finger are joined together. Pressure on the left hand can be given by the right hand and on the right hand by the left hand thumb and the index finger. This is considered to be one of the most effective acupressure and acupuncture points to relieve headache and pain in other parts of the body, to relax muscles and it also balances the flow of energy in the lower and upper part of the body. It also activates the bowel movement. This point is being recommended here for the reason that the pathway of this meridian passes directly through the neck Pregnant women should not press this point as it can cause miscarriage.

Li 11, known as 'Pool at the Crook' it is located at the outside end of the crease that is formed in case we bend our hand to touch our shoulder. Give pressure on both hands with the help of opposite hands. This point becomes very tender on pressing therefore, utmost caution has to be exercised while pressing this point which is very useful in clearing the excess heat and dampness from the body and is as such helpful for clearing heat from the throat too. Used in conjunction with Li 4, this point is

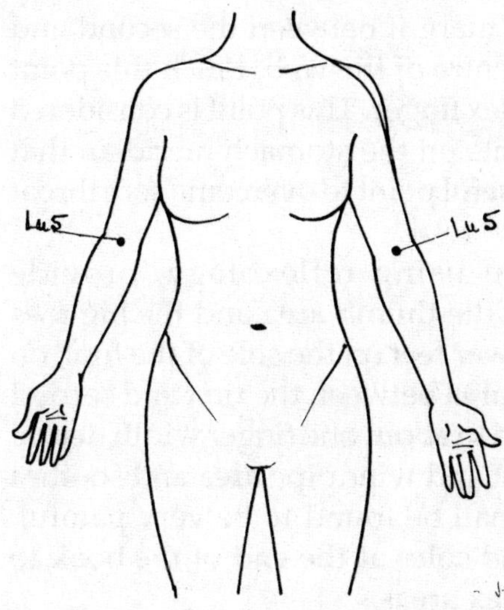

very helpful for this condition.

Lu 10 is located on the palm side of the hand in the centre of the pad of the thumb. It is called 'Fish Border' and it relieves breathing, coughing and swollen throat.

Kd 6, called 'Shining Sea', is located about a thumb width below the ankle bone (big toe side), towards the sole of the feet. Apply firm pressure. Because stagnation of kidney 'yin' is involved in menopause symptoms, pressing this point helps strengthen the kidney 'yin' and has a moistening and cooling effect on the throat.

Lu 5, 'Cubit Marsh', is located in the elbow crease towards the thumb side about a thumb width from Li 11. This point helps clear the heat from the throat and moisten it. It is very useful for chronic sore throat.

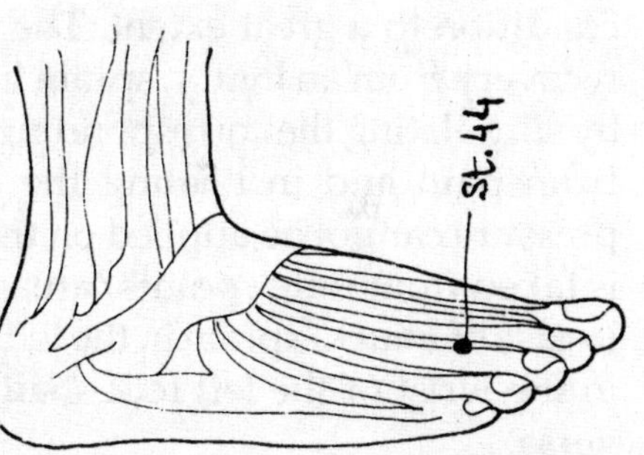

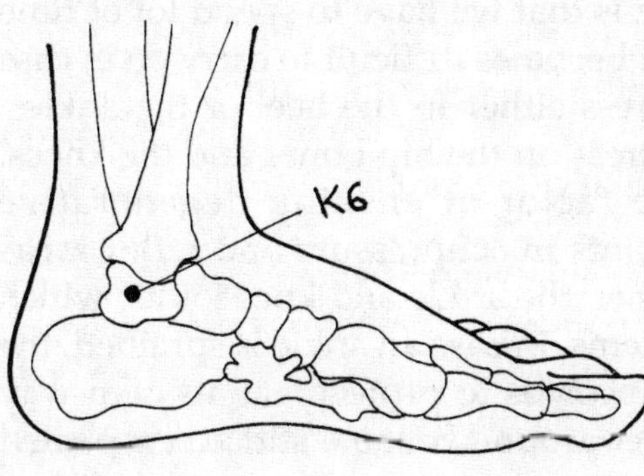

Lu 11, called 'Lesser Metal' is located on the thumb at the corner of the thumb nails bottom. This point too clears excess heat from the body and thus helps chronic sore throat condition.

St 44, 'Inner Courtyard', is located on

the top of the foot in the web margin between the second and third toes; it lies right in the centre of the web. Pinch this point between the thumb and the index finger. This point is considered to be one of the powerful points on the stomach meridian that helps clear the excess heat. A useful point to overcome sore throat condition.

Treating this condition using reflexology, provide stimulation below the joint of the thumb area and the big toes where the big toe meets the lower feet on the sole of the foot, on both sides. Also stimulate the area between the first and second toes in the 'V' like formation up to about one finger width depth. This area pertains to the throat and windpipe area and soothes the throat, though this area shall be found to be very painful. Refer to the figure of palm and soles at the end of the book to see the location of various reflex areas.

Q. 92: Can acupressure/reflexology help overcome the tendency to get sprains? Can it also cure a sprained ankle?

A. 92: Acupressure and reflexology can help overcome the condition to a great extent. The principle behind both is to aid recovery from an injury, sprain in this situation, by easing stress, by stimulating the corresponding reflex areas to provide comfort from pain and in healing the affected portion. Since direct pressure cannot be applied on the affected part of the limb, help is taken from reflex points/areas in the corresponding limb, i.e. in case of injury/sprain in the left foot ankle, corresponding areas in the wrist of the left foot shall get the desired relief and vice versa.

Our body weight is mostly supported by our heel and the ankles. Another fact of life is that we have to spend lot of time standing or walking and it becomes difficult to carry on in case there is pain, injury or stress either in the heel or the ankles. Weak ankles put undue stress on the hip bones and the knees. This can be a causative factor of ensuing degenerative osteoarthritis. Pressure points in acupressure and reflex areas in reflexology can strengthen the ankle and knee joints, which in turn prevent such problems. In case an ankle is sprained, the natural reaction from the body is to protect it in its own way and we see that the muscles around become stiff accompanied

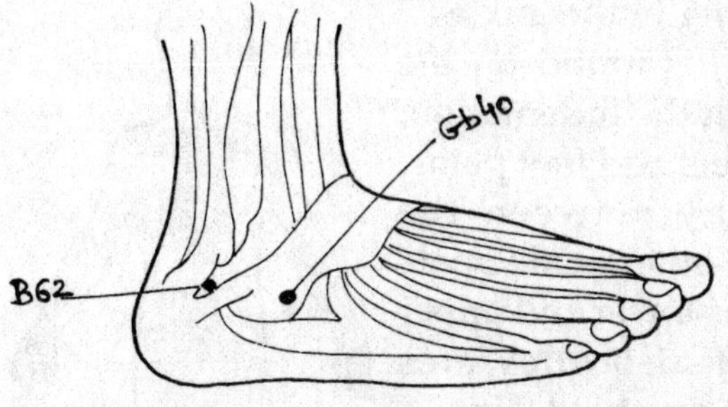

with swelling in the area that almost immobilizes the ankle joint. That is perhaps what a medical practitioner would recommend in case you go to him for advice in such a condition and may be he would wrap it with a crepe bandage too, to further immobilise the ankle, besides prescribing some anti-inflammatory and painkilling medicines.

Both, acupressure and reflexology can provide enough relief in this condition. The best part is that both ways you can strengthen the ankle area so that this condition does not recur frequently, as is the case with some people who have a tendency to twist their ankles and get sprained every now and then due to some weakness in these joints. The following schedule of pressure points may be followed:

GB 40, known by the name 'Wilderness Mound', is located in the hollow in front of the outer ankle bone. This point relieves ankle sprain, toe cramps, etc.

Kd 3 lies midway between the inside of the ankle bone and the Achilles tendon in the back of the ankle. This point relieves ankle pain, swelling in the feet as also strengthens the ankle joints.

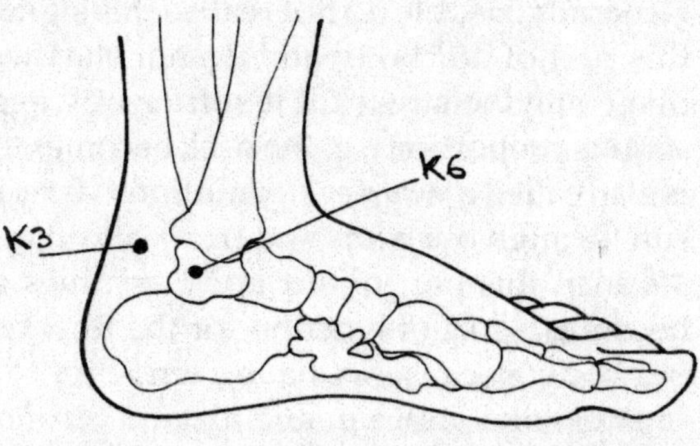

Kd 6, called 'Shining Sea', is located about a thumb width below the ankle bone (big toe side), towards the sole of the feet. Apply firm pressure. Because stagnation of kidney yin is involved in menopause symptoms, pressing this point helps strengthen the kidney yin, the heel and ankle pain, and also alleviate swelling in the ankles.

B 62, 'Calm Sleep', is found on the outer side of the ankle in the indentation. It relieves back, ankle, heel and foot pains.

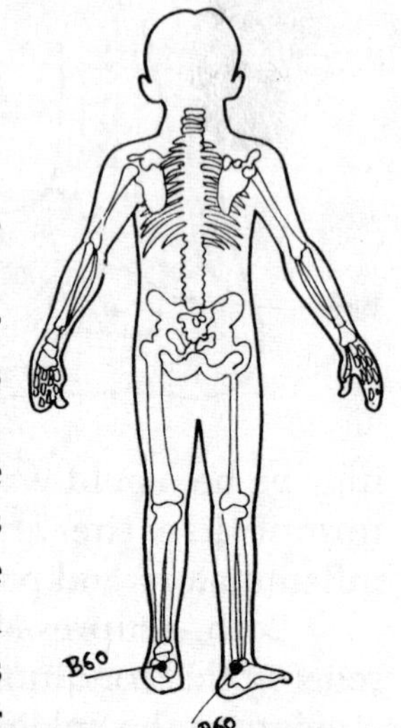

B 60 lies half way between the Achilles tendon and the outer ankle bone. It relieves back pain in the lower and upper back, and the legs. It also alleviates swelling and ankle pain due to sprain.

In case tenderness or swelling in the affected ankle area is so severe that it does not allow the area to be touched, give stimulation on the wrist area of the affected side on both sides of the wrist as well as on the bony prominence on the little finger side, giving a thorough massage like pressure. Hot and cold compresses alternately on the affected ankle shall also provide much relief. After fomentation, pat dry the affected part and apply some muscle relaxant before wrapping a crepe bandage for quick relief. Keep movement restricted to the minimum for some period to strengthen the ankle and feet to avert frequent spraining tendency.

Q. 93: Discuss the causes of stiffness in the neck. Can acupressure/reflexology help overcome this condition?

A. 93: Neck tension, stiffness and pain in this area and the shoulders is a very common and usually neglected condition. Generally, people do not realise this signal from nature through this part of our body and do not start working on this area to overcome the stress till it sufficiently aggravates and assumes serious proportion e.g. the neck becomes totally immobile, which is also called a wry neck condition. Many meridians in our body run through our arms and trunk and they converge at the neck. As such this part of our body assumes great importance as it becomes a sort of junction for the flow of Ch'i or life energy in our body. Because we have a tendency to move around with lot of stress and strain in and around our neck and shoulders, the flow of Ch'i gets easily blocked and this blockage becomes the cause of stiffness and pain. We do feel the tension, but we keep on accumulating it by involuntary contraction of the muscles in the shoulder area that leads to stress, strain and tightening of the muscles around the neck and shoulders. This, in course of time results in muscle rigidity, which may adversely affect the curvature and alignment of the cervical spine. We should get wiser and take timely action to avert this sort of a situation and overcome the tension and stress that comes simultaneously than allowing it to accumulate over a period of time and convert into a much painful condition.

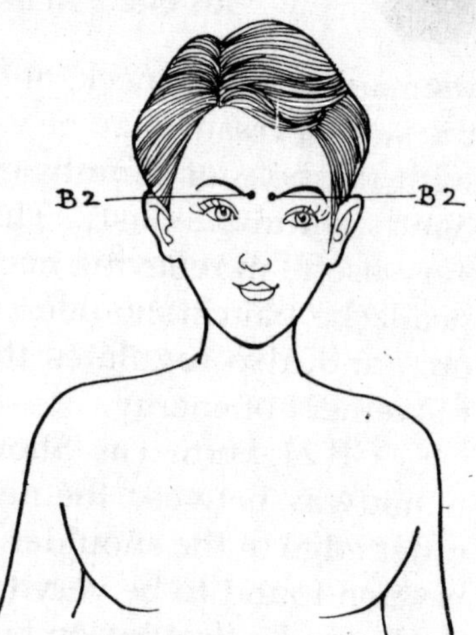

The following schedule of pressure points and stimulation of reflex areas falling in certain zones shall be found to be of much help:

Li 4, known as 'Adjoining Valley', is known for its ability to relieve pain and circulating Ch'i. It lies on the end of the crease that is formed when the thumb and index finger are joined together. It stimulates elimination of toxins through bowels. It relieves stagnation of Ch'i too. Pregnant women should not use this point.

GV 16, 'Wind Mansion' is located in the centre of the back of the head in the hollow under the base of the skull. It relieves mental stress and stiffness in the neck.

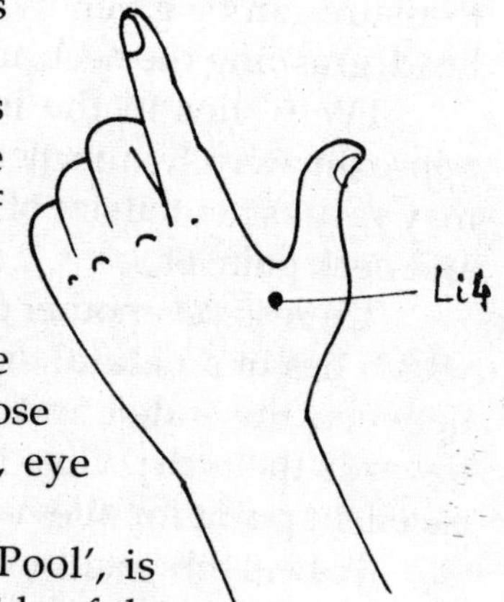

B 2, 'Drilling Bamboo', lies in the indentation over the bridge of the nose between the eyebrows. It relieves, eye fatigue, neck pain and headache.

Gb 20, also called the 'Wind Pool', is located in the depression on either side of the vertebra of your neck, one thumb width above the hairline of the neck, at the base of the skull. Pressure can be easily given with the help of thumbs of both the hands simultaneously. This point is very useful in relieving neck stiffness, headache, pain in shoulders/heaviness etc., and also regulates the internal movement of energy.

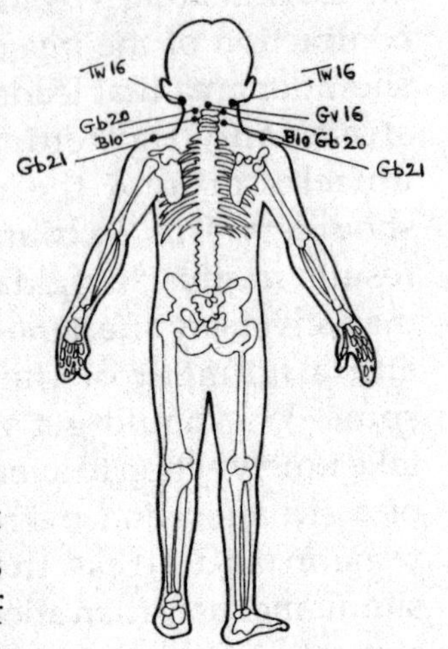

GB 21, known as 'Shoulder Well' is midway between the neck and the outer edge of the shoulder. This point is often found to be very tender. This point can be pressed on both sides of the shoulders simultaneously. It becomes even more beneficial in case the patient takes slow and deep breaths as you press various points. This points restores normal flow of Ch'i in the lungs (the upper part of the body). It relieves shoulder tension, nervousness and fatigue. Pregnant women should not press this point.

B 10 is located about one and a half inch below the base of the skull, one half an inch on either side of the spine. It has been given the name 'Heavenly Pillars' and it relieves allergic reactions, e.g. swollen eyes, headache, stress and stiff neck, etc. Pressure can be given by interlacing your fingers behind your head, grasping the neck and pressing firmly for about a minute.

TW16, lies in the indentation at the base of the skull, approximately two inches on the back of the earlobe, location may vary as per the size of the skull. It relieves stiff neck, shoulder and neck pain, etc.

There is yet another point which is known as, an extra point which lies in a natural depression on the hands in the channel between the index and middle finger about a finger width towards the wrist. Give firm pressure for a minute. This is an excellent point for alleviating neck pain and stiffness.

To heal this condition using reflexology, stimulate the reflex areas around and under the big toes, give rolling or kneading type stimulation on the pad of the sole below the big toe and also stimulate the upper part of the sole towards the little toe, an area of approximately two inches from the little toe. This area pertains to the region of the shoulders.

Q. 94: Stress is considered to be one of the major factors behind many ailments. What causes stress in our life? Can acupressure/reflexology help overcome stress factor?

A. 94: It is a fact that stress is one of the major factors behind most of our ailments and putting it in terms of percentage, perhaps on a vague estimate more than 60-70 per cent of our physical and emotional problems are caused by the stress factor. Besides the physical causes, viz., fatigue, prolonged exposure to extreme temperatures in our work situation, vehicle and noise pollution and pressure of work, exams, family problems, disappointment, loss of someone close to you, etc., may be some of the emotional causes responsible for this condition. At times we have to work under pressure to attain targets and deadlines. However, the effect of this type of stress varies from person to person depending upon the stamina and temperament of each individual.

To add to this, reaction of our body's biochemical response further aggravates its intensity and may result in certain health problems e.g. it may trigger an asthma attack, disturbance in the digestive system, high blood pressure, disturbance in the menstrual cycle, diabetes, and at times if the stress level is too high, it can attribute to dreadful diseases like a heart attack or even insanity. No doubt it affects the overall immune system also.

Depending upon the temperament, some of us can avoid stressful situations, whereas under the same set of circumstances others tend to break down. One of the steps to avert such a situation is to learn the art of stress management to minimise its harmful effect. This can be achieved through exercise, relaxation techniques, meditation, Yoga, etc. Pressure point therapy has also been found to be of great benefit in managing stress since, as per the Chinese medicine, the main effect of stress on the body is disruption of the smooth flow of Ch'i, the life energy. Since acupressure is capable of eliminating this blockage effectively and restoring the balance in the flow of life force, it can easily overcome this condition. The following schedule of points shall be helpful:

Pc 6, is known by the name 'Inner Gate'. It is located on the palm side of the wrist, about three finger widths above the wrist crease in the centre of the arm. It helps restore proper functioning of the diaphragm and consequently the hiccups. It is known for its harmonising effect on the stomach. Use medium pressure for about a minute, building up slowly and releasing gradually at the end of the session. Repeat on the other hand too.

Lv 3, lies between the big and second toes on the top of the foot. It regulates and tonifies the liver and the flow of Ch'i in the liver meridian, which is considered to be the most powerful organ for detoxification.Thus it is helpful in reducing stress.

Li 4, known as 'Adjoining Valley', is known for its ability to relieve pain and help circulate Ch'i. It lies on the end of the crease that is formed when the thumb and index finger are joined together. It stimulates elimination of toxins through bowels. It helps reduce the muscular tension also. Pregnant women should not use this point.

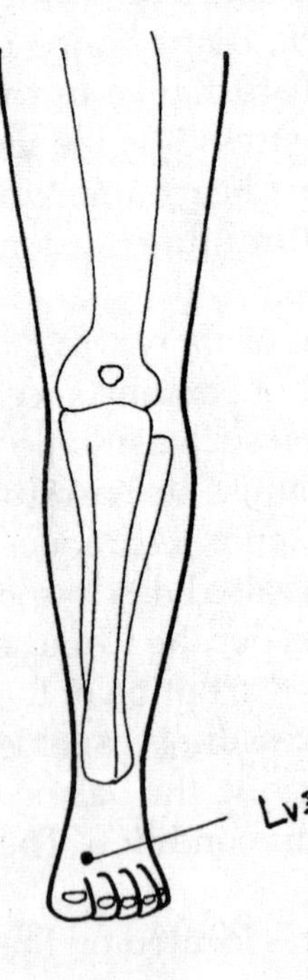

Yin Tang, is an extra point which lies above the bridge of the nose between the eyebrows, almost the same position as that of GV 24.5 and is known for its calming effect. Press with mild to moderate pressure for about a minute.

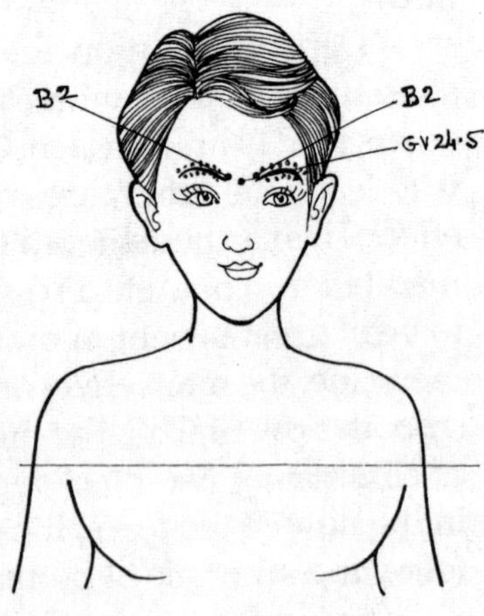

H 7, 'Spirit Gate' is located on the inside of the wrist crease towards the little finger side. It relieves anxiety which causes insomnia and is thus very useful. Press for about half a minute and release gradually. This has a calming effect on the mind and emotions and is considered to be an effective stress remover.

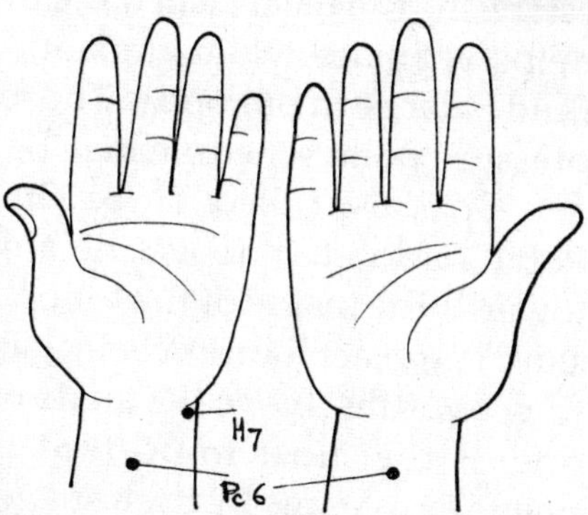

To handle this problem with reflexology, the reflex areas of brain, sinuses, all endocrine glands, digestive system, liver, kidneys, and heart need to be stimulated by giving pressure on the reflex areas belonging to them, in the soles as well as in the palms. To get the maximum benefit special emphasis needs to be given on and around the reflexes on the big toes and the thumbs as the nerves from the cervical area nourish the head and neck part of the body.

Q. 95: What is the cause behind swelling (oedema/water retention) in our body? Can acupressure help overcome this condition?

A. 95: Swelling/oedema due to water retention can affect any part of the body. Feet and ankles generally swell. Women, during or before their monthly cycle may find their belly or thighs bloated or their breasts also tender. This condition is caused due to water retention in the space between the cells. Swelling could be caused by other factors also, e.g. sprains, fracture, some sort of infection in our body, etc. However, in this part we are dealing with swelling or oedema due to water retention only. As per TCM, spleen and kidney are the main organs that govern water metabolism in our body. Thus, to overcome this condition, stimulating various pressure points connected with these two organs as well as certain other points which directly interact with these two organs helps overcome water retention problem, as

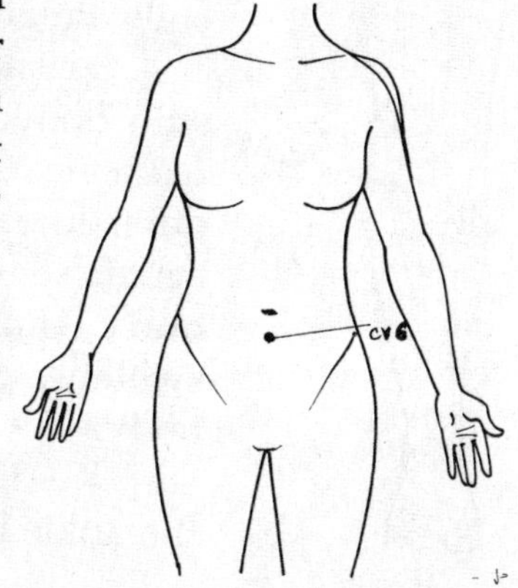

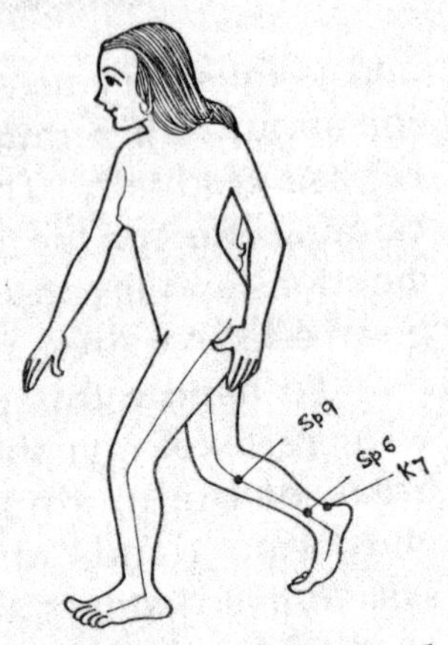

establishing a balance in these meridians helps regulate water metabolism and fluid balance in our body. The following pressure point schedule may be helpful:

Sp 6, also called 'Three Yin Meeting Point', is located above the ankle bone towards the inside of the leg on the back side. The exact location being about four finger widths above the ankle bone. It is one of the most important pressure points as its name by itself suggests since it strengthens the Yin of three meridians, viz. spleen, liver and kidney at a time. It helps flush Ch'i and blood through the body. Is considered one of the best pressure points to regulate any gynecological problem. Pregnant women should not press this point

St 36, lies four finger widths below the kneecap, one finger width on the outside of the shin bone. This point strengthens the whole body, tones the muscles particularly in combination with Sp 6, it strongly revitalises the entire body.

CV 6, 'Sea of Energy', lies three finger widths below the navel. It relieves reproductive problems, irregular periods and impotency. It strengthens the overall reproductive system. Use moderate pressure, hold for a minute, breathe deeply and then gradually release. It has a powerful effect on strengthening Ch'i in the entire body and in circulating the same in the body. Pregnant women should not use this point.

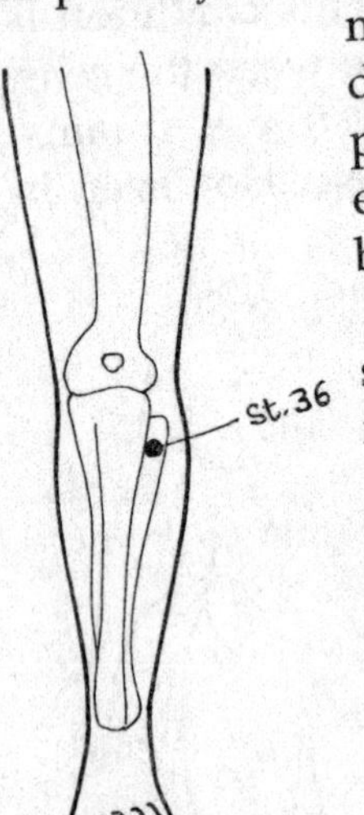

Sp 9 lies on the inside of the leg, under the shin bone, just below the bulge. It helps in reducing oedema, water retention, swelling and other knee problems, as this point is highly beneficial in regulating water metabolism in our body and thereby overcoming oedema/ swelling, particularly in the lower part of our body.

Kd 3, lies midway between the inside of the ankle bone and the Achilles tendon in the

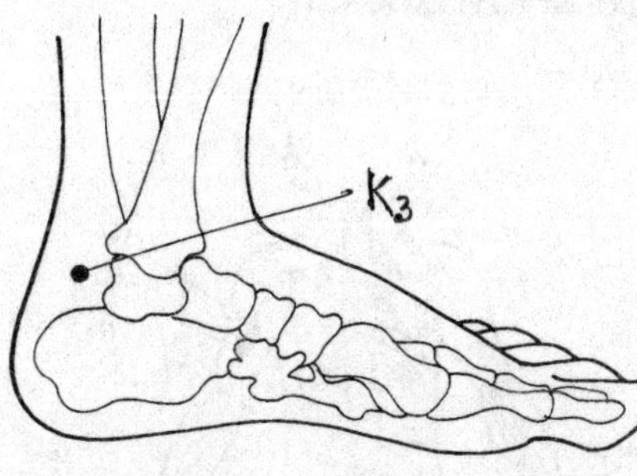

back of the ankle. It helps overcome sexual tensions, menstrual irregularity, etc. From this point, three finger widths above towards the knees is the Kd 7 point. Press for about a minute with thumb pressure. This point is specific to Yang aspect of kidney's Ch'i, which is required to be strengthened in overcoming this condition.

Q. 96: What is tennis elbow and how is it caused? Can acupressure help?

A. 96: Some muscles fixed to their tendons on a bone on the outside of the elbow are responsible for the movement of the fingers and the wrist. Due to overuse of these muscles continuously over a period of time, the tendons may become overstressed and thereby result in pain in the elbow, which may radiate towards the wrist. This problem can occur even in housewives who carry out a lot of activity in their kitchen, cleaning house and washing clothes, etc., manually, or in people working in factories using hammers and other tools, carpenters; badminton and baseball players also suffer from this condition at times. Since this problem is commonly faced by tennis players, the ailment has been named tennis elbow. This stabbing sort of pain caused in this problem is very distressful and is not easily controllable.

This condition can be corrected by balancing the circulation of the life force, Ch'i in the elbow area. The following schedule of pressure points shall be found to be useful in alleviating and curing this difficult to heal condition:

Li4

Li 4 is also known by the name 'Adjoining Valley' and is located at the crease of the mound that pops up when the thumb and index finger are joined together. Pressure on the left hand can be given by the right hand and on the right hand by the left hand thumb and the index finger. This is considered to be one of the most effective acupressure and acupuncture points to relieve headache and pain in other parts of the body, and to relax muscles. Balances the flow of energy in the lower and upper part of the body. It also activates the bowel movement. Pregnant women should not press this point as it can cause miscarriage.

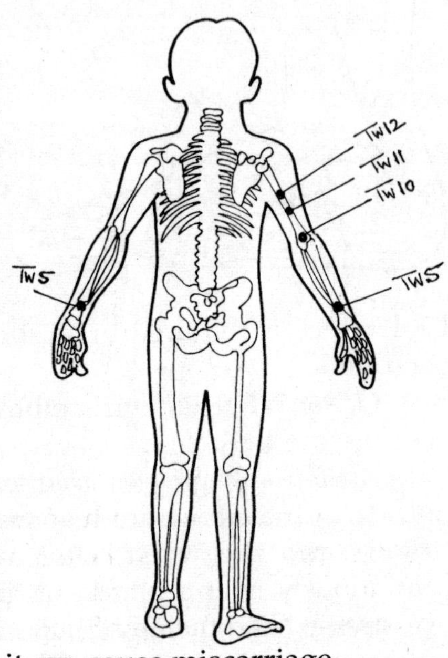

Li 11, known as 'Pool at the Crook' it is located at the outside end of the crease that is formed when we bend our hand to touch our shoulder. Give pressure on both hands with the help of opposite hands. This point becomes very tender on pressing, therefore utmost caution has to be exercised while pressing this point which is very useful in clearing excess heat and dampness from the body, and also pain in the elbow, arm and shoulders. It is also an important point to combat allergy and to treat tennis elbow.

TW 5, called the 'Outer Gate' is located midway between the ulna and radius about three finger widths above the wrist crease towards the elbow bone on the outside of the wrist (back side). Give pressure on this point for about a minute. The

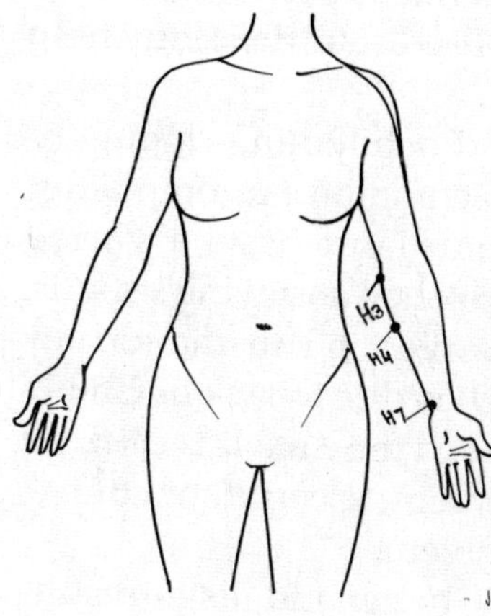

Triple Warmer channel runs up the back of the arm to the shoulder and neck, then moves around to the side of the neck. This point is extensively used to treat any type of problem with the arm, shoulder and neck.

TW 10, 'Heavenly Well' is located one thumb width directly above the tip of the elbow, towards the shoulder. It helps relieve elbow pain, stiffness in the elbow and the shoulder. Press firmly for about a minute with your thumb or middle finger then release gradually. Deep breathing simultaneously shall further improve the effect of this point.

St 36 lies four finger widths below the kneecap, one finger width on the outside of the shinbone. This point strengthens the whole body, tones the muscles particularly in combination with Sp 6, it strongly revitalises the entire body.

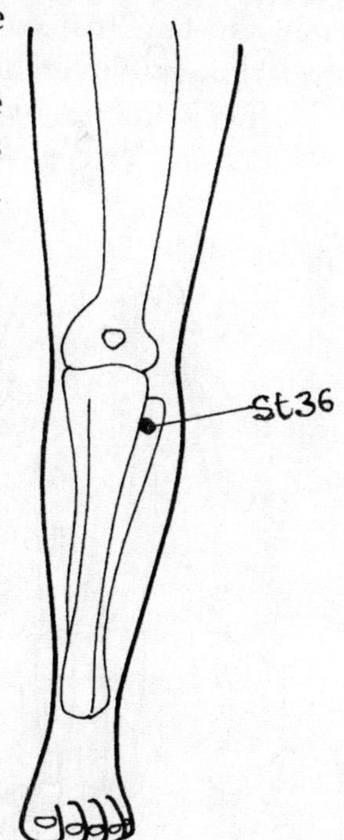

H 3 lies on the inside crease of the elbow on little finger side. This point is very tender and should be stimulated with mild massage like pressure. It is particularly useful for alleviating pain in the ulnar nerve located in the elbow area.

H 4 is located on the palm side of the arm about one and a half thumb widths or say two finger widths above the wrist crease, towards the little finger. Is helpful in reducing arm pain and muscle spasms.

TW 11, is located on the back of the arm in the tendon of the triceps muscle, three finger widths from the point of elbow towards the shoulder. It is used for pain in the arm, shoulder and shoulder blades.

TW12, is located midway between the elbow and the shoulder in the triceps muscle. This point also relieves pain in the upper arm.

Q. 97: What is tinnitus? Can acupressure/reflexology help alleviate this condition?

A. 97: Tinnitus is a distracting and debilitating ringing or rushing sound in the ears. It is one of the common ear complaints. The patients suffering from this complaint have a varied experience ranging from shrill to high pitched annoying sounds, which is commonly caused by excessive Ch'i in the kidney meridian or a low pitched sound which is due to lack of Ch'i in the kidney meridian, in either one or both the ears. It is difficult to pinpoint the cause behind this problem, it could, of course, be the symptom of a more serious problem.

Using acupressure or reflexology, better and faster results can be achieved in excess type, i.e. conditions due to excess of Ch'i in the kidney meridian, for the reason that it is easier to drain out excess Ch'i than to overcome the deficiency. However, in the deficiency type also results do come though it may require more patience and faith in the therapy and continued practice it for a comparatively longer duration. Be sure you will get positive results. The following pressure point schedule may be undertaken to overcome this annoying condition:

TW 7, known by the name 'Ancestral Gathering' is located on the back of the arm, one palm width from the crease of the wrist on the outside tendon and is useful for alleviating deafness, tinnitus and other ear disorders.

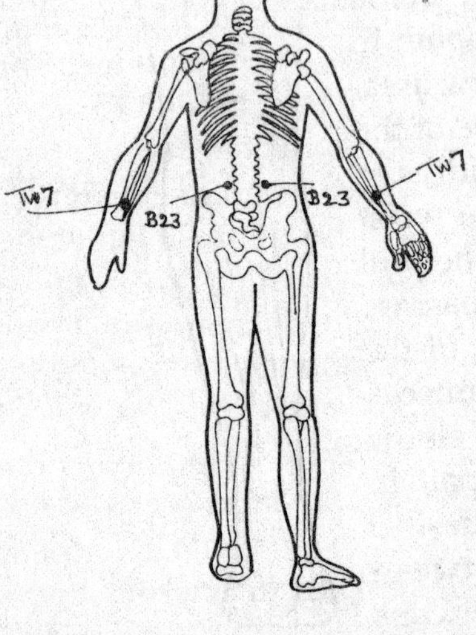

TW16, 'Celestial Window', lies in the muscle, slightly behind the ear lobe on the lower side. Is useful in sudden deafness, swollen face and dizziness.

TW17, 'Wind Screen', is found under the ear lobe on the skull bone where it meets the jaw bone. This point is used for overcoming deafness, tinnitus and vertigo, etc.

TW 21, 'Ear Gate', lies in the front, at the top of the ear. It is used for overcoming deafness, tinnitus, ear infections and earaches.

TW 22, 'Harmony Bone-hole' as shown in the figure, is located in front of the opening of the ear about two finger widths on the bone and about one thumb width in the muscle above the cheekbone. A useful point for tinnitus and earaches.

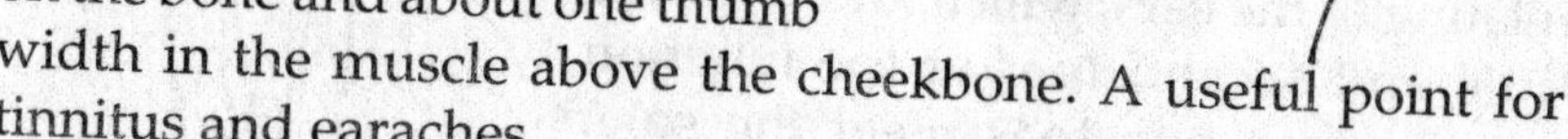

SI 19, 'Hearing Palace', lies in front of the opening of the ear, in the depression. It is used for all ear disorders, deafness, tinnitus, ear infections and vertigo, etc.

GB 2, 'Hearing Meeting', is just below SI 19. This point is also used for tinnitus, deafness and other ear ailments.

Kd 3, is located in the middle of the ankle bone and the Achilles tendon on the back edge of the ankle. This point is known by the name 'Supreme Stream'. It is known as the root of the Yin and Yang of the entire body and is considered to be the prime source point in respect of the kidney meridian. This point has a powerful tonifying effect on the meridian and the entire body. Pressing this point shall be very useful in this condition.

B 23 can be located in the middle of the waist, half way between the rib cage and the hip bone on the inner edge. This point in association with Kd 3 strengthens the kidney Ch'i.

Lv 2, lies at the junction of the big and the second toes. This point is considered to be the best point for draining out excess energy from the Liver meridian.

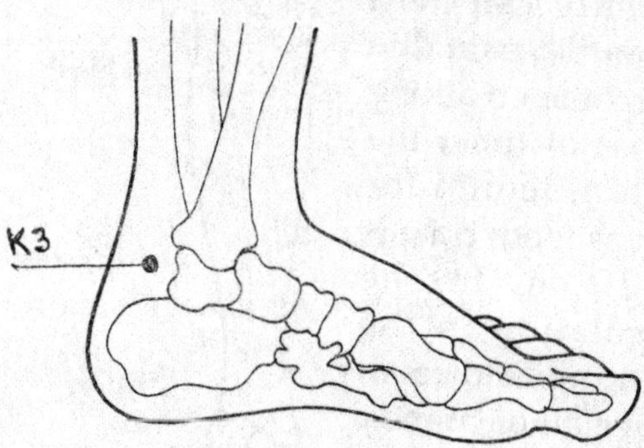

GB 43, 'Clamped Stream', is located in the web margin between the fourth and fifth toes. Excess of energy in the gall bladder meridian is also one of the prime causes responsible for this condition. Pressing this point is the best option for draining out excess energy from the gall bladder meridian and to get relief.

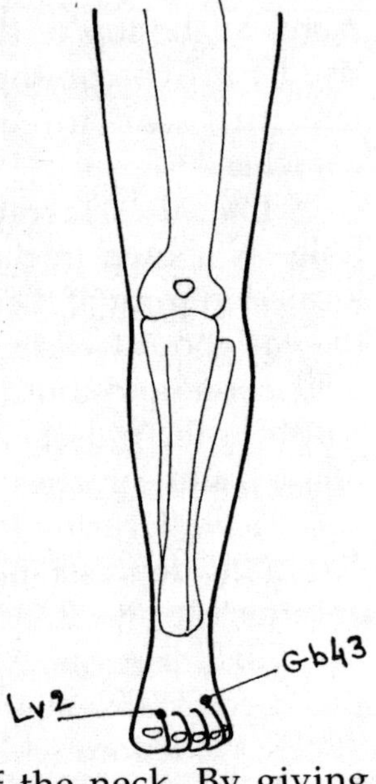

For handling this condition using reflexology, stimulate the reflex areas relating to the ears, which are below the little and second toes at the junction where these two toes meet the sole. Besides give thorough stimulation on and around both the big toes and the crease below the big toes, as this area stimulates the nerves in the region of the neck and ears. At times, deafness is also caused because of some stagnation in the free flow of life force in the region of the neck. By giving stimulation in this area the stagnant flow is revived and that helps in overcoming certain problems relating to ears too.

Q. 98: What are the causes of toothache? Can acupressure help alleviate the condition?

A. 98: Tooth pain may be caused by tooth decay, or an injury that may expose the nerves in the roots. It may also occur because of coming up of a wisdom tooth or some infection or inflammation in the gums. Whereas acupressure can help alleviating the pain temporarily, pain due to infection cannot be overcome on a long term basis, so without loss of time, the patient should approach a dentist for getting the right treatment as tooth pain is a very agonising condition. In the meantime, to avoid escalation in the intensity of pain, avoid eating cold food, sweets, etc., a swab of clove oil or brandy over the affected tooth, may also give

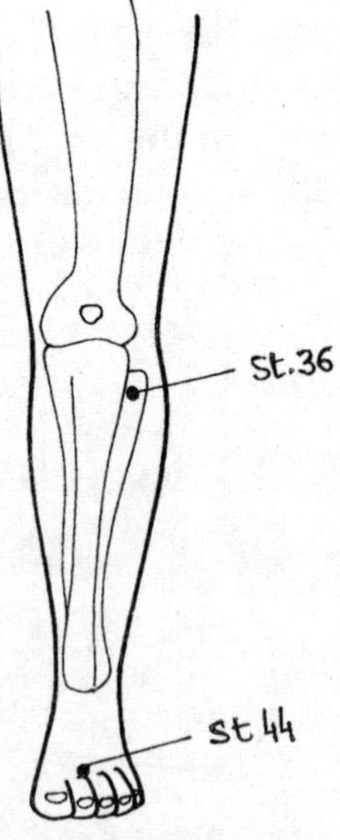

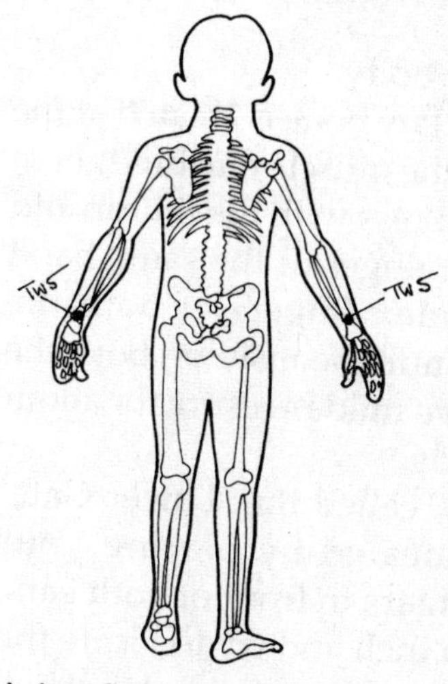

temporary relief and allow you to sleep by alleviating the pain substantially.

It is believed that toothaches are caused due to excess heat in the Stomach meridian. Acupressure points on the large intestine meridian are therefore used to overcome toothache. The following pressure point schedule may be used:

Li 4 is also known by the name 'Adjoining Valley', and is located at the crease of the mound that pops up when the thumb and index finger are joined together. Pressure on the left hand can be given by the right hand and on the right hand by the left hand thumb and the index finger. This is considered to be one of the most effective acupressure and acupuncture points to relieve headache and pain in other parts of the body, and to relax muscles. It also balances the flow of energy in the lower and upper part of the body. It also activates the bowel movement. Pregnant women should not press this point as it can cause miscarriage.

TW 5, called the 'Outer Gate' is located midway between the ulna and radius about three finger widths above the wrist crease towards the elbow bone on the outside of the wrist (back side). Give pressure on this point for about a minute. The Triple Warmer channel runs up the back of the arm to the shoulder and neck, then moves around to the side of the neck. This point is extensively used to treat any type of problem with the arm, shoulder and neck.

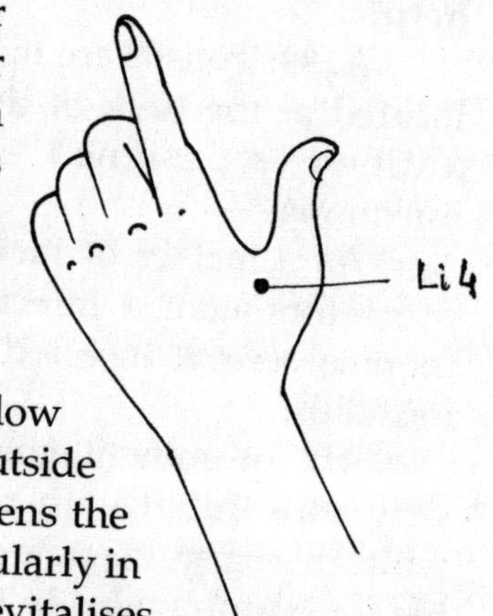

St 36, lies four finger widths below the kneecap, one finger width on the outside of the shin bone. This point strengthens the whole body, tones the muscles particularly in combination with Sp 6, it strongly revitalises

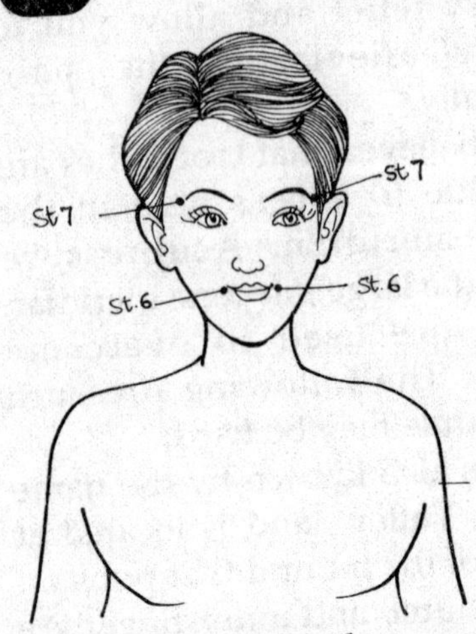

the entire body.

St 6, Jaw bone is located at the centre of the muscle that buldges at the jaws. Press with the thumb and the index finger of the same hand or the index fingers of both the hands simultaneously on both the sides. Give mild pressure for about 30 seconds.

St 7, called the 'Lower Gate' can be located by placing your index fingers in front of both ears, about an inch and try to locate the hard bony ridge that goes across your face around the cheek bone. St.7 is right below this ridge, in the natural depression. This point helps overcome tooth pain temporarily.

St 44, called the, 'Inner Court' lies on the edge of the skin between the second and third toes. It helps overcome infections in the nose, throat, toothaches and headaches.

LI 1, 'Metal Yang', lies on the bottom and thumb facing edge of the nail of the index finger. Helps overcome acute infections in the mouth and throat area, sore throat, gum infection, etc.

Q. 99: What is tonsillitis? Can acupressure/reflexology help?

A. 99: Tonsils are masses of lymphatic tissue located at the back of the throat. They produce antibodies designed to help our body fight infections.

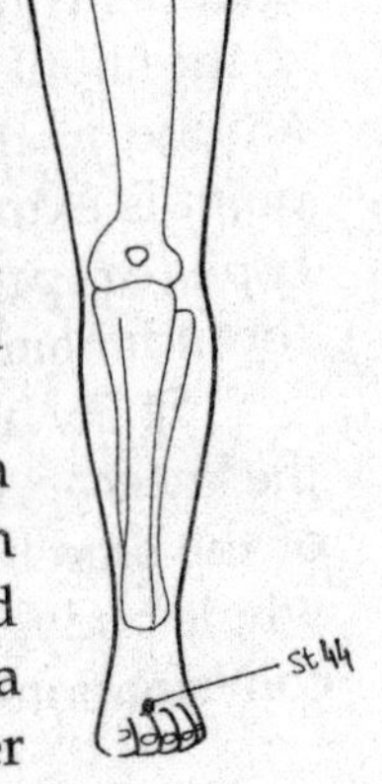

As a matter of fact, tonsils are the body's protectors against infection. When these tissues themselves get infected, the condition is called tonsillitis.

The prominent symptoms of tonsillitis are a very sore throat with red, swollen tonsils with white discharge or spots on the tonsils; swollen and tender lymph nodes in the neck under the jaw; a low grade fever and headache accompanying other symptoms, e.g. difficulty in swallowing, earache, etc. This condition may be helped by reflexology to a great extent. However, in case the incidence of attacks of tonsillitis are very frequent and severe, they may affect the health of the child. In such a condition, surgical removal of the tonsils may be the best alternative.

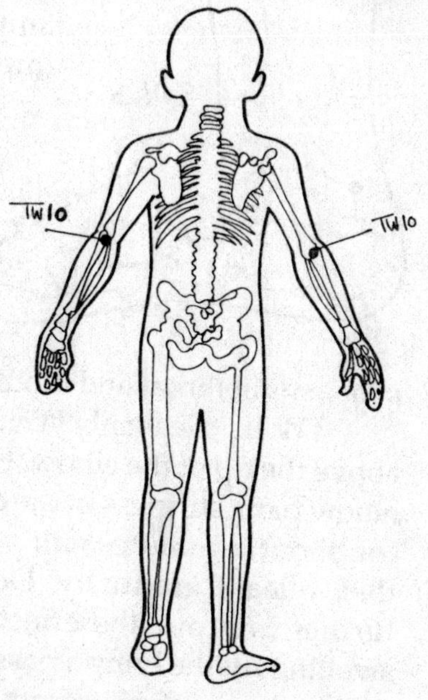

Handling this condition using acupressure, pressure points schedule discussed below may be useful:

Li 4 is also known by the name 'Adjoining Valley', and is located at the crease of the mound that pops up when the thumb and the index finger are joined together. Pressure on the left hand can be given by the right hand and on the right hand by the left hand thumb and the index finger. This is considered to be one of the most effective acupressure points to treat infections in the mouth and throat area. Pregnant women should not press this point as it can cause miscarriage.

Li 11 known as 'Pool at the Crook' it is located at the outside end of the crease that is formed in case we bend our hand to touch our shoulder. Give pressure on both hands with the help of opposite hands. This point becomes very tender on pressing, therefore, utmost caution has to be exercised while pressing this point which is very

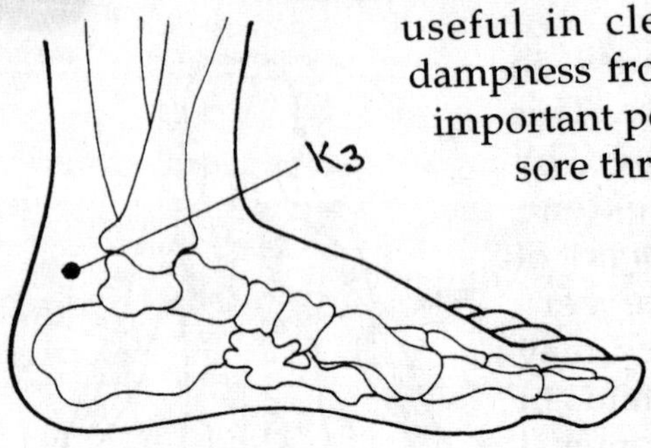

useful in clearing excess heat and dampness from the body. It is also an important point to combat allergy and sore throat.

Kd 3, lies midway between the inside of the ankle bone and the Achilles tendon in the back of the ankle. It is helpful in overcoming problems in throat and mouth and is helpful in healing tonsillitis.

TW 10, 'Heavenly Well' is located one thumb width directly above the tip of the elbow, towards the shoulder. It helps relieve elbow pain, stiffness in the elbow and the shoulder. Press firmly for about a minute with your thumb or middle finger firmly then release gradually. Deep breathing simultaneously shall further improve the effect of this point. It helps in reducing swellings of the lymph passage in the neck and throat. A helpful point when suffering from tonsillitis.

St 44, called the 'Inner Court' lies on the edge of the skin between the second and third toes. Helps overcome infections in the nose and throat, toothaches and headaches.

LI 1, 'Metal Yang', lies on the bottom and thumb facing edge of the nail of the index finger. It helps overcome acute infections in the mouth and throat area, sore throat, gum infection, etc.

LI 14, 'Upper Arm' on the outside of the upper arm, helps in problems with lymph drainage in the neck and throat, the armpit; and eye problems.

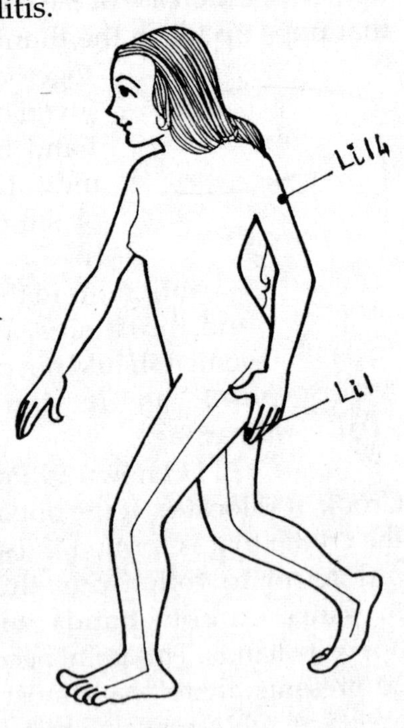

St 9, 'Man's prognosis', is located about a thumb width on either side of the adam's apple. Checks infection in the throat and the mouth.

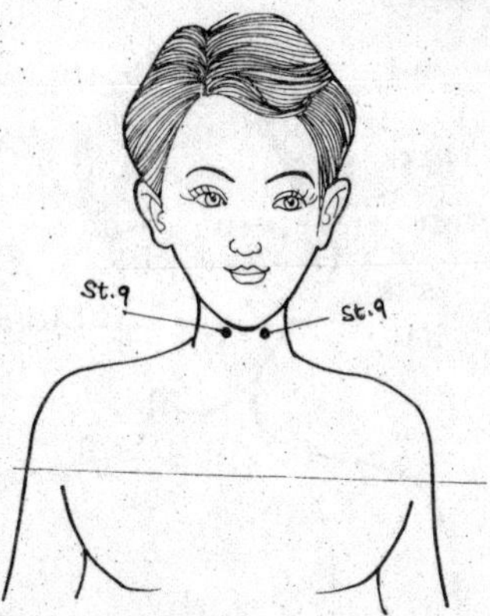

Using reflexology, focus on the following reflex points for treating this condition, stimulate the reflex areas pertaining to the throat, tonsils, lymphatic system, ears, head, brain, adrenals, solar plexus, diaphragm, the neck and the lungs. Pressure can be given on each of the areas from one to two minutes. Special attention may be paid to the lymphatic system, adrenals, ears, neck and throat areas.

Q. 100: What are the symptoms of trigeminal neuralgia? Can acupressure alleviate this condition?

A. 100: Neuralgia, or nerve pain as the name suggests, is a nerve pain, occurring when a nerve is irritated or inflamed. The pain spreading along neural pathways may be acute or chronic and may range from mild to unbearable. Neuralgia accompanied with facial pain is called trigeminal neuralgia after the multi branched cranial nerve that is affected. This condition occurs mostly in people above the age of 50 and women are more prone to this ailment. Nerves of the buttocks and legs are also vulnerable. Irritation of the sciatic nerve produces neuralgia known as sciatica. Another type is post herpetic neuralgia, which often strikes after the type of herpes infection which has continuous burning sensation as its typical symptom.

This nerve pain may be sudden, shooting, sharp, burning or stabbing. At times it is also accompanied by a burning sensation, itching or aching. It occurs only in one part of our body (only on one side). The pain may be intermittent or continuous. It may last for days or weeks and may recur off and on. Facial neuralgia spreads to any eye, this could even damage the eye if not treated properly. The pain becomes too much to bear.

One should not try to handle this type of ailments by depending only upon alternative therapies. However,

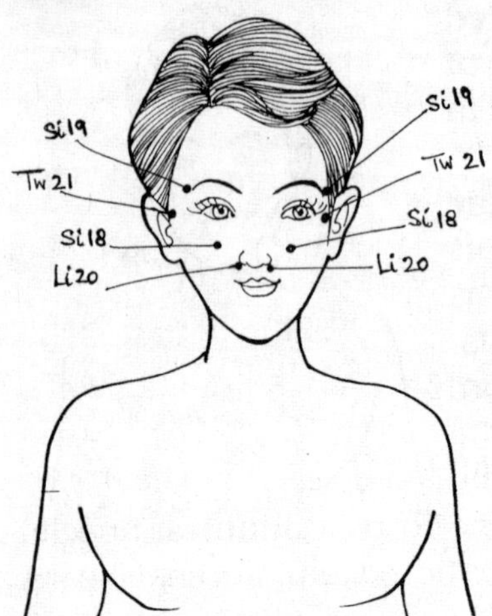

acupressure in complement to traditional medicine would be found to be very helpful in alleviating the condition of the patient. The following pressure point schedule may be followed:

Li 4 is also known by the name 'Adjoining Valley' and is located at the crease of the mound that pops up when the thumb and index finger are joined together. Pressure on the left hand can be given by the right hand and on the right hand by the left hand thumb and the index finger. This is considered to be one of the most effective acupressure points to treat infections in the mouth and throat area and also very helpful by its pain killing effect also. Pregnant women should not press this point as it can cause miscarriage.

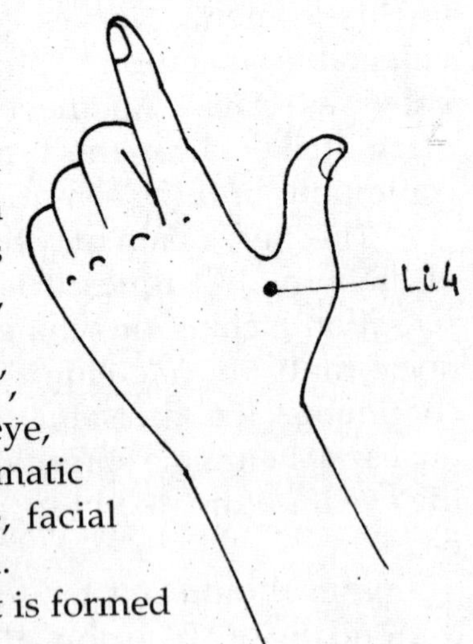

St 44, called the 'Inner Court' lies on the edge of the skin between the second and third toes. It helps overcome infections in the nose, throat, toothaches and headaches.

Si 18, called 'Cheek Bone Hole', lies below the outside edge of the eye, in an indentation below the zygomatic bone. It relieves pain in the face, facial paralysis and trigeminal neuralgia.

Si 19 is in the depression that is formed

when the mouth is opened. Stimulate this point with your mouth open. Make sure that you are pressing in the centre of the depression thus formed. Apply pressure on this point using the three fingers of your hand joined together so that two more points about half inch above and below this point are also pressed simultaneously. This is the crossing point of the gall bladder and Triple Warmer meridians and has a beneficial effect on the hearing power of the ears and over the trigeminal nerve. It overcomes nerve pain.

LI 20 is located outside each nostril on the cheeks. Nasal congestion, sinus and facial swelling is overcome by giving pressure on these points.

TH 21, called 'Ear Gate', is located at the front of the ear at the point where the upper edge of the zygomatic bone meets the ear. It corrects ear problems (both infection and sound), besides infections of the trigeminal nerve.

Q. 101: What is urinary tract infection (UTI), how is it caused? Can acupressure/reflexology help?

A. 101: The main components of the urinary tract are the kidneys, ureter, bladder and urethra. Bladder infection is the most frequent condition in this area. This condition is known as Cystitis. This ailment is generally caused by an infection of the mucus membranes of the bladder by bacteria that moves in from the intestines or the anus. The symptoms comprise a frequent desire to urinate; the quantum of urine passed on each occasion may be low in volume accompanied with lot of pain during urination.

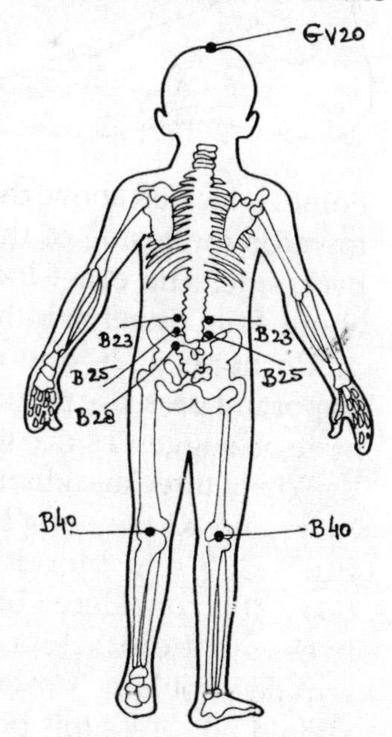

One reason why women suffer from UTI more frequently than men is that as the urethra is shorter in women than men, bacteria travel more quickly from anus to the bladder. Bladder infections are

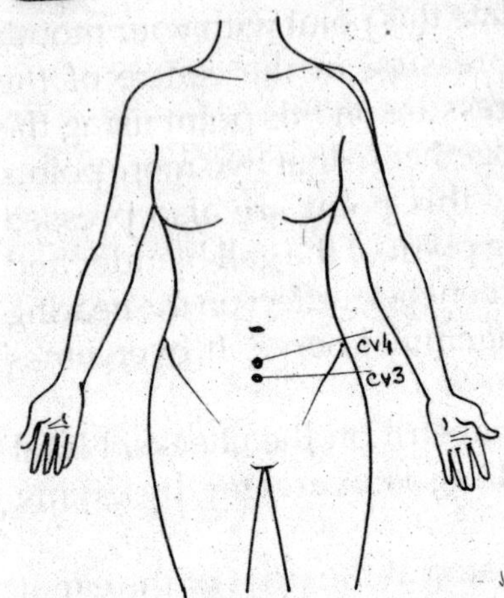

particularly more frequent in those people who do not drink enough fluids. The result, their bladders are not well rinsed.

Since the urinary bladder meridian runs along the outside of the feet and the kidney meridian along the inside of the feet, pressure points on these meridians have a harmonising effect on the urinary tract. In this way acupressure can be an effective complementary measure to conventional medical treatment. The following pressure point schedule shall be found to be beneficial:

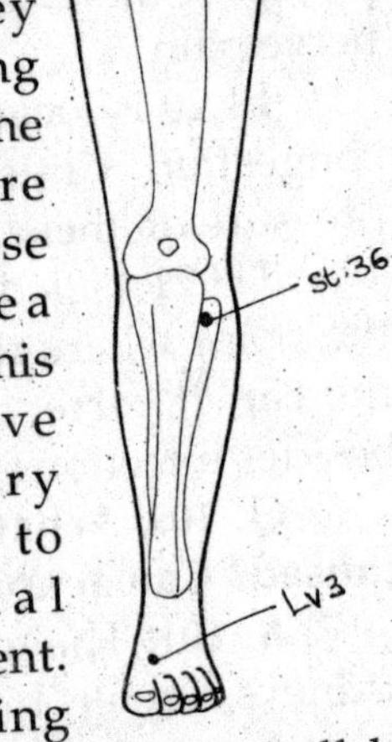

K3

Sp 6, also called 'Three Yin Meeting Point', is located above the ankle bone towards the inside of the leg on the back side. The exact location being about four finger widths above the ankle bone. It is one of the most important pressure points as its name by itself suggests since it strengthens the Yin of three meridians viz. Spleen, Liver and Kidney at a time. It helps flush Ch'i and blood through the body. It is considered one of the best pressure points to regulate any female problem. Pregnant women should not press this point

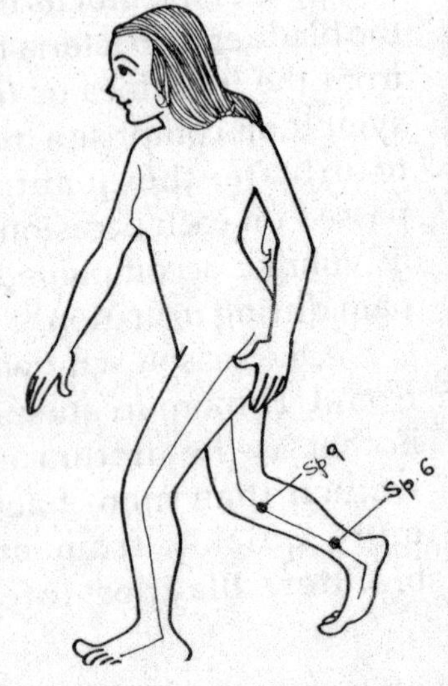

St 36, lies four finger widths below the kneecap, one finger width on the outside of the shin bone. This point strengthens the whole body, tones the muscles particularly in combination with Sp 6, it strongly revitalises the entire body.

Lv 3, lies between the big and second toes on the top of the foot. It regulates and tonifies the liver and the flow of Ch'i in the Liver meridian, which is considered to be the most powerful organ for detoxification.

□□□

REFLEX CENTRES ON THE FEET

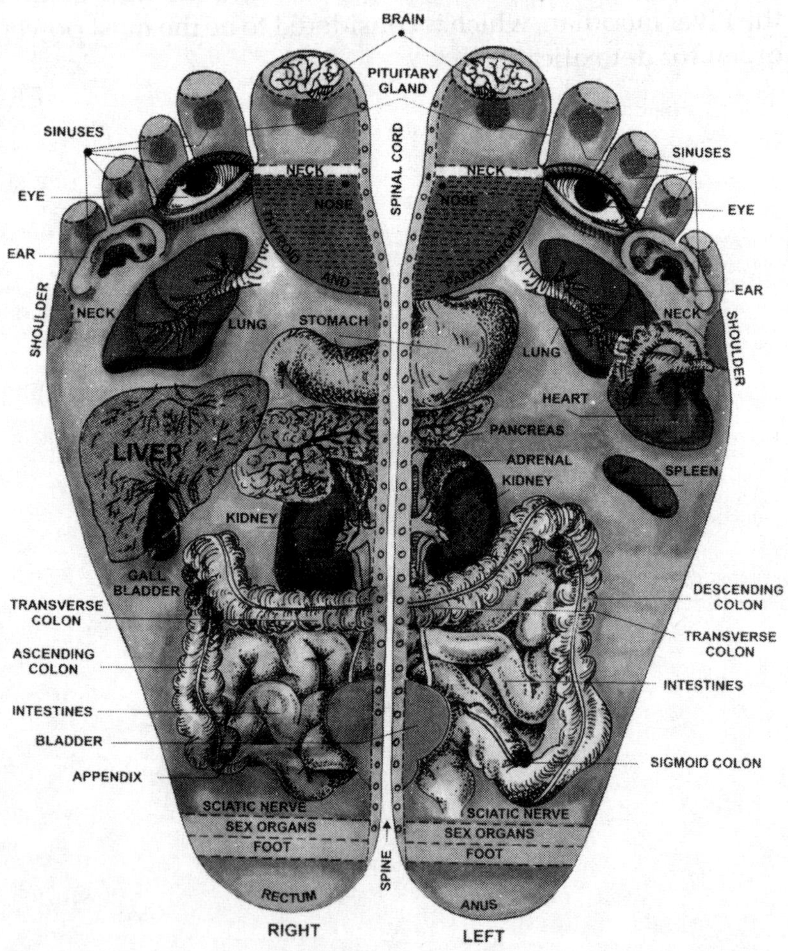

Adopted with Thanks from the books
'Acupressure Do-it-yourself therapy' by my guruji Dr. Attar Singh.

REFLEX CENTRES ON THE HANDS

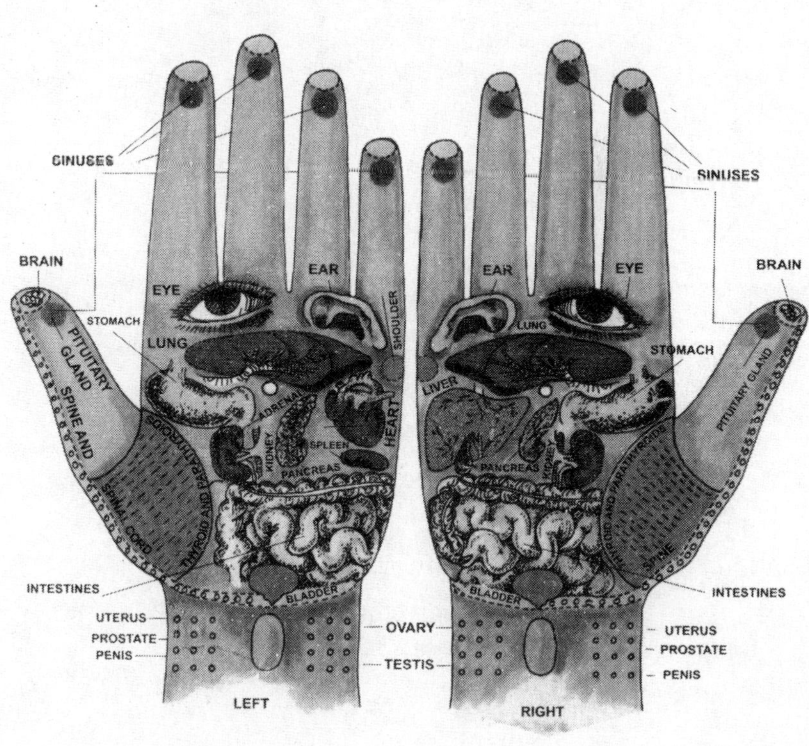

Adopted with Thanks from the books
'Acupressure Do-it-yourself therapy' by my guruji Dr. Attar Singh.